AF597432

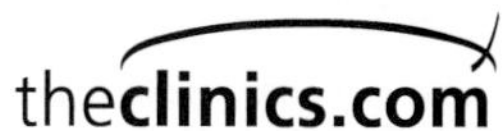

NEUROLOGIC CLINICS

Dementia

GUEST EDITOR
Neill R. Graff-Radford, MBBCh, FRCP

August 2007 • Volume 25 • Number 3

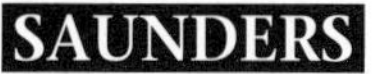

An Imprint of Elsevier, Inc.
PHILADELPHIA LONDON TORONTO MONTREAL SYDNEY TOKYO

W.B. SAUNDERS COMPANY
A Division of Elsevier Inc.

1600 John F. Kennedy Blvd., Suite 1800, Philadelphia, PA 19103-2899

http://www.theclinics.com

NEUROLOGIC CLINICS
August 2007
Editor: Donald Mumford

Volume 25, Number
ISSN 0733-861
ISBN 1-4160-5092-
978-1-4160-5092-

Neurologic Clinics (ISSN 0733-8619) is published quarterly by Elsevier Inc., 360 Park Avenue South, New Yor
NY 10010–171. Months of issue are February, May, August, and November. Business and editorial offices: 16
John F. Kennedy Blvd., Suite 1800, Philadelphia, PA 19103-2899. Customer Service Office: 6277 Sea Harb
Drive, Orlando, FL 32887–4800. Accounting and circulation offices: 6277 Sea Harbor Drive, Orlando, F
32887-4800. Periodicals postage paid at New York, NY, and additional mailing offices. Subscription pric
are $198.00 per year for US individuals, $313.00 per year for US institutions, $99.00 per year for US student
$248.00 per year for Canadian individuals, $367.00 per year for Canadian institutions, $259.00 per year for i
ternational individuals, $367.00 per year for international institutions and $132.00 for Canadian and foreig
students/residents. To receive student/resident rate, orders must be accompanied by name of affiliated inst
tution, date of term, and the *signature* of program/residency coordinator on institution letterhead. Orders w
be billed at individual rate until proof of status is received. Foreign air speed delivery is included in all *Clini*
subscription prices. All prices are subject to change without notice. POSTMASTER: Send address changes t
Neurologic Clinics, Elsevier Periodicals Customer Service, 6277 Sea Harbor Drive, Orlando, FL 32887-480
Customer Service: 1-800-654-2452 (US). From outside of the US, call 1-407-345-4000.

Neurologic Clinics is also published in Spanish by Nueva Editorial Interamericana S.A., Mexico City, Mexic

Neurologic Clinics is covered in *Current Contents/Clinical Medicine, Index Medicus, EMBASE/Excerpta Medica,* a
PsycINFO, and *ISI/BIOMED.*

Printed in the United States of America.

GUEST EDITOR

NEILL R. GRAFF-RADFORD, MBBCh, FRCP, Professor of Neurology, Mayo College of Medicine, Mayo Clinic Jacksonville, Jacksonville, Florida

CONTRIBUTORS

BRADLEY F. BOEVE, MD, Divisions of Behavioral Neurology and Movement Disorders, Department of Neurology, Mayo Clinic, Rochester; Associate Professor of Neurology, Mayo Clinic College of Medicine, Rochester, Minnesota

HELENA C. CHUI, MD, McCarron Professor and Chair, Department of Neurology, University of Southern California, Keck School of Medicine, Los Angeles, California

ELIZABETH A. ECKMAN, PhD, Assistant Professor and Associate Consultant, Department of Neuroscience, Mayo Clinic College of Medicine, Jacksonville, Florida

CHRISTOPHER B. ECKMAN, PhD, Associate Professor and Consultant, Department of Neuroscience, Mayo Clinic College of Medicine, Jacksonville, Florida

ERIC EGGENBERGER, DO, FAAN, Associate Chairman, Department of Neurology and Ophthalmology, Michigan State University, East Lansing, Michigan

NILÜFER ERTEKIN-TANER, MD, PhD, Assistant Professor of Neuroscience, Departments of Neurology and Neuroscience, Mayo Clinic Rochester, Rochester, Minnesota

TANIS J. FERMAN, PhD, Department of Psychiatry and Psychology, Mayo Clinic College of Medicine, Jacksonville, Florida

MICHAEL D. GESCHWIND, MD, PhD, Assistant Professor, Department of Neurology, University of California San Francisco, San Francisco, California

NEILL R. GRAFF-RADFORD, MBBCh, FRCP, Professor of Neurology, Mayo College of Medicine, Mayo Clinic Jacksonville, Jacksonville, Florida

AISSA HAMAN, MD, Research Analyst, Department of Neurology, University of California San Francisco, San Francisco, California

KRISTOFFER HAUGARVOLL, MD, Department of Neuroscience, Mayo Clinic College of Medicine, Jacksonville, Florida; Department of Neurology, Mayo Clinic College of Medicine, Jacksonville, Florida; and Department of Neuroscience, NTNU—Norwegian University of Science and Technology, Trondheim, Norway

MICHAEL HUTTON, PhD, Department of Neuroscience, Mayo Clinic College of Medicine, Jacksonville, Florida

CLIFFORD R. JACK Jr, MD, Professor of Radiology, Department of Radiology, Mayo Clinic, Rochester, Minnesota

KEITH A. JOSEPHS, MST, MD, Associate Professor of Neurology, Department of Neurology, Divisions of Behavioral Neurology and Movement Disorders, Mayo Clinic and Mayo Foundation, Rochester, Minnesota

BRENDAN J. KELLEY, MD, Mayo Clinic, Department of Neurology, Rochester, Minnesota

BRUCE L. MILLER, MD, Professor, Department of Neurology, University of California San Francisco, San Francisco, California

RONALD C. PETERSEN, MD, PhD, Mayo Clinic, Department of Neurology, Rochester, Minnesota

JENNIFER L. WHITWELL, PhD, Research Fellow, Department of Radiology, Mayo Clinic, Rochester, Minnesota

ZBIGNIEW K. WSZOLEK, MD, Department of Neurology, Mayo Clinic College of Medicine, Jacksonville, Florida

CONTENTS

Preface **xi**
Neill R. Graff-Radford

Alzheimer's Disease and Mild Cognitive Impairment **577**
Brendan J. Kelley and Ronald C. Petersen

As our society ages, age-related diseases assume increasing prominence as both personal and public health concerns. Disorders of cognition are particularly important in both regards, and Alzheimer's disease is by far the most common cause of dementia of aging. In 2000, the prevalence of Alzheimer's disease in the United States was estimated to be 4.5 million individuals, and this number has been projected to increase to 14 million by 2050. Although not an inevitable consequence of aging, these numbers speak to the dramatic scope of its impact. This article focuses on Alzheimer's disease and the milder degrees of cognitive impairment that may precede the clinical diagnosis of probable Alzheimer's disease, such as mild cognitive impairment.

Genetics of Alzheimer's Disease: A Centennial Review **611**
Nilüfer Ertekin-Taner

Alzheimer's disease (AD) genetics may be one of the most prolifically published areas in medicine and biology. Three early-onset AD genes with causative mutations (*APP, PSEN1, PSEN2*) and one late-onset AD susceptibility gene, apolipoprotein E (*APOE*), exist with ample biologic, genetic, and epidemiologic data. Evidence suggests a significant genetic component underlying AD that is not explained by the known genetic risk factors. This article summarizes the evidence for the genetic component in AD and the identification of the early-onset familial AD genes and *APOE*, and examines the current state of knowledge about additional AD susceptibility loci and alleles. The future directions for genetic research in AD as a common and complex condition are also discussed.

An Update on the Amyloid Hypothesis **669**
Christopher B. Eckman and Elizabeth A. Eckman

Alzheimer's disease (AD) is a devastating neurodegenerative disease. To rationally develop novel therapeutic and/or preventative agents for AD, an understanding of the etiology and pathogenesis of this complex disease is necessary. This article examines the evidence for the amyloid hypothesis of AD pathogenesis and discusses how it relates to the neurological and neuropathological features of AD, the known genetic risk factors and causative mutations, and the heightened risk associated with advanced age.

Frontotemporal Lobar Degeneration **683**
Keith A. Josephs

Frontotemporal lobar degeneration (FTLD) is a syndromic diagnosis that encompasses at least three different variants. Imaging modalities are clinically useful in FTLD, although pathology remains the gold standard for definitive diagnosis. To date, four different genes have been identified that account for FTLD.

The Genetics of Frontotemporal Dementia **697**
Kristoffer Haugarvoll, Zbigniew K. Wszolek, and Michael Hutton

This article describes the remarkable progress that has been made over the past decade in identifying the genetic contribution to frontotemporal dementia. The clinical and neuropathologic features of frontotemporal dementia with parkinsonism linked to chromosome 17 and the nature of the mutations in the progranulin and microtubule-associated protein tau genes are emphasized.

Subcortical Ischemic Vascular Dementia **717**
Helena C. Chui

Subcortical ischemic vascular dementia (SIVD) has been proposed as a subtype of vascular cognitive impairment. MRI often discloses "silent" hyperintensities in 20% to 40% of community-dwelling elderly. Efforts to relate MRI-measured lacunes and white matter changes to cognitive impairment have not been straightforward. The possibility that Alzheimer's disease pathology contributes to cognitive impairment increases with age. A rare disorder known as cerebral autosomal dominant arteriopathy with subcortical infarctions and leukoencephalopathy (CADASIL) provides an opportunity to study SIVD in the absence of Alzheimer's disease. Lacunes and deep white matter changes are associated with dysexecutive syndrome. Hypertension, the leading risk factor for sporadic SIVD, is treatable. High priority must be given to reducing vascular risk profiles.

Dementia with Lewy Bodies 741

Tanis J. Ferman and Bradley F. Boeve

The advent of new immunostains have improved the ability to detect limbic and cortical Lewy bodies, and it is evident that dementia with Lewy bodies (DLB) is the second most common neurodegenerative dementia, after Alzheimer's disease (AD). Distinguishing DLB from AD has important implications for treatment, in terms of substances that may worsen symptoms and those that may improve them. Neurocognitive patterns, psychiatric features, extrapyramidal signs, and sleep disturbance are helpful in differentiating DLB from AD early in the disease course. Differences in the severity of cholinergic depletion and type/distribution of neuropathology contribute to these clinical differences.

Parkinson-Related Dementias 761

Bradley F. Boeve

Recent advances in neurogenetics, molecular biology, and immunocytochemical staining methods have expanded the spectrum of neurodegenerative disorders now known to cause dementia associated with parkinsonism. This review concentrates on those rare disorders in which cognitive impairment/dementia and parkinsonism coexist: corticobasal syndrome/corticobasal degeneration, progressive supranuclear palsy, multiple system atrophy, and frontotemporal dementia with parkinsonism linked to chromosome 17. The clinical, neuropsychologic, neuroradiologic, and neuropathologic similarities and differences in these disorders are compared and contrasted with each other and with Alzheimer's disease, Parkinson's disease, Parkinson's disease with dementia, and dementia with Lewy bodies, highlighting the features critical for identifying the correct diagnosis.

Rapidly Progressive Dementia 783

Michael D. Geschwind, Aissa Haman, and Bruce L. Miller

Rapidly progressive dementias (RPDs) are neurologic conditions that develop subacutely over weeks to months or, rarely, acutely over days. In contrast to most dementing conditions that take years to progress to death, RPD quickly can be fatal. It is critical to evaluate patients who have RPD without delay, usually in a hospital setting, as they may have a treatable condition. This review discusses a differential diagnostic approach to RPD, emphasizing neurodegenerative, toxic and metabolic, infectious, autoimmune, neoplastic, and other conditions to consider.

Normal Pressure Hydrocephalus 809

Neill R. Graff-Radford

Doctors find the management of normal pressure hydrocephalus (NPH) difficult because their diagnosis often is uncertain and the treatment with shunt surgery carries a significant risk. With the aim of bringing to the attention of physicians the useful, but largely anecdotal, information available regarding this problem, this article discusses the epidemiology, reasons why the diagnosis is difficult, differential diagnosis, features of the history, examination, neuropsychologic assessment, radiologic evaluation, and special tests that may help clinicians with management.

Prion Disease **833**
Eric Eggenberger

Prion diseases are a unique group of neurologic diseases caused by an abnormal protein conformation. Prion diseases encompass genetic, sporadic, iatrogenic, and acquired conditions in humans and other mammals. Although they are relatively rare, they produce a diverse array of symptoms, uniformly are fatal, and provide important information about proteins and degenerative neurobiology in addition to lessons about animal and human food chains.

Neuroimaging in Dementia **843**
Jennifer L. Whitwell and Clifford R. Jack Jr

Neuroimaging has become increasingly important in the clinical assessment and diagnosis of dementia. Structural imaging with MRI and functional imaging techniques, such as positron emission tomography and single photon emission CT, increasingly are used to aid in the differential diagnosis and early detection of dementia. Imaging techniques also can track disease progression over time and may be useful to monitor treatment effects. The most important development in the field over the past decade is the ability to image amyloid in the brain. This technique will revolutionize patient management and care.

Index **859**

FORTHCOMING ISSUES

November 2007

Brain Tumors in Adults
Patrick Y. Wen, MD, and
David Schiff, MD, *Guest Editors*

February 2008

Neurovirology
Christopher Power, MD, and
Richard Johnson, MD, *Guest Editors*

May 2008

Sports Neurology
Cory Toth, MD, *Guest Editor*

RECENT ISSUES

May 2007

Neck and Back Pain
Kerry H. Levin, MD, *Guest Editor*

February 2007

Peripheral Neuropathies
Yadollah Harati, MD, *Guest Editor*

November 2006

Preoperative and Perioperative Issues in Cerebrovascular Disease
José Biller, MD, *Guest Editor*

August 2006

Psychoneuroimmunology
Gregory G. Freund, MD, *Guest Editor*

May 2006

Neurology Case Studies
Randolph W. Evans, MD, *Guest Editor*

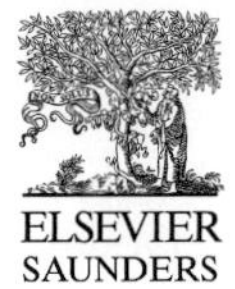

NEUROLOGIC CLINICS

Neurol Clin 25 (2007) xi–xii

Preface

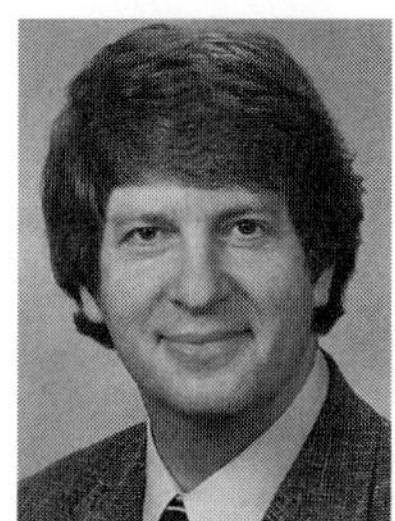

Neill R. Graff-Radford, MBBCh, FRCP
Guest Editor

The field of dementia has seen some important recent developments and this issue updates the reader in many areas. The first three articles address the area of Alzheimer's disease. Drs. Kelly and Petersen lead off, covering a wide array of clinical topics. Dr. Tanner then provides an update on the fast-moving genetics of this disease, and Dr. Eckman discusses the molecular basis of the amyloid beta protein as an important therapeutic target. The topic then switches to frontotemporal dementia, and Dr. Josephs begins by writing about the improved understanding of the clinical, pathologic, and biochemical factors of this disease; Drs. Haugervoll, Wszolek, and Hutton then place the new genetic findings in perspective and also discuss mouse models. Dr. Chui covers the very complicated topic of subcortical vascular dementia in her scholarly style, and Dr. Ferman provides a broad overview of Lewy body disease. Dr. Boeve then writes about other Parkinson-related dementias such as corticobasal degeneration, progressive supranuclear palsy, and multiple system atrophy. Dr. Geschwind provides a unique perspective on the group of dementias that present acutely and subacutely. My article focuses on a practical approach to normal pressure hydrocephalus, and Dr. Eggenberger presents an overview of Creutzfeldt-Jakob disease. In the last article, Drs. Whitwell and Jack present an overview of imaging in dementia that relates to many of the earlier articles.

0733-8619/07/$ - see front matter
doi:10.1016/j.ncl.2007.05.001 *neurologic.theclinics.com*

It has been my privilege to work with such outstanding coauthors, whom I thank sincerely for their hard work. I would also like to thank Donald Mumford and Sarah Fowler for their professionalism, support, and excellent editing throughout this project.

Neill R. Graff-Radford, MBBCh, FRCP
Mayo Clinic
4500 San Pablo Road
Jacksonville, FL 32224, USA

E-mail address: graffradford.neill@mayo.edu

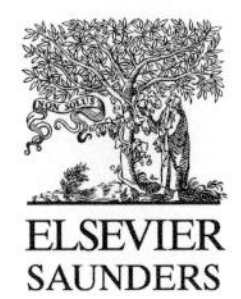

ELSEVIER
SAUNDERS

Neurol Clin 25 (2007) 577–609

NEUROLOGIC
CLINICS

Alzheimer's Disease and Mild Cognitive Impairment

Brendan J. Kelley, MD, Ronald C. Petersen, PhD, MD*

Mayo Clinic, Department of Neurology, 200 First Street SW, Rochester, MN 55905, USA

As our society ages, age-related diseases assume increasing prominence as personal and public health concerns. Disorders of cognition are particularly important in both regards, and Alzheimer's disease (AD) is by far the most common cause of dementia associated with aging. In 2000, the prevalence of AD in the United States was estimated to be 4.5 million individuals, and this number has been projected to increase to 14 million by 2050 [1]. Although AD is not an inevitable consequence of aging, these numbers speak to the dramatic scope of its impact. This article focuses on AD and the milder degrees of cognitive impairment that may precede the clinical diagnosis of probable AD, such as mild cognitive impairment (MCI) [2].

One presumes a gradual pathologic progression, which begins with normal aging, evolves through clinically probable AD, and culminates in neuropathologically proven AD [3]. It is likely that individuals pass through a transitional stage between normal aging and clinically probable AD, as illustrated in Fig. 1. This phase of MCI may be characterized by memory impairment associated with minimal or no functional decline. These individuals do not meet the criteria for clinically probable AD, yet are worthy of identification and monitoring.

In 2001, the American Academy of Neurology (AAN) published three practice parameters, evidence-based medicine analyses of the extant literature on dementia [4–6]. One paper dealt with MCI [5], the second with diagnostic issues concerning AD and other dementias [4], and the third reviewed treatment recommendations for AD and other dementias [6]. These

The authors would like to acknowledge the support for preparation of this article and research reported herein from the National Institute on Aging P50 AG16574, U01 AG06786, and the Robert H. and Clarice Smith and Abigail van Buren Alzheimer's Disease Research Program.

* Corresponding author.

E-mail address: peter8@mayo.edu (R.C. Petersen).

doi:10.1016/j.ncl.2007.03.008 ***neurologic.theclinics.com***

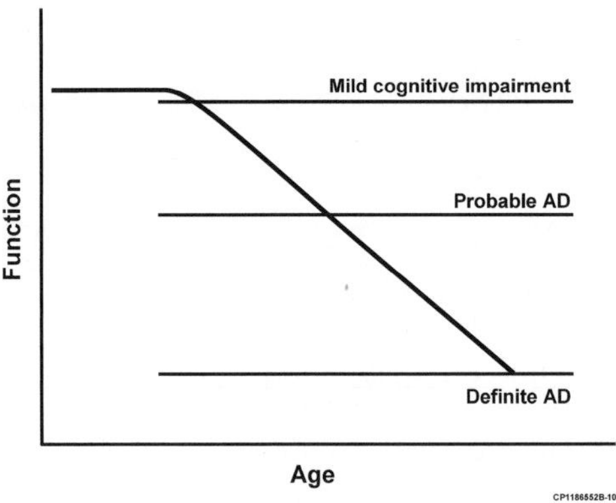

Fig. 1. Theoretic progression of cognitive function from normal, through MCI, to probable and definite AD in persons destined to develop AD. (*From* Petersen RC. Aging, mild cognitive impairment, and Alzheimer's disease. Neurol Clin 2000;10(4):789–805; with permission.)

documents provide current assessments of diagnostic and management issues regarding AD.

Normal aging

Implicit to a discussion of AD and MCI is knowledge about the cognitive changes of normal aging. Characterization of these cognitive changes remains an active area of research, with no agreement on the nature or degree of impairment or the pathologic substrate of that clinical picture. Consequently, the characterization of early changes of MCI remains difficult [7]. Normative data on various neuropsychologic tests for individuals up to age 100 years exist, as do criticisms of these data [8,9]. Some argue that existent normative data are contaminated by the inclusion of persons who would meet current definitions of MCI, and consequently, the norms reflect more impairment than should be expected as a consequence of "normal aging" [9]. Exclusion of these individuals from the normative data presents a conundrum, and the recursive logic necessary to solve it makes doing so impractical, if not impossible.

A meta-analysis investigating cognitive impairment before the diagnosis of AD indicated that preclinical deficits in global functioning, episodic memory, perceptual speed, and executive functioning were indicative of the subsequent development of AD [10]. Among episodic memory parameters, delayed recall procedures produced the largest effect sizes, and the investigators concluded that deficits in multiple cognitive domains preceded the clinical development of AD.

Research to delineate more precisely the cognitive changes associated with normal aging may allow a more accurate interpretation of very early cognitive changes and prediction of their pathologic substrates. At present, clinical judgment remains the best means of assessing MCI.

Dementia

Dementia implies a cognitive decline of sufficient severity to compromise a person's daily function. Although diagnostic criteria vary depending on dementia subtype, general features such as those found in the Diagnostic and Statistical Manual, 3rd edition, revised (DSM-III-R), remain useful [11]. In general, they require memory impairment beyond what would be normal for aging, and impairment of at least one other cognitive domain, such as attention, language, visuospatial skills, or problem solving. These deficits are of sufficient severity to compromise daily functional activities and do not occur in the setting of altered sensorium, such as delirium, or an acute confusional state. Once this type of cognitive impairment has been determined, the clinician must then determine the underlying nature of the dementia. In the DSM-III-R definition, memory impairment is an essential feature of dementia. Although this is true of many dementias, it is conceivable that patients who have frontotemporal dementia or a Lewy body dementia might present with significant impairment of nonmemory cognitive domains early in the disorder. Nevertheless, the DSM-III-R criteria provide a practical reference point, particularly for AD.

In an elderly person with gradually progressive amnestic disorder that has advanced to involve nonmemory cognitive domains to a degree that these changes affect daily functioning, AD is the most likely diagnosis.

Alzheimer's disease

This dementia is slowly progressive, with prominent memory disturbance appearing early in the clinical presentation [12]. As the disease progresses, other cognitive domains become involved and behavioral alterations arise [13–16]. AD is a degenerative disorder, and definitive diagnosis can only be made by postmortem examination of the brain. The classic neuropathologic features are neuritic plaques and neurofibrillary tangles [17].

Epidemiology

AD is an age-related phenomenon, and is the most common cause of dementia in the United States. The incidence of AD increases dramatically with age, doubling every 5 years after age 65 [18]. The prevalence of AD rises dramatically with age, becoming quite common in the 70s and more so into the 80s. It is uncertain whether the incidence of AD continues to rise into the 90s; however, the incidence of dementia increases rapidly in that age range. The prevalence of AD doubles every 5 years, and it occurs more often in women, likely reflecting their greater longevity [19–25].

Clinical diagnosis

The most commonly used clinical criteria for diagnosis of AD are those listed in the Diagnostic and Statistical Manual, 4th edition (DSM-IV), [26] or those established by the National Institute of Neurologic, Communicative Disorders and Stroke/Alzheimer's Disease and Related Disorders Association (NINCDS-ADRDA) work group [27]. The DSM-IV criteria for dementia of the Alzheimer's type (Box 1) involve the development of memory impairment, accompanied by impairment of one or more other cognitive domains, including aphasia, apraxia, agnosia, or disturbance of executive functioning. The cognitive impairments are gradually progressive, of sufficient severity to impair functional abilities, and cannot be accounted for by other neurologic or psychiatric disturbances. The AAN practice parameter found these criteria to be reliable [4].

An adequate history is essential to establishing the diagnosis of dementia. It is critical to take the history from the patient and an informant who knows the patient well. Simple inquiry regarding changes in the patient's ability to carry out typical activities of daily living provide a valuable gauge of the severity of cognitive impairment.

In addition to the history, instruments designed to screen for cognitive impairment, such as the Mini-Mental State Examination (MMSE) [28], the Modified Mini-Mental State Examination (3MS) [29], the Blessed Orientation Memory Concentration Test [30], the Kokmen Short Test of Mental Status [31], or the Clinical Dementia Rating scale (CDR) [32], can be quite useful. None has been demonstrated to be superior to the others.

Box 1. Diagnostic criteria for dementia of the Alzheimer's type

A Memory impairment
   Learning or recall
B One or more of the following
   i. Aphasia
   ii. Apraxia
   iii. Agnosia
   iv. Dysexecutive function (planning, organizing, sequencing, abstracting)
C Cognitive deficits of sufficient severity to affect social or occupational functioning, representing a change from previous level
D Clinical course with gradual onset and progression
E Not caused by delirium
F No alternative central nervous system explanation (eg, stroke, Parkinson's disease)

General neurologic examination

In early AD, the general neurologic examination is typically normal, with the exception of the mental status evaluation. Abnormalities such as parkinsonism, focal neurologic deficits, or deficits in other parts of the nervous system, may suggest an alternative diagnosis. It is important to assess sensory functions because sensory deprivation can affect the mental status and neurologic examination. Finally, the neurologic examination should be complemented by a general medical examination looking for medical conditions that may contribute to cognitive impairment.

Laboratory tests

The usefulness of various laboratory tests in evaluating a patient who has dementia was assessed in the AAN practice parameter [4]. The investigators concluded that vitamin B-12 levels and thyroid functions should be assessed routinely in cases of dementia.

In practice, various tests may be considered in the evaluation of dementia, as outlined in Box 2. Although few of these have been demonstrated to

Box 2. Evaluation of patients who have dementia

Routine
Electrolytes
Complete blood count
Vitamin B_{12} level[a]
Thyroid function studies[a]
Syphilis serology
CT/MRI[a]

Optional
Sedimentation rate
Drug levels
HIV testing
Lyme serology
Urinalysis
24-urine for heavy metal
Cerebrospinal fluid
Chest radiograph
Electrocardiogram
Electroencephalogram
Positron emission tomography/single photon emission computed tomography

[a] Suggested by the AAN [4]

actually have an impact on improving the dementia, they can be helpful in the appropriate clinical setting because medical conditions may impact cognitive function.

Neuroimaging

The AAN practice parameter recommended that a CT or MRI be done in most circumstances at the initial dementia assessment to exclude potentially treatable structural lesions, such as subdural hematoma, neoplasm, and stroke [4].

Atrophy of medial temporal lobe structures (eg, the hippocampus) has been found in patients who have AD, but this atrophy may be nonspecific and, although consistent with AD, it may also be seen in other conditions [33]. Longitudinal volumetric measurements of the hippocampal formation have indicated more rapid progression of atrophy among persons with AD than among normal controls [34]. The usefulness of volumetric measurements of the entorhinal cortex remains controversial [35–37]. Although atrophy of the hippocampus, amygdala, and entorhinal cortex is established in AD, the role of these findings in the diagnostic evaluation of people having, or at risk for developing, AD remains to be defined [38].

Functional neuroimaging has been studied in AD, and although several studies have suggested that single photon emission computed tomography (SPECT) imaging augments the clinician's acumen [39–43], added discriminability has not been demonstrated definitively. Positron emission tomography (PET) scanning has shown promise in differentiation among dementias [44], and ^{18}F-2-deoxyglucose (FDG)-PET may be a useful adjunct in the diagnosis of AD [45]. Literature validates the usefulness of FDG-PET in differentiating AD from frontotemporal dementia, and the Centers for Medicare and Medicaid have approved for reimbursement the use of FDG-PET for this purpose. Some evidence suggests that FDG-PET may be useful in assessing people at risk for developing AD, but longitudinal outcome data are not available [45].

Proton MR spectroscopy has also shown promise in evaluating incipient cases of AD [46], and possibly in differentiating among the various types of dementias [47]. This technique may be useful in assisting in the diagnosis of dementia in the future.

Recently, exciting new imaging techniques have been developed that allow antemortem detection of amyloid deposition in the brain through the use of the radioligand PET imaging studies [48–50]. Pittsburgh compound-B, although not ready for clinical use, provides the potential for detecting the onset of amyloid deposition before the development of clinical symptoms, and the opportunity of following amyloid-targeted therapies [51,52]. Another compound, FDDNP, which binds to both amyloid and tau, was recently reported to differentiate between normal controls, MCI, and AD [50]. These developments may lead to important new research opportunities in the early diagnosis and treatment of AD [52].

Neuropsychologic testing

Neuropsychologic testing can help determine if reported cognitive changes represent normal aging or MCI, or signify AD. In early AD, subjects commonly have deficits in delayed verbal recall and learning, and may also exhibit impaired naming. A depressed subject may generate a flat learning curve over multiple trials to learn a list of words, but will be able to retain the amount learned after a delay. Frontotemporal dementia patients may have profound difficulties with executive function, sustained attention, and speed of processing, with relative sparing of naming and memory. Although not diagnostic, these neuropsychologic profiles can help distinguish among various dementias. Neuropsychologic testing can also provide a baseline against which to compare future evaluations. Consequently, depending on the particular clinical situation, neuropsychologic testing can be an important adjunct.

Lumbar puncture

Several retrospective studies have found little evidence to recommend spinal fluid analysis in the routine evaluation of dementia in elderly patients [53]. Dementia characterized by a subacute mental status change, fever, nuchal rigidity, or in the setting of possible contributing processes such as systemic cancer or collagen vascular disease, may warrant cerebrospinal fluid (CSF) analysis. Positive syphilis serology may be evaluated further by CSF examination. In immunocompromised patients, syphilis, fungal infections, lymphoma, and other opportunistic infections must be considered. Individuals having a rapidly progressive or atypical clinical course and those presenting younger than age 60 may also prompt CSF analysis. Obviously, one must ascertain that no contraindications to the procedure exist.

Genetic testing

Individuals presenting in their 30s, 40s, or 50s with a family history suggestive of an autosomal dominant disease may merit testing for mutations on chromosomes 1, 14, or 21 [54]. Testing should be undertaken only in the setting of appropriate genetic counseling, because the results may have a significant impact on the patient and family members. Typically, genetic testing for specific mutations is not useful in typical late-onset AD.

Among susceptibility polymorphisms for AD, the most recognized is the lipid-carrying protein, apolipoprotein E (Apo E) [55,56]. A large neuropathologic study investigating the usefulness of Apo E genotyping found that Apo E ϵ4 presence increased diagnostic accuracy for AD by about 4%, and its absence increased the diagnostic accuracy of something other than AD by 8% [57]. These percentages augmented the clinician's diagnostic accuracy. Apo E testing is not recommended currently for asymptomatic individuals who feel they may be at risk by virtue of a positive family history

[56,58]. The AAN does not recommend evaluation of any genetic markers for AD at this time [4].

Biomarkers

Several studies have found that CSF levels of amyloid beta (Aβ) 1-42 are reduced in AD subjects, relative to normal controls [59–62], but the usefulness of these measurements for early diagnosis remains unclear. Low Aβ 1-42 levels were not found to correlate with degree of cognitive impairment [63]. A recent study found CSF Aβ 1-42 useful in distinguishing AD with white matter lesions from vascular dementia, with the acknowledgment that Aβ 1-42 serves simply as a surrogate marker in this context [64].

CSF tau levels in AD have been shown to be elevated, relative to controls [65–68]. Few studies have compared the CSF Aβ or tau levels to a clinical diagnosis. One study found that in 26 neuropathologically confirmed AD cases, CSF phosphorylated tau (p-tau) and brain homogenate p-tau correlated, as did the score of neuritic plaques [69]. The combination of CSF Aβ 1-42 and tau, and in particular the species of tau phosphorylated at threonine 181 or 231 (p-tau), may be useful, and studies have indicated sensitivities and specificities of 85% and 87%, respectively [60,62,70–72]. However, it is not known if these biomarkers augment the diagnostic accuracy of the clinician.

Another CSF marker, AD7c-NTP (neuronal thread protein), has shown high sensitivities and specificities, but because of technical limitations and the absence of studies of well-delineated patient populations, the usefulness of quantitative measurement of this marker in CSF or urine is unclear [73–76].

The AAN practice parameter states that no biomarkers have emerged as being appropriate for routine use in the clinical evaluation of patients who have suspected AD [4].

Alzheimer's disease pathophysiology

Most investigators believe that AD is caused completely, or in part, by abnormal processing or deposition of amyloid. The pathogenic form of amyloid is generated by abnormal cleavage of amyloid precursor protein (APP), and is referred to as Aβ 1-42. Normally, APP is cleaved by α-secretase. Aβ 1-42 is formed when APP is cleaved by β- and γ-secretases and then deposited in the brain as an insoluble aggregate. This deposition presumably initiates a cascade of events that result in inflammatory responses and cell destruction. Although this pathologic process may not be the only one, it is believed to be an important component of the degenerative cascade, and is the target for many new treatment interventions.

The other primary pathologic feature of AD involves the abnormal processing of tau and neurofibrillary tangle formation. The recent development of animal models exhibiting both Aβ deposition and neurofibrillary tangles holds the promise of providing a better model of the fundamental pathologic elements involved in human AD.

Mild cognitive impairment

Conceptual framework

Elderly individuals who feel that their memory has changed from a previous level of functioning are frequently concerned about developing AD. Clinicians must then face the dilemma of trying to determine the significance of a patient's forgetfulness. MCI refers to the clinical state in which a subject is cognitively impaired, usually in the memory domain, but not demented.

The AAN practice parameter addressing MCI concluded that persons with memory impairment, who meet the criteria for MCI, have an increased risk for progressing to clinically probable AD and should be counseled and followed accordingly [5]. Ideally, identification of these individuals would allow an effective treatment intervention to reduce this risk of progression to dementia, but, at present, no treatment exists that does so. Candidate treatments include cholinesterase inhibitors, antioxidants, anti-inflammatories, and nootropics [77].

Clinical criteria

Although the diagnosis of MCI has no accepted criteria, most investigators have used a variation of those presented in Box 3. Longitudinal clinical studies indicate that subjects with amnestic MCI have an increased rate of progression to clinically probable AD [78]. These criteria for MCI are clinical. Although neuropsychologic testing may help differentiate these individuals from those who experience normal aging, MCI is not a neuropsychologic diagnosis. A recent study from France demonstrated the unreliability of retrospective application of a neuropsychologic test–based definition of MCI [79]. This study found that application of arbitrary neuropsychologic cutoffs in the absence of clinical judgment eliminated the predictive

Box 3. Clinical criteria for mild cognitive impairment

1. Cognitive complaint (usually memory), preferably corroborated by an informant
2. Cognitive impairment (usually memory) for age and education
3. Essentially normal general cognitive function
4. Largely preserved activities of daily living
5. Not demented

value of the MCI diagnosis. However, diagnosis based on neuropsychologic data used in conjunction with the clinical criteria shown in Box 3 can be reliable and predictive of eventual progression [80].

The first diagnostic criterion is a cognitive complaint. Typically, subjects are mildly affected and are aware of their deficit, and corroboration by an informant is particularly useful [81]. The second criterion requires objective demonstration of cognitive impairment by the clinician and neuropsychologist, relative to the subjects' age- and education-matched peers [82,83]. As discussed, no particular reference point for normal aging is entirely accurate, but normative data on subjects of similar demographic characteristics may be useful. MCI subjects tend to fall 1.5 standard deviations below their age- and education-matched mates on measures of learning and recall, but these are only guidelines and not cutoff scores for assisting in the diagnosis of MCI. Some subjects who fall within the normal range of memory function may, in fact, have experienced a decline from their prior level of function, and it may be appropriate to diagnose MCI.

The third criterion refers to relatively normal general cognition. Put simply, cognitive domains outside the one primarily impaired are relatively preserved. Close inspection of these subjects may demonstrate subtle deficits in other cognitive domains, but they are not of sufficient severity to suggest that the person is demented [80]. Again, this judgment is clinical. Similarly, activities of daily living are largely preserved. Subjects may experience minor difficulties caused by memory deficits so, technically, their activities of daily living are slightly impaired. However, the degree of impairment is insufficient to constitute dementia.

The last criterion is perhaps the most important. The clinician does not feel that the patient meets the criteria for dementia or clinically probable AD. These individuals function independently in the community and carry out their routine daily activities. Most clinicians feel that it would be a disservice to label these patients with the diagnosis of AD at this very mild stage of impairment, and the concept of MCI has been developed to identify them.

More recently, the construct of MCI has been extended beyond just memory deficit [84]. As shown in Fig. 2, the person can now have any type of cognitive complaint, although memory is the most common. In the estimation of the clinician, this person is not normal for age, but not demented, based on the clinical history from the patient and an informant, and an office examination, possibly supplemented with additional cognitive testing. Despite the cognitive decline, the activities of daily living remain essentially normal. Patients meeting these criteria merit consideration for the diagnosis of MCI. As Fig. 2 illustrates, the major subtypes of MCI are amnestic MCI or nonamnestic MCI. Memory function is assessed by the mental status examination, which may be supplemented with neuropsychologic testing. If memory impairment is present, cognitive testing can help determine whether only memory is affected (amnestic MCI, single domain)

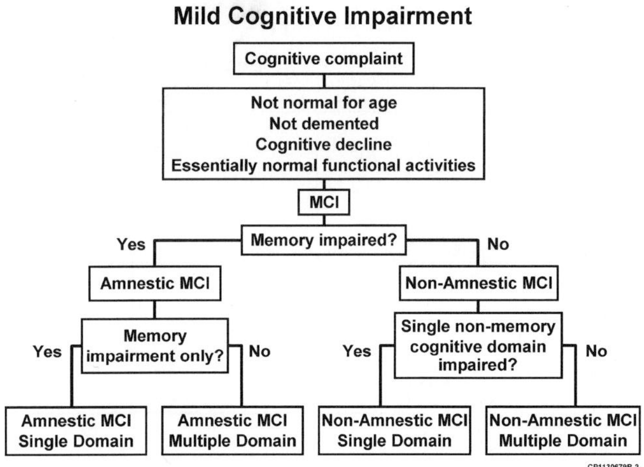

Fig. 2. Flow diagram for diagnosing MCI. The cardinal feature is cognitive impairment intermediate between the cognitive changes of normal aging and those of early dementia. Subtyping of MCI is first made along the dimension of memory, into amnestic and nonamnestic. These subtypes are further classified into single cognitive domain or multiple cognitive domains.

or whether other cognitive domains are also impaired (amnestic cognitive impairment, multiple domain). The other cognitive domains typically evaluated include language, attention/executive function, and visuospatial skills. If the person meets MCI criteria and memory is not impaired, other cognitive domains need to be assessed to determine if it is an isolated problem (nonamnestic MCI, single domain) or if multiple nonmemory domains are involved (nonamnestic MCI, multiple domain).

Similar to the evaluation of dementia, historical and neuroimaging data may suggest the cause of MCI to be degenerative, vascular, psychiatric, or traumatic, or secondary to medical illnesses, as illustrated in Fig. 3. In reality, part of the scheme shown in Fig. 3 is theoretic and not validated, whereas other aspects are well documented in the literature [85–87]. Amnestic MCI with a degenerative cause is highly likely to progress to AD, and the AAN endorsed this construct in its practice parameter [5]. The corresponding outcome of nonamnestic MCI subjects is currently under investigation.

Evaluation

The clinical evaluation of suspected MCI is virtually identical to that described earlier for clinically probable AD. As mentioned, the history is of particular importance and should be verified by an informant, if at all possible. The clinician should perform a mental status examination, in addition to a general neurologic examination. Most of the commonly used instruments available, MMSE, 3MS, Kokmen Short Test of Mental Status [28,29,31], are relatively insensitive in this range of cognitive function, and, in all likelihood, performance on these measures will appear more

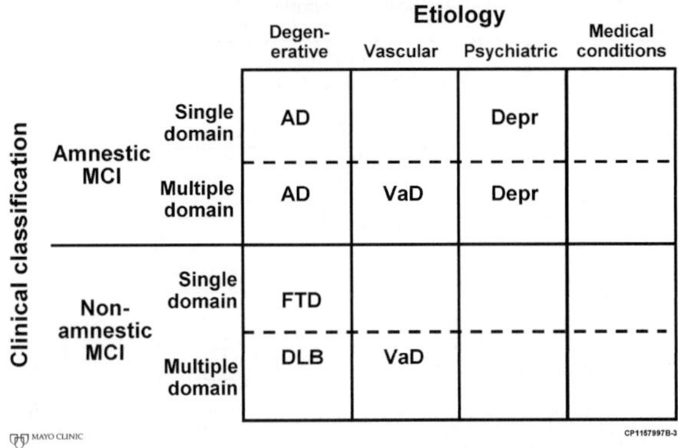

Fig. 3. The four clinical subtypes of MCI are then combined with the presumed cause of the clinical syndrome. For example, amnestic MCI of single or multiple domain subtypes can be combined with the presumed degenerative cause to result in the likely outcome of AD when the condition progresses to dementia. The other suggested clinical outcomes are theoretic; other outcomes may be possible. Depr, depression; DLB, diffuse Lewy body disease; FTD, frontotemporal dementia; VaD, vascular dementia.

normal than not. Subjects with MCI often score in the 26-to-28 range on the MMSE, which is typically reported as normal. If the mental status examination instrument does not have a significant memory component, subjects with relatively isolated memory impairment will not be differentiated from those who are aging normally. Consequently, the clinician may consider augmenting the clinical examination with an additional memory test [88,89].

The medical laboratory tests are also similar to those described earlier for clinically probable AD (see Box 2). One should pay particular attention to subtle medical issues that could affect cognitive function. Although depression often can be differentiated from clinically probable AD, it could present with subtle memory impairment in its early stages. Consequently, the clinician should also remain attuned to possible psychiatric components of subtle memory impairments.

Neuroimaging

Several recent MRI studies involving volumetric assessments of the medial temporal lobe have been informative [33–36,90]. Discussion is ongoing about the relative usefulness of volumetric measurements of the hippocampal formation versus entorhinal cortex volumes [35–37]. Measurements of whole-brain atrophy are under investigation, although it remains to be determined if whole-brain volume changes will be useful in assessing the early stages of AD. A 2001 study suggested that this may be the case [91] and was supported by a subsequent prospective study [92], although precise delineation of the rate of atrophy in early AD requires further study.

The usefulness of other imaging modalities, such as MR spectroscopy, SPECT, and PET, has not been demonstrated definitively in this population [93]. Nevertheless, in selected instances, particularly in the setting of a normal structural imaging scan, functional imaging modalities may provide additional useful information [94]. Patients who have amnestic MCI are at an increased risk for progression to AD, and imaging agents such as Pittsburgh compound-B or FDDNP may augment this prognostic information, although this has not yet been verified.

Neuropsychologic testing

Neuropsychologic testing can aid in differentiating subjects with MCI from those with normal aging impairments, but the testing battery must involve sufficiently difficult learning and recall tasks to tease apart these subtle deficits. Neuropsychologic testing will not make the diagnosis of MCI, but can be suggestive in the appropriate clinical context [95]. Fig. 4 presents typical neurocognitive profiles of subjects with MCI, normal aging, and very mild clinically probable AD (CDR 0.5). On measures of general cognitive function, such as the MMSE and full-scale IQ, the individual with MCI performs more like the normal elderly subject, whereas memory function on delayed verbal recall (Logical Memory II) and delayed nonverbal recall (Visual Reproductions II) more closely resembles mild AD [80].

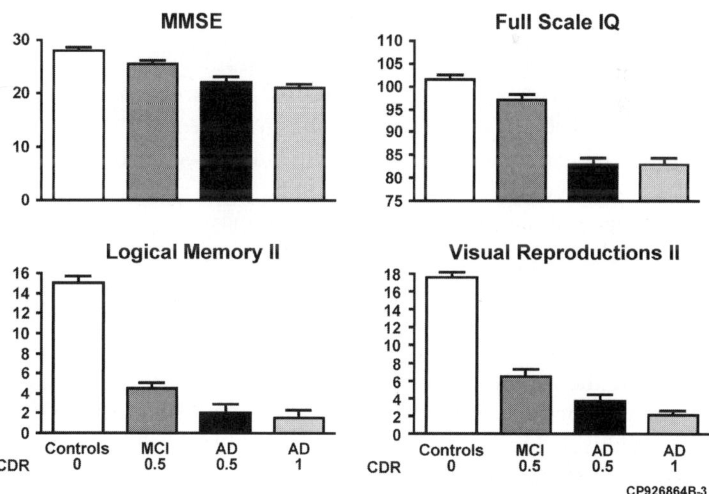

Fig. 4. Cognitive profile of persons with an MCI. The top two panels, MMSE and full-scale IQ, represent measures of general intellectual function. The bottom two panels represent memory function for verbal memory (Logical Memory II) and nonverbal memory (Visual Reproductions II). (*From* Petersen RC, Smith GE, Waring SC, et al. Mild cognitive impairment: clinical characterization and outcome. Arch Neurol 1999;56(3):303–8; with permission.)

Biomarkers

As in AD, biomarkers are in the early stages of development. It is possible that the CSF measures of Aβ and tau may be useful in differentiating subjects with MCI from normal aging [60,66,96]. These markers may have usefulness in predicting progression from MCI to AD [63,97]. A multinational study found that baseline CSF levels of tau phosphorylated at threonine 231, but not total tau protein levels, correlated with cognitive decline and conversion from MCI to AD [72]. Another recent study that investigated the usefulness of CSF concentrations of Aβ 1-42, total tau (t-tau), and tau phosphorylated at threonine 181 (p-tau) in predicting progression from MCI to AD reported a sensitivity of 95% and a specificity of 83% using the combination of elevated t-tau and lowered Aβ 1-42 [98]. This area of research is exciting, but the present data are insufficient to recommend use of CSF biomarkers in the evaluation of MCI.

Genetics

The genetic features of MCI are similar to those of clinically probable AD. MCI appears to have a higher representation of Apo E ϵ4 carriers, and some studies suggest that the presence of the ϵ4 allele may predict a higher rate of progression [99,100]. However, these data are only weakly positive, and Apo E genotyping is not recommended currently as a diagnostic or prognostic indicator in MCI.

Neuropathology

Several studies have reported on the neuropathology of subjects who died with the clinical classification of MCI [101,102]. Neuropathology in subjects with MCI in the Religious Orders Study was intermediate, between the neuropathologic changes of normal aging and fully developed AD [101]. This study also indicated that vascular features were present and suggested that neurodegenerative and vascular changes may account for the clinical features of MCI. Another report, from the Nun Study, indicated that individuals who were retrospectively classified as having MCI primarily had neuropathologic changes of AD at autopsy [103]. This study found that patients who had MCI had significantly more neuritic plaques relative to controls, and that these findings were more similar to those of early AD than normal aging. However, a study from the Mayo Clinic on MCI demonstrated that subjects had intermediate neuropathologic changes significantly different from both controls and AD [102]. MCI subjects in this series more closely resembled normal control subjects than AD subjects, implying that these MCI subjects were diagnosed at an earlier stage in the disease process. Two small neuropathologic studies demonstrated neurofibrillary tangle pathology in the nucleus basalis [104] and locus caeruleus [105] in MCI and early AD.

A Washington University study found that when dementia subjects classified as having AD and a CDR of 0.5 progressed, 84% of them had the neuropathologic features of AD [106]. A Mayo Clinic study of 34 subjects previously diagnosed with MCI who had progressed to dementia demonstrated that although approximately 75% of these subjects went on to have AD, the other 25% developed other forms of dementia [107]. Therefore, although amnestic MCI criteria are predictive of developing AD, they are not absolute, and when patients are diagnosed at an early stage of impairment, neuropathologic features do not correspond to AD at that point in time.

Summary

The construct of MCI identifies individuals at increased risk of developing AD. The early identification of these more subtle impairments may allow clinicians to counsel and follow their patients more effectively. Many subjects with amnestic MCI will ultimately progress to probable AD. Identification at this earlier point in the progression may ultimately allow intervention to slow or halt progression. MCI is an important area for clinical research, and work characterizing the clinical features of these subjects and documenting their outcome is progressing at a rapid rate.

Treatments

Alzheimer's disease

Symptomatic

Five drugs are approved by the Food and Drug Administration (FDA) for the treatment of clinically probable AD (Table 1), although only four are used commonly. Three of these four are acetylcholinesterase inhibitors, used in response to various lines of research which implicate a cholinergic deficit in AD [108]. Acetylcholine is involved in many aspects of cognition, including memory and attention. Cholinergic neurons in the basal forebrain project to many regions of the neocortex and to the medial temporal lobe, including the hippocampus. Anticholinergic drugs, such as scopolamine, can impair learning and recall, reminiscent of the cognitive changes seen in AD [109]. Choline acetyltransferase, the synthetic enzyme for acetylcholine, is reduced in the brains of patients who have AD [110,111]. In the past decade, acetylcholinesterase inhibitors have been shown to be effective at modulating the symptoms of AD and currently form the mainstay of treatment in clinically probable AD.

The first compound approved was tacrine (Cognex), which led the way for treatment of AD. However, tacrine required dosing four times a day and liver toxicity necessitated regular monitoring of liver enzymes. Newer drugs without these limiting features were introduced, and tacrine is now used only rarely for the treatment of AD.

Table 1
Symptomatic medications for Alzheimer's disease

Drug	Mechanism	Initial dose	Target dose	Titration interval	Side effects
Donepezil (Aricept)	AchEI	5 mg qd	10 mg qd	4–6 wk	Nausea, vomiting, diarrhea, muscle cramps, anorexia, vivid dreaming
Rivastigmine (Exelon)	AchEI	1.5 mg bid	6 mg bid	2–4 wk	Nausea, vomiting, diarrhea, weight loss, dizziness
Galantamine (Reminyl)	AchEI	4 mg bid	12 mg bid	4 wk	Nausea, vomiting, diarrhea, anorexia, dizziness
Tacrine (Cognex)	AchEI	10 mg qid	40 mg qid	4 wk	Liver function test evaluations, diarrhea, anorexia, nausea, vomiting, myalgia
Memantine (Namenda)	NMDA-A	5 mg qd	10 mg bid	1–2 wk	Dizziness, confusion, headache, constipation, nausea, agitation, hallucination, seizure

Abbreviations: AChEI, acetylcholinesterase inhibitor; NMDA-A, NMDA antagonist.

Donepezil (Aricept) became available in the mid-1990s as the next acetylcholinesterase inhibitor approved by the FDA. It is administered once daily and does not require any laboratory monitoring. It is heavily bound to plasma proteins, and has a half-life of approximately 70 hours. Typically, it is started at 5 mg daily and the dose is increased to 10 mg daily after 4 to 6 weeks, if the drug is well tolerated. The most common side effects include nausea, increased bowel frequency, and vomiting. Occasionally, patients experience vivid dreaming, which may be reduced by morning administration of the drug. Cholinesterase inhibitors could theoretically influence cardiac rhythm, but this is not commonly encountered in the absence of an underlying disturbance of cardiac conduction. They may also have an effect on respiratory conditions such as chronic obstructive pulmonary disease or asthma, and could theoretically interfere with the administration of anesthesia during surgery. The absorption of donepezil is not influenced by food intake.

Several studies of the efficacy of donepezil show a modest improvement in cognitive function as measured by scales such as the Alzheimer's Disease Assessment Scale–Cognitive Subscale (ADAS-Cog) and the Clinician's Interview-Based Impression of Change (CIBIC Plus) [6]. The drug is approved for mild to moderate AD. The length of the response has been documented up to 52 weeks but it is uncertain if the benefit persists longer. Studies indicate that performance of the subject returns to the same as in the untreated state when donepezil is discontinued, suggesting that donepezil has a symptomatic effect on the disease but does not affect the underlying pathophysiologic process.

A large study of donepezil in amnestic MCI found a reduced rate of progression to AD during the first 12 months of the study, but no overall impact on rate of progression at the 3-year end point [112]. This finding suggests a transient symptomatic benefit without modification of disease course in amnestic MCI, similar to its effect in AD.

Rivastigmine (Exelon) is another acetylcholinesterase inhibitor approved by the FDA [113]. Rivastigmine is a pseudo-irreversible inhibitor of acetylcholinesterase and dissociates from the enzyme slowly. Dosing begins with 1.5 mg twice a day and increases in increments of 1.5 mg per dose, to a maximum of 6 mg twice daily. This dosing offers greater flexibility; however, the twice-daily dosing may make it more difficult for memory-impaired patients to adhere to therapy. It may provide greater cholinesterase inhibition at the highest dose, but it is also prone to an increased frequency of side effects, possibly related to its inhibition of butyrylcholinesterase. Side effects are similar to those of donepezil, although with a somewhat higher incidence of gastrointestinal side effects [113]. To encourage adherence to dose increases, titration is recommended, to be advanced on a 2- to 4-week basis. The effect size of rivastigmine on the ADAS-Cog and the CIBIC Plus is approximately the same as that of donepezil [6].

The fourth cholinesterase inhibitor approved by the FDA, galantamine (Reminyl), is a reversible inhibitor of cholinesterase that also has some nicotinic receptor activity. This mechanism has been proposed to provide an additional benefit over the other cholinesterase inhibitors. The initial starting dose of galantamine is 4 mg twice daily, which is increased to 8 mg twice daily, and ultimately 12 mg twice daily, if tolerated. This dose escalation is done at 4-week intervals to minimize side effects. Galantamine has similar potential for GI, cardiac, and pulmonary concerns as the other cholinesterase inhibitors. The effect size of galantamine on the ADAS-Cog and the CIBIC Plus is similar to those of donepezil and rivastigmine. One study found that galantamine had an effect on the activities of daily living and behavior [114]. Concern about an increase in mortality, presumably from cardiac deaths, has arisen in clinical trials of galantamine in MCI. The FDA has expressed caution about the use of galantamine for that indication.

Memantine (Namenda) is an N-methyl-D-aspartate (NMDA) antagonist that has been approved by the FDA for the treatment of moderate to severe AD. This drug can be used either alone or in combination with a cholinesterase inhibitor to help improve the symptoms of AD, but has not been shown to have an effect on the underlying disease process.

In summary, donepezil, rivastigmine, galantamine, and memantine are the most commonly used drugs in the treatment of AD. They appear to be equally efficacious and have similar side effect profiles, their cost is approximately equivalent, and little evidence recommends one over the other. They appear to provide a modest enhancement of cognitive function in subjects with AD but do not seem to have a significant impact on the underlying pathophysiology of AD. The AAN practice parameter on treatment of dementia recommended that cholinesterase inhibitors be considered in mild to moderate AD patients, although the effect size is modest [6]. The gastrointestinal side effects can be minimized with slow titration of the drug. Their role in MCI is defined incompletely, with a large trial suggesting transient symptomatic benefit in amnestic MCI, but no lasting impact on progression to AD [112].

The cost effectiveness of cholinesterase inhibitors has been debated, with one study suggesting a modest cost savings in favor of donepezil over placebo, with a reduction in the use of residential care [115], and another study coming to the opposite conclusion [116]. Comparable studies have not been done with the other cholinesterase inhibitors or with memantine. Thus, the long-term benefit remains questionable from an economic perspective.

Disease modifying

Vitamin E. Considerable research supports a role of oxidative damage in the pathophysiology of AD, and the use of antioxidants as a treatment of AD remains an area of active research. Epidemiologic data suggest that antioxidants may be associated with a lower incidence of AD [117–121]. A large clinical trial of moderate AD patients found that vitamin E and selegiline were effective at slowing the progression of moderate AD [122]. The primary end points of this study were death, institutionalization, loss of basic activities of daily living, or a progression on the CDR from 2 to 3, and both vitamin E and selegiline reduced the rate of progression. The dosage of vitamin E was 1,000 IU twice daily and that of selegiline was 10 mg daily. Because of selegiline's drug interactions and other potential toxicities, and as a suggestion of a very mild superiority of vitamin E, the AAN practice parameter recommended that vitamin E at 1000 IU twice daily be considered as a treatment to slow the progression of AD [6]. This finding has not been replicated, nor has the optimal dose of vitamin E been determined by additional studies. A single large study that investigated vitamin E in amnestic MCI found no benefit over placebo [112]. Theoretic concerns of gastrointestinal toxicity and bleeding exist with vitamin E, but generally it is well tolerated.

This single positive study for vitamin E needs to be interpreted in the context of a recent meta-analysis that suggests an increased risk of death among those taking vitamin E at 400 IU or more per day [123]. These deaths were mostly cardiovascular, and the overall medical condition of the participants in the studies pooled for meta-analysis may not accurately represent typical AD patients.

Under investigation

Anti-inflammatory medications. Research implicates an inflammatory component to the neurodegenerative process in AD [124,125], and epidemiologic studies have suggested that nonsteroidal anti-inflammatory drug (NSAID) use may protect against developing AD [126–130]. Given this background, it is not surprising that several studies have been undertaken to determine the possible efficacy of anti-inflammatories in treating AD [131–133].

Studies using glucocorticoids such as prednisone or NSAIDs have been negative to date [131,134]. The cyclooxygenase (COX)-2 inhibitors have not been demonstrated to be beneficial, and cardiovascular concerns exist regarding the prolonged use of these medications [135–139]. Thus, although the epidemiologic data and theoretic considerations remain intriguing, the benefit of anti-inflammatory agents for the treatment or prevention of AD has not been demonstrated [140].

It has been speculated that some NSAIDs may have specific Aβ-lowering properties and hence might be useful in the treatment of AD through an alternative mechanism, and research is ongoing in this area [141–143].

Estrogen replacement therapy. Some epidemiologic evidence suggests that postmenopausal women who take estrogen replacement may be protected from developing AD [144–147]. More recently, however, the Women's Health Initiative Memory Study has demonstrated that postmenopausal estrogen use might actually be a risk factor for developing AD and MCI, rather than a protective factor [148–151]. Longitudinal studies are underway concerning a possible prophylactic effect of estrogen in reducing the risk of developing dementia, but the data from these studies are pending [152,153]. A large trial of estrogen replacement in mild to moderate AD failed to demonstrate benefit over the course of 12 months [154]. A smaller, 16-week trial was also negative [155]. A case-control study found no overall correlation between estrogen replacement and incident cases of AD, although it did suggest that this factor interacted with smoking history [156]. At present, no data suggest that estrogen is useful as a treatment or prophylactic for AD and it is currently not recommended for that purpose.

Amyloid treatments. Deposition of Aβ is considered to be intrinsic to the pathophysiology of AD, and several research strategies are underway that address this mechanism [157]. Aβ is a major component of the neuritic plaques in AD, and fibrillar Aβ has been shown to be neurotoxic. Aβ is processed by several proteases to various amylogenic and nonamylogenic pathways [158]. The protease α-secretase produces the nonamylogenic fragments and is the preferred pathway, whereas β-secretase and γ-secretase cleavage results in the generation of Aβ. Consequently, strategies that attempt to inhibit the activities of β-secretase and γ-secretase have been developed [159–162]. The β-secretase enzyme BACE is one target [163] and γ-secretase is another [164–167]. A 12-month clinical trial of an NSAID-derived γ-secretase inhibitor suggested benefit in daily activities and psychiatric events [168], and a larger phase III trial of this agent is ongoing. Thus, although candidate compounds have been identified, only limited clinical trial data are currently available.

Immunization was proposed as a treatment in 1999, based on mouse data that suggested that immunization with Aβ in early life reduced Aβ plaque formation later in life [169]. Midlife immunization of these mice showed a reduced progression of the disease and suggested some regression of the underlying pathology [169].

A multicenter phase II clinical trial of active immunotherapy with a vaccine against Aβ-42 (AN1792) plus adjuvant QS-21 in humans began in 2001. This study was halted in early 2002 after a subacute meningoencephalitis developed in approximately 5% of the immunized subjects [170]. Active immunization was discontinued; however, it was suggested that the subset of subjects who developed sufficient antibody levels may have had a reduced progression of the disease [171]. The few autopsies performed on trial participants have suggested some clearance of neuritic plaques [172]. Subjects who produced antibody showed more brain volume reduction on MRI, hinting that some degree of amyloid clearing process may have affected brain volumes [173].

Polyclonal antibodies against Aβ can be found in human immunoglobulins, and intravenous immunoglobulin (IVIg) has been advanced as a method of passive immunization for the treatment of AD [174,175]. One study of five patients suggested that monthly IVIg reduced CSF Aβ concentrations while increasing serum levels of Aβ [175]. A phase I trial of IVIg in eight patients suggested sustained cognitive benefit among some patients [176], and a small phase II trial is currently underway. Passive immunization using monoclonal antibodies produced in cell culture has also been proposed, and a phase IIa trial of bapineuzumab (a humanized antibody against Aβ) is expected to be completed in 2008.

Noncognitive symptoms

Noncognitive symptoms of AD, such as anxiety, depression, psychosis, and sleep disturbances, may prove more bothersome to the patient and family than cognitive impairment and can cause considerable stress on both the patient and the caregiver. These noncognitive symptoms often require ongoing active management by the physician and are the motivating factor for many telephone calls. Many of these symptoms can be ameliorated, and consequently, they deserve significant attention on the part of the treating physician. Increased recognition of these noncognitive symptoms has fostered increasing research attention in this area [177].

An increased risk of cardiovascular symptoms, glucose intolerance, stroke, and death has been associated with the use of atypical antipsychotics in some psychiatric disorders, resulting in an FDA "black box warning" on the use of atypical antipsychotics in older subjects with dementia [178]. Caution should be exercised in using these drugs, but their judicious use can have a dramatically positive impact on problematic behavioral symptoms [6].

Frequency of symptoms. Estimates of the frequency of noncognitive symptoms in AD vary from virtually absent to more than 80% (Table 2) [179–183]. One study using the Neuropsychiatric Inventory (a questionnaire established to assess an array of neuropsychiatric symptoms and their impact as estimated by caregivers), found apathy to be the most common symptom, followed by agitation, anxiety, irritability, dysphoria, disinhibition, delusions, hallucinations, and euphoria, respectively [182]. Co-occurrence of noncognitive symptoms is also common, and the symptom complexes tend to fluctuate. Consequently, treatment strategies require ongoing adjustment.

Assessment. It should not be presumed that all noncognitive symptoms in an AD patient are a result of progression of the underlying neurodegenerative process. Medical problems may manifest as a behavioral change, and screening for urinary tract infection, pneumonia, congestive heart failure, and electrolyte abnormality should be considered. Treatment of the underlying medical issues may improve or eliminate the problematic behaviors.

Behavioral management. Nonpharmacologic methods should be considered, and can avoid the potential side effects of additional medications [16]. Environmental changes, such as family crises, new caregivers, or altered surroundings, may exacerbate or cause behavioral problems. Often, simple strategies, such as distraction, redirection, or exercise, can ameliorate the behaviors.

Pharmacologic treatments. Behaviors of sufficient severity to disrupt a patient's (or caregiver's) quality of life may require pharmacologic intervention. Accurate assessment of the underlying condition is a crucial first step [182] and several scales exist to assist the clinician in addressing these behaviors, including the BEHAVE-AD [183], the Cohen-Mansfield Agitation Inventory (CMAI) [184], and the Neuropsychiatric Inventory (NPI) [185]. The NPI is one of the most commonly used instruments, and assesses

Table 2
Frequency of behavioral disorders in Alzheimer's disease

Behavioral disorder	Frequency
Agitation	50%–70%
Anxiety	30%–50%
Depression	25%–50%
Disinhibition	20%–35%
Aggression	25%
Delusions	15%–50%
Hallucinations	10%–25%
Sexual disinhibition	5%–10%

Adapted from Reisberg B, Borenstein J, Salob SP, et al. Behavioral symptoms in Alzheimer's disease: phenomenology and treatment. J Clin Psychiatry 1987;48(Suppl):9–15.

10 commonly encountered behaviors, including delusions, hallucinations, agitation, dysphoria, anxiety, apathy, irritability, euphoria, disinhibition, and aberrant motor behavior. The frequency and severity of the symptoms are reported by a caregiver, allowing computation of a final index for each behavior. The impact on the caregiver is also assessed. The NPI-Q is an abbreviated version designed for assessment in the office setting [186]. Table 2 shows the frequency of noncognitive behaviors in AD.

Depression. Depression or dysphoria is common in AD, and can herald the onset of the disorder [187] or develop as the dementia progresses [182]. It commonly worsens cognitive symptoms and places greater stress on the caregiver. Selective serotonin reuptake inhibitors are the preferred treatments for depression in AD. Tricyclic antidepressants may also be effective, but anticholinergic side effects may worsen cognition and act at a cross-purpose to cholinesterase inhibitors (Table 3).

Psychosis. Delusions are common in AD, often with coexistent paranoia [188,189]. Hallucinations can be seen in AD, particularly if Lewy bodies are present, and misidentification syndromes can occur when the right hemisphere is predominantly involved. Psychosis can also indicate a more rapid decline in function [15,190].

Nonpharmacologic interventions are the preferable first-line treatment for psychosis, agitation, aggression, and other problematic behaviors that may compromise the health and safety of patients and those around them. Atypical antipsychotic medications remain the preferred treatment of psychosis in AD. Risperidone was demonstrated to improve psychosis and aggression, but did produce somnolence and extrapyramidal symptoms [191]. Quetiapine has been shown to reduce psychotic symptoms with relatively few side effects [192], as has olanzapine [193]. The results of the CATIE-AD trial generated significant publicity by suggesting that the potential adverse effects of atypical antipsychotics may offset the potential benefits from these agents [194]. A subsequent meta-analysis of placebo-controlled trials of atypical neuroleptic medications found only modest group efficacy and echoed the concerns about potential adverse effects [195]. In this analysis, the investigators recommend that deliberate consideration and discussion with patients and their families should precede initiation of antipsychotic medications. These medications should be discontinued if improvement has not been seen within 10 to 12 weeks and should be adjusted to the minimum effective dosage. Periodic medication withdrawal trials may be used to evaluate for continued necessity. These investigators also caution against the imprudence of prescribing alternative medications as first-line agents because of a perception that they are safer than, or as effective as, antipsychotics. Atypical antipsychotics can be expensive, but generally are felt to be preferable to typical antipsychotic agents such as haloperidol (see Table 3).

Table 3
Medications for noncognitive symptoms in dementia

Class	Agents	Usual daily dose
Delusions	Risperidone (Risperdal)	1 mg (0.05–2 mg)
	Olanzapine (Zyprexa)	5 mg (5–10 mg)
	Quetiapine (Seroquel)	400 mg (50–400 mg)
	Aripiprazole (Abilify)	5 mg (5–20 mg)
	Haloperidol (Haldol)	1 mg (0.5–3 mg)
Agitation/aggression	Risperidone (Risperdal)	1 mg (0.05–2 mg)
	Olanzapine (Zyprexa)	5 mg (5–10 mg)
	Quetiapine (Seroquel)	400 mg (50–400 mg)
	Aripiprazole (Abilify)	5 mg (5–20 mg)
	Haloperidol (Haldol)	1 mg (0.5–3 mg)
	Trazodone (Desyrel)	100 mg (100–400 mg)
	Buspirone (Buspar)	15 mg (15–30 mg)
	Propranolol (Inderal)	120 mg (80–240 mg)
	Carbamazepine (Tegretol)	400 mg (200–1200 mg)
	Divalproex (Depakote)	500 mg (250–2000 mg)
	Lorazepam (Ativan)	1 mg (0.5–6 mg)
Depression	Fluoxetine (Prozac)	20 mg (20–40 mg)
	Sertraline (Zoloft)	50 mg (50–200 mg)
	Paroxetine (Paxil)	20 mg (10–50 mg)
	Citalopram (Celexa)	20 mg (10–30 mg)
	Venlafaxine (Effexor)	100 mg (50–225 mg)
	Nefazodone (Serzone)	400 mg (200–600 mg)
	Mirtazapine (Remeron)	15 mg (7.5–30 mg)
	Duloxetine (Cymbalta)	20 mg (20–60 mg)
	Nortriptyline (Pamelor)	50 mg (50–100 mg)
	Trazodone (Desyrel)	50 mg (100–400 mg)
Anxiety	Oxazepam (Serax)	30 mg (20–60 mg)
	Lorazepam (Ativan)	1 mg (0.5–6 mg)
	Buspirone (Buspar)	30 mg (15–45 mg)
	Propranolol (Inderal)	120 mg (80–240 mg)
Insomnia	Trazodone (Desyrel)	50 mg (50–200 mg)
	Zolpidem (Ambien)	10 mg (5–10 mg)
	Temazepam (Restoril)	15 mg (15–30 mg)
	Zaleplon (Sonata)	10 mg
Apathy	Donepezil (Aricept)	10 mg (5–10 mg)
	Rivastigmine (Exelon)	9 mg (6–12 mg)

Adapted from Cummings JL, Mega M, Gray K, et al. The Neuropsychiatric Inventory: comprehensive assessment of psychopathology in dementia. Neurology 1994;44(12):2308–14; with permission.

Apathy. Apathy may be the most common noncognitive symptom in AD [177,182] and causes diminished quality of life for both the patient and caregiver. Acetylcholinesterase inhibitors may be useful, but pharmacologic management of these symptoms is not well developed. Other medications, such as methylphenidate, bromocriptine, pramipexole, or ropinirole, or activating antidepressants such as fluoxetine may theoretically be useful, although benefit has not been established in the literature [196].

Agitation. Agitation can be quite bothersome to caregivers because the patient appears to be in distress [197]. Trazodone can useful, and has a better side effect profile than haloperidol [198]. Atypical antipsychotic agents such as risperidone, olanzapine, and quetiapine can be considered, as can anticonvulsants such as carbamazepine or valproic acid [199,200].

Summary. Noncognitive symptoms of AD can be responsible for significant distress for both patients and caregivers; however, their impact can be ameliorated by using pharmacologic and behavioral interventions. Interventions are being studied more extensively, with the recognition that successful intervention can result in significant improvement of the quality of life for all involved.

References

[1] Brookmeyer R, Gray S, Kawas C. Projections of Alzheimer's disease in the United States and the public health impact of delaying disease onset. Am J Public Health 1998;88(9): 1337–42.

[2] Petersen RC. Aging, mild cognitive impairment, and Alzheimer's disease. Neurol Clin 2000; 18(4):789–805.

[3] Petersen RC. Mild cognitive impairment: transtion from aging to Alzheimer's disease. In: Iqbal K, Sisodia SS, Winblad B, editors. Alzheimer's disease: advances in etiology, pathogenesis and therapeutics. West Sussex (England): J Wiley & Sons, Ltd.; 2001. p. 141–51.

[4] Knopman DS, DeKosky ST, Cummings JL, et al. Practice parameter: diagnosis of dementia (an evidence-based review). Report of the Quality Standards Subcommittee of the American Academy of Neurology. Neurology 2001;56(9):1143–53.

[5] Petersen RC, Stevens JC, Ganguli M, et al. Practice parameter: early detection of dementia: mild cognitive impairment (an evidence-based review). Report of the Quality Standards Subcommittee of the American Academy of Neurology. Neurology 2001;56(9):1133–42.

[6] Doody RS, Stevens JC, Beck C, et al. Practice parameter: management of dementia (an evidence-based review). Report of the Quality Standards Subcommittee of the American Academy of Neurology. Neurology 2001;56(9):1154–66.

[7] Ivnik RJ, Smith GE, Lucas JA, et al. Testing normal older people three or four times at 1- to 2-year intervals: defining normal variance. Neuropsychology 1999;13(1):121–7.

[8] Petersen RC. Mild cognitive impairment: aging to Alzheimer's disease. Oxford (UK): Oxford University Press; 2003.

[9] Siwinski M, Lipton RB, Buschke H, et al. The effects of preclinical dementia on estimates of normal cognitive functioning in aging. J Gerontol B Psychol Sci Soc Sci 1996;51(4):P217–25.

[10] Backman L, Jones S, Berger AK, et al. Cognitive impairment in preclinical Alzheimer's disease: a meta-analysis. Neuropsychology 2005;19(4):520–31.

[11] American Psychiatric Association. Diagnostic and statistical manual of mental disorders. 3rd edition, revised. Washington, DC: American Psychiatric Association; 1987.

[12] Fleming KC, Adams AC, Petersen RC. Dementia: diagnosis and evaluation. Mayo Clin Proc 1995;70(11):1093–107.

[13] Burns A, Jacoby R, Levy R. Psychiatric phenomena in Alzheimer's disease. IV: disorders of behaviour. Br J Psychiatry 1990;157:86–94.

[14] Drevets WC, Rubin EH. Psychotic symptoms and the longitudinal course of senile dementia of the Alzheimer type. Biol Psychiatry 1989;25(1):39–48.

[15] Rosen J, Zubenko GS. Emergence of psychosis and depression in the longitudinal evaluation of Alzheimer's disease. Biol Psychiatry 1991;29(3):224–32.

[16] Teri L, Larson EB, Reifler BV. Behavioral disturbance in dementia of the Alzheimer's type. J Am Geriatr Soc 1988;36(1):1–6.
[17] The National Institute on Aging, and Reagan Institute Working Group on Diagnostic Criteria for the Neuropathological Diagnosis of Alzheimer's Disease. Consensus recommendations for the postmortem Diagnosis of Alzheimer's disease. Neurobiol Aging 1997; 18(4 Suppl):S1–2.
[18] Kukull WA, Ganguli M. Epidemiology of dementia: concepts and overview. Neurol Clin 2000;18(4):923–50.
[19] Bachman DL, Wolf PA, Linn R, et al. Prevalence of dementia and probable senile dementia of the Alzheimer type in the Framingham Study. Neurology 1992;42(1):115–9.
[20] Canadian Study of Health and Aging Working Group. Study methods and prevalence of dementia. CMAJ 1994;150(6):899–913.
[21] Evans DA, Funkenstein HH, Albert MS, et al. Prevalence of Alzheimer's disease in a community population of older persons. Higher than previously reported. JAMA 1989;262(18): 2551–6.
[22] Hendrie HC, Osuntokun BO, Hall KS, et al. Prevalence of Alzheimer's disease and dementia in two communities: Nigerian Africans and African Americans. Am J Psychiatry 1995; 152(10):1485–92.
[23] Hofman A, Ott A, Breteler MM, et al. Atherosclerosis, apolipoprotein E, and prevalence of dementia and Alzheimer's disease in the Rotterdam Study. Lancet 1997;349(9046):151–4.
[24] Kokmen E, Beard CM, Offord KP, et al. Prevalence of medically diagnosed dementia in a defined United States population: Rochester, Minnesota, January 1, 1975. Neurology 1989;39(6):773–6.
[25] White L, Petrovitch H, Ross GW, et al. Prevalence of dementia in older Japanese-American men in Hawaii: The Honolulu-Asia Aging Study. JAMA 1996;276(12):955–60.
[26] American Psychiatric Association. Diagnostic and statistical manual of mental disorders. 4th edition text revision (DSM-IV-TR). Washington, DC: American Psychiatric Association; 2000.
[27] McKhann G, Drachman D, Folstein M, et al. Clinical diagnosis of Alzheimer's disease: report of the NINCDS-ADRDA Work Group under the auspices of Department of Health and Human Services Task Force on Alzheimer's Disease. Neurology 1984;34(7):939–44.
[28] Folstein M, Folstein S, McHugh P. "Mini-mental state." A practical method for grading the cognitive state of patients for the clinician. J Psychiatr Res 1975;12:189–98.
[29] Teng EL, Chui HC. The modified mini-mental state (3MS) examination. J Clin Psychiatry 1987;48(8):314–8.
[30] Katzman R, Brown T, Fuld P, et al. Validation of a short orientation-memory-concentration test of cognitive impairment. Am J Psychiatry 1983;140(6):734–9.
[31] Kokmen E, Smith GE, Petersen RC, et al. The short test of mental status. Correlations with standardized psychometric testing. Arch Neurol 1991;48(7):725–8.
[32] Morris JC. The Clinical Dementia Rating (CDR): current version and scoring rules. Neurology 1993;43(11):2412–4.
[33] Jack CR Jr, Petersen RC, Xu YC, et al. Medial temporal atrophy on MRI in normal aging and very mild Alzheimer's disease. Neurology 1997;49(3):786–94.
[34] Jack CR Jr, Petersen RC, Xu YC, et al. Prediction of AD with MRI-based hippocampal volume in mild cognitive impairment. Neurology 1999;52(7):1397–403.
[35] Killiany RJ, Gomez-Isla T, Moss M, et al. Use of structural magnetic resonance imaging to predict who will get Alzheimer's disease. Ann Neurol 2000;47(4):430–9.
[36] Xu Y, Jack CR Jr, O'Brien PC, et al. Usefulness of MRI measures of entorhinal cortex versus hippocampus in AD. Neurology 2000;54(9):1760–7.
[37] Wahlund LO, Almkvist O, Blennow K, et al. Evidence-based evaluation of magnetic resonance imaging as a diagnostic tool in dementia workup. Top Magn Reson Imaging 2005; 16(6):427–37.

[38] Ramani A, Jensen JH, Helpern JA. Quantitative MR imaging in Alzheimer disease. Radiology 2006;241(1):26–44.
[39] Van Gool WA, Walstra GJ, Teunisse S, et al. Diagnosing Alzheimer's disease in elderly, mildly demented patients: the impact of routine single photon emission computed tomography. J Neurol 1995;242(6):401–5.
[40] Claus JJ, van Harskamp F, Breteler MM, et al. The diagnostic value of SPECT with Tc 99m HMPAO in Alzheimer's disease: a population-based study. Neurology 1994;44(3 Pt 1): 454–61.
[41] Johnson KA, Kijewski MF, Becker JA, et al. Quantitative brain SPECT in Alzheimer's disease and normal aging. J Nucl Med 1993;34(11):2044–8.
[42] Johnson KA, Holman BL, Rosen TJ, et al. Iofetamine I 123 single photon emission computed tomography is accurate in the diagnosis of Alzheimer's disease. Arch Intern Med 1990;150(4):752–6.
[43] Bartenstein P, Minoshima S, Hirsch C, et al. Quantitative assessment of cerebral blood flow in patients with Alzheimer's disease by SPECT. J Nucl Med 1997;38(7):1095–101.
[44] Mielke R, Heiss WD. Positron emission tomography for diagnosis of Alzheimer's disease and vascular dementia. J Neural Transm Suppl 1998;53:237–50.
[45] Silverman DH, Small GW, Chang CY, et al. Positron emission tomography in evaluation of dementia: regional brain metabolism and long-term outcome. JAMA 2001;286(17):2120–7.
[46] Kantarci K, Jack CR Jr, Xu YC, et al. Regional metabolic patterns in mild cognitive impairment and Alzheimer's disease: A 1H MRS study. Neurology 2000;55(2):210–7.
[47] Kantarci K, Petersen RC, Boeve BF, et al. 1H MR spectroscopy in common dementias. Neurology 2004;63(8):1393–8.
[48] Klunk WE, Engler H, Nordberg A, et al. Imaging brain amyloid in Alzheimer's disease with Pittsburgh compound-B. Ann Neurol 2004;55(3):306–19.
[49] Shoghi-Jadid K, Small GW, Agdeppa ED, et al. Localization of neurofibrillary tangles and beta-amyloid plaques in the brains of living patients with Alzheimer disease. Am J Geriatr Psychiatry 2002;10(1):24–35.
[50] Small GW, Kepe V, Ercoli LM, et al. PET of brain amyloid and tau in mild cognitive impairment. N Engl J Med 2006;355(25):2652–63.
[51] Nordberg A. PET imaging of amyloid in Alzheimer's disease. Lancet Neurol 2004;3(9): 519–27.
[52] Johnson KA. Amyloid imaging of Alzheimer's disease using Pittsburgh Compound B. Curr Neurol Neurosci Rep 2006;6(6):496–503.
[53] Becker PM, Feussner JR, Mulrow CD, et al. The role of lumbar puncture in the evaluation of dementia: the Durham Veterans Administration/Duke University Study. J Am Geriatr Soc 1985;33(6):392–6.
[54] Hardy J, Gwinn-Hardy K. Genetic classification of primary neurodegenerative disease. Science 1998;282(5391):1075–9.
[55] Roses AD, et al. Apolipoprotein E and Alzheimer's disease. In: Rosenberg RN, Prusiner SB, DiMaur OS, editors. The molecular and genetic basis of neurological disease. 2nd edition. Boston: Butterworth-Heinemann; 1997. p. 1019–36.
[56] Farrer LA, Cupples LA, Haines JL, et al. Effects of age, sex, and ethnicity on the association between apolipoprotein E genotype and Alzheimer disease. A meta-analysis. APOE and Alzheimer disease meta analysis consortium. JAMA 1997;278(16):1349–56.
[57] Mayeux R, Saunders AM, Shea S, et al. Utility of the apolipoprotein E genotype in the diagnosis of Alzheimer's disease. Alzheimer's disease centers consortium on apolipoprotein E and Alzheimer's disease. N Engl J Med 1998;338(8):506–11.
[58] Roses AD, et al. The predictive value of APOE genotyping in the early diagnosis of dementia of the Alzheimer type: data from three independent series. In: Iqbal K, Winblad B, Nishimura T, editors. Alzheimer's disease: biology, diagnosis and therapeutics. West Sussex (England): John Wiley & Sons; 1997. p. 85–91.

[59] Andreasen N, Hesse C, Davidsson P, et al. Cerebrospinal fluid beta-amyloid(1-42) in Alzheimer disease: differences between early- and late-onset Alzheimer disease and stability during the course of disease. Arch Neurol 1999;56(6):673–80.
[60] Galasko D, Chang L, Motter R, et al. High cerebrospinal fluid tau and low amyloid beta42 levels in the clinical diagnosis of Alzheimer disease and relation to apolipoprotein E genotype. Arch Neurol 1998;55(7):937–45.
[61] Hulstaert F, Blennow K, Ivanoiu A, et al. Improved discrimination of AD patients using beta-amyloid(1-42) and tau levels in CSF. Neurology 1999;52(8):1555–62.
[62] Shoji M, Matsubara E, Kanai M, et al. Combination assay of CSF tau, A beta 1-40 and A beta 1-42(43) as a biochemical marker of Alzheimer's disease. J Neurol Sci 1998;158(2):134–40.
[63] Stefani A, Martorana A, Bernardini S, et al. CSF markers in Alzheimer disease patients are not related to the different degree of cognitive impairment. J Neurol Sci 2006;251(1–2):124–8.
[64] Stenset V, Johnsen L, Kocot D, et al. Associations between white matter lesions, cerebrovascular risk factors, and low CSF Abeta42. Neurology 2006;67(5):830–3.
[65] Arai H, Higuchi S, Sasaki H. Apolipoprotein E genotyping and cerebrospinal fluid tau protein: implications for the clinical diagnosis of Alzheimer's disease. Gerontology 1997;43(Suppl 1):2–10.
[66] Galasko D, Clark C, Chang L, et al. Assessment of CSF levels of tau protein in mildly demented patients with Alzheimer's disease. Neurology 1997;48(3):632–5.
[67] Kurz A, Riemenschneider M, Buch K, et al. Tau protein in cerebrospinal fluid is significantly increased at the earliest clinical stage of Alzheimer disease. Alzheimer Dis Assoc Disord 1998;12(4):372–7.
[68] Andreasen N, Minthon L, Clarberg A, et al. Sensitivity, specificity, and stability of CSF-tau in AD in a community-based patient sample. Neurology 1999;53(7):1488–94.
[69] Buerger K, Ewers M, Pirttila T, et al. CSF phosphorylated tau protein correlates with neocortical neurofibrillary pathology in Alzheimer's disease. Brain 2006;129(Pt 11):3035–41.
[70] Clark CM, Xie S, Chittams J, et al. Cerebrospinal fluid tau and beta-amyloid: how well do these biomarkers reflect autopsy-confirmed dementia diagnoses? Arch Neurol 2003;60(12):1696–702.
[71] Schoonenboom NS, Pijnenburg YA, Mulder C, et al. Amyloid beta(1-42) and phosphorylated tau in CSF as markers for early-onset Alzheimer disease. Neurology 2004;62(9):1580–4.
[72] Buerger K, Teipel SJ, Zinkowski R, et al. CSF tau protein phosphorylated at threonine 231 correlates with cognitive decline in MCI subjects. Neurology 2002;59(4):627–9.
[73] de la Monte SM, Volicer L, Hauser SL, et al. Increased levels of neuronal thread protein in cerebrospinal fluid of patients with Alzheimer's disease. Ann Neurol 1992;32(6):733–42.
[74] de la Monte SM, Wands JR. The AD7c-ntp neuronal thread protein biomarker for detecting Alzheimer's disease. Front Biosci 2002;7:d989–96.
[75] Monte SM, Ghanbari K, Frey WH, et al. Characterization of the AD7C-NTP cDNA expression in Alzheimer's disease and measurement of a 41-kD protein in cerebrospinal fluid. J Clin Invest 1997;100(12):3093–104.
[76] Ghanbari K, Ghanbari HA. A sandwich enzyme immunoassay for measuring AD7C-NTP as an Alzheimer's disease marker: AD7C test. J Clin Lab Anal 1998;12(4):223–6.
[77] Geda YE, Petersen RC. Clinical trials in mild cognitive impairment. In: Gauthier S, Cummings JL, editors. Alzheimer's disease and related disorders annual 2001, vol 103. London: Martin Dunitz; 2001. p. 69–83.
[78] Petersen RC, Doody R, Kurz A, et al. Current concepts in mild cognitive impairment. Arch Neurol 2001;58(12):1985–92.
[79] Ritchie K, Artero S, Touchon J. Classification criteria for mild cognitive impairment: a population-based validation study. Neurology 2001;56(1):37–42.

[80] Petersen RC, Smith GE, Waring SC, et al. Mild cognitive impairment: clinical characterization and outcome. Arch Neurol 1999;56(3):303–8.
[81] Daly E, Zaitchik D, Copeland M, et al. Predicting conversion to Alzheimer disease using standardized clinical information. Arch Neurol 2000;57(5):675–80.
[82] Smith GE, Petersen RC, Parisi JE, et al. Definition, course, and outcome of mild cognitive impairment. Aging Neuropsychology & Cognition 1996;3(2):141–7.
[83] Ivnik RJ, Malec JF, Smith GE, et al. Mayo's older Americans normative studies: WAIS-R, WMS-R and AVLT norms for ages 56 to 97. Clin Neuropsychol 1992;6(Suppl):1–104.
[84] Petersen RC. Mild cognitive impairment as a diagnostic entity. J Intern Med 2004;256(3): 183–94.
[85] Bennett DA, Wilson RS, Schneider JA, et al. Natural history of mild cognitive impairment in older persons. Neurology 2002;59(2):198–205.
[86] Ganguli M, Dodge HH, Shen C, et al. Mild cognitive impairment, amnestic type: an epidemiologic study. Neurology 2004;63(1):115–21.
[87] Lopez OL, Jagust WJ, DeKosky ST, et al. Prevalence and classification of mild cognitive impairment in the Cardiovascular Health Study Cognition Study: part 1. Arch Neurol 2003;60(10):1385–9.
[88] Knopman DS, Ryberg S. A verbal memory test with high predictive accuracy for dementia of the Alzheimer type. Arch Neurol 1989;46(2):141–5.
[89] Petersen RC. Memory assessment at the bedside. In: Yanagihara T, Petersen RC, editors. Memory disorders. New York: Dekker; 1991. p. 137–52.
[90] Fox NC, Warrington EK, Freeborough PA, et al. Presymptomatic hippocampal atrophy in Alzheimer's disease. A longitudinal MRI study. Brain 1996;119(Pt 6):2001–7.
[91] Fox NC, Crum WR, Scahill RI, et al. Imaging of onset and progression of Alzheimer's disease with voxel-compression mapping of serial magnetic resonance images. Lancet 2001; 358(9277):201–5.
[92] Schott JM, Price SL, Frost C, et al. Measuring atrophy in Alzheimer disease: a serial MRI study over 6 and 12 months. Neurology 2005;65(1):119–24.
[93] Small GW, Mazziotta JC, Collins MT, et al. Apolipoprotein E type 4 allele and cerebral glucose metabolism in relatives at risk for familial Alzheimer disease. JAMA 1995; 273(12):942–7.
[94] Reiman EM, Caselli RJ, Yun LS, et al. Preclinical evidence of Alzheimer's disease in persons homozygous for the epsilon 4 allele for apolipoprotein E. N Engl J Med 1996; 334(12):752–8.
[95] Petersen RC. Mild cognitive impairment: transition between aging and Alzheimer's disease. Neurologia 2000;15(3):93–101.
[96] Growdon JH. Biomarkers of Alzheimer disease. Arch Neurol 1999;56(3):281–3.
[97] Sunderland T, Wolozin B, Galasko D, et al. Longitudinal stability of CSF tau levels in Alzheimer patients. Biol Psychiatry 1999;46(6):750–5.
[98] Hansson O, Zetterberg H, Buchhave P, et al. Association between CSF biomarkers and incipient Alzheimer's disease in patients with mild cognitive impairment: a follow-up study. Lancet Neurol 2006;5(3):228–34.
[99] Petersen RC, Smith GE, Ivnik RJ, et al. Apolipoprotein E status as a predictor of the development of Alzheimer's disease in memory-impaired individuals. JAMA 1995; 273(16):1274–8.
[100] Tierney MC, Szalai JP, Snow WG, et al. A prospective study of the clinical utility of ApoE genotype in the prediction of outcome in patients with memory impairment. Neurology 1996;46(1):149–54.
[101] Bennett DA, Schneider JA, Bienias JL, et al. Mild cognitive impairment is related to Alzheimer disease pathology and cerebral infarctions. Neurology 2005;64(5):834–41.
[102] Petersen RC, Parisi JE, Dickson DW, et al. Neuropathologic features of amnestic mild cognitive impairment. Arch Neurol 2006;63(5):665–72.

[103] Riley KP, Snowdon DA, Markesbery WR. Alzheimer's neurofibrillary pathology and the spectrum of cognitive function: findings from the Nun Study. Ann Neurol 2002;51(5): 567–77.
[104] Mesulam M, Shaw P, Mash D, et al. Cholinergic nucleus basalis tauopathy emerges early in the aging-MCI-AD continuum. Ann Neurol 2004;55(6):815–28.
[105] Grudzien A, Shaw P, Weintraub S, et al. Locus coeruleus neurofibrillary degeneration in aging, mild cognitive impairment and early Alzheimer's disease. Neurobiol Aging 2007; 28(3):327–35.
[106] Morris JC, Storandt M, Miller JP, et al. Mild cognitive impairment represents early-stage Alzheimer disease. Arch Neurol 2001;58(3):397–405.
[107] Jicha GA, Parisi JE, Dickson DW, et al. Neuropathologic outcome of mild cognitive impairment following progression to clinical dementia. Arch Neurol 2006;63(5):674–81.
[108] Whitehouse PJ, Price DL, Clark AW, et al. Alzheimer disease: evidence for selective loss of cholinergic neurons in the nucleus basalis. Ann Neurol 1981;10(2):122–6.
[109] Petersen RC. Scopolamine induced learning failures in man. Psychopharmacology (Berl) 1977;52(3):283–9.
[110] Bowen DM, Smith CB, White P, et al. Neurotransmitter-related enzymes and indices of hypoxia in senile dementia and other abiotrophies. Brain 1976;99(3):459–96.
[111] Davies P, Maloney AJ. Selective loss of central cholinergic neurons in Alzheimer's disease. Lancet 1976;2(8000):1403.
[112] Petersen RC, Thomas RG, Grundman M, et al. Vitamin E and donepezil for the treatment of mild cognitive impairment. N Engl J Med 2005;352(23):2379–88.
[113] Rosler M, Anand R, Cicin-Sain A, et al. Efficacy and safety of rivastigmine in patients with Alzheimer's disease: international randomised controlled trial. BMJ 1999;318(7184):633–8.
[114] Tariot PN, Solomon PR, Morris JC, et al. A 5-month, randomized, placebo-controlled trial of galantamine in AD. The Galantamine USA-10 Study Group. Neurology 2000;54(12): 2269–76.
[115] Feldman H, Gauthier S, Hecker J, et al. Economic evaluation of donepezil in moderate to severe Alzheimer disease. Neurology 2004;63(4):644–50.
[116] Courtney C, Farrell D, Gray R, et al. Long-term donepezil treatment in 565 patients with Alzheimer's disease (AD2000): randomised double-blind trial. Lancet 2004;363(9427):2105–15.
[117] Gale CR, Martyn CN, Cooper C. Cognitive impairment and mortality in a cohort of elderly people. BMJ 1996;312(7031):608–11.
[118] Goodwin JS, Goodwin JM, Garry PJ. Association between nutritional status and cognitive functioning in a healthy elderly population. JAMA 1983;249(21):2917–21.
[119] La Rue A, Koehler KM, Wayne SJ, et al. Nutritional status and cognitive functioning in a normally aging sample: a 6-y reassessment. Am J Clin Nutr 1997;65(1):20–9.
[120] Morris MC, Beckett LA, Scherr PA, et al. Vitamin E and vitamin C supplement use and risk of incident Alzheimer disease. Alzheimer Dis Assoc Disord 1998;12(3):121–6.
[121] Perrig WJ, Perrig P, Stahelin HB. The relation between antioxidants and memory performance in the old and very old. J Am Geriatr Soc 1997;45(6):718–24.
[122] Sano M, Ernesto C, Thomas RG, et al. A controlled trial of selegiline, alpha-tocopherol, or both as treatment for Alzheimer's disease. The Alzheimer's Disease Cooperative Study. N Engl J Med 1997;336(17):1216–22.
[123] Miller ER 3rd, Pastor-Barriuso R, Dalal D, et al. Meta-analysis: high-dosage vitamin E supplementation may increase all-cause mortality. Ann Intern Med 2005;142(1):37–46.
[124] Aisen PS, Davis KL. Inflammatory mechanisms in Alzheimer's disease: implications for therapy. Am J Psychiatry 1994;151(8):1105–13.
[125] McGeer PL, Rogers J. Anti-inflammatory agents as a therapeutic approach to Alzheimer's disease. Neurology 1992;42(2):447–9.
[126] Andersen K, Launer LJ, Ott A, et al. Do nonsteroidal anti-inflammatory drugs decrease the risk for Alzheimer's disease? The Rotterdam Study. Neurology 1995;45(8):1441–5.

[127] Breitner JC, Welsh KA, Helms MJ, et al. Delayed onset of Alzheimer's disease with nonsteroidal anti-inflammatory and histamine H2 blocking drugs. Neurobiol Aging 1995; 16(4):523–30.

[128] Breitner JC, Gau BA, Welsh KA, et al. Inverse association of anti-inflammatory treatments and Alzheimer's disease: initial results of a co-twin control study. Neurology 1994;44(2): 227–32.

[129] Canadian Study of Health and Aging Working Group. Risk factors for Alzheimer's disease in Canada. Neurology 1994;44(11):2073–80.

[130] Stewart WF, Kawas C, Corrada M, et al. Risk of Alzheimer's disease and duration of NSAID use. Neurology 1997;48(3):626–32.

[131] Aisen PS, Davis KL, Berg JD, et al. A randomized controlled trial of prednisone in Alzheimer's disease. Alzheimer's Disease Cooperative Study. Neurology 2000;54(3):588–93.

[132] Rogers J, Kirby LC, Hempelman SR, et al. Clinical trial of indomethacin in Alzheimer's disease. Neurology 1993;43(8):1609–11.

[133] Scharf S, Mander A, Ugoni A, et al. A double-blind, placebo-controlled trial of diclofenac/misoprostol in Alzheimer's disease. Neurology 1999;53(1):197–201.

[134] Aisen PS, Schafer KA, Grundman M, et al. Effects of rofecoxib or naproxen vs placebo on Alzheimer disease progression: a randomized controlled trial. JAMA 2003;289(21): 2819–26.

[135] Ho L, Pieroni C, Winger D, et al. Regional distribution of cyclooxygenase-2 in the hippocampal formation in Alzheimer's disease. J Neurosci Res 1999;57(3):295–303.

[136] Pasinetti GM, Aisen PS. Cyclooxygenase-2 expression is increased in frontal cortex of Alzheimer's disease brain. Neuroscience 1998;87(2):319–24.

[137] Sainati SM, Ingram DM, Talwalker S, et al. Results of a double-blind, randomized, placebo-controlled study of celecoxib in the treatment of progression of Alzheimer's disease. Paper presented at the Sixth International Stockholm/Springfield Symposium on Advances in Alzheimer Therapy. Stockholm (Sweden), April 5–8, 2000.

[138] Mukherjee D, Nissen SE, Topol EJ. Risk of cardiovascular events associated with selective COX-2 inhibitors. JAMA 2001;286(8):954–9.

[139] Topol EJ. Failing the public health–rofecoxib, Merck, and the FDA. N Engl J Med 2004; 351(17):1707–9.

[140] Launer L. Nonsteroidal anti-inflammatory drug use and the risk for Alzheimer's disease: dissecting the epidemiological evidence. Drugs 2003;63(8):731–9.

[141] in t' Veld BA, Ruitenberg A, Hofman A, et al. Nonsteroidal antiinflammatory drugs and the risk of Alzheimer's disease. N Engl J Med 2001;345(21):1515–21.

[142] Weggen S, Eriksen JL, Das P, et al. A subset of NSAIDs lower amyloidogenic Abeta42 independently of cyclooxygenase activity. Nature 2001;414(6860):212–6.

[143] Weggen S, Eriksen JL, Sagi SA, et al. Evidence that nonsteroidal anti-inflammatory drugs decrease amyloid beta 42 production by direct modulation of gamma-secretase activity. J Biol Chem 2003;278(34):31831–7.

[144] Henderson VW, Paganini-Hill A, Emanuel CK, et al. Estrogen replacement therapy in older women. Comparisons between Alzheimer's disease cases and nondemented control subjects. Arch Neurol 1994;51(9):896–900.

[145] Kawas C, Resnick S, Morrison A, et al. A prospective study of estrogen replacement therapy and the risk of developing Alzheimer's disease: the Baltimore longitudinal study of aging. Neurology 1997;48(6):1517–21.

[146] Paganini-Hill A, Henderson VW. Estrogen deficiency and risk of Alzheimer's disease in women. Am J Epidemiol 1994;140(3):256–61.

[147] Paganini-Hill A, Henderson VW. Estrogen replacement therapy and risk of Alzheimer disease. Arch Intern Med 1996;156(19):2213–7.

[148] Shumaker SA, Legault C, Rapp SR, et al. Estrogen plus progestin and the incidence of dementia and mild cognitive impairment in postmenopausal women: the Women's Health Initiative Memory Study: a randomized controlled trial. JAMA 2003;289(20):2651–62.

[149] Rapp SR, Espeland MA, Shumaker SA, et al. Effect of estrogen plus progestin on global cognitive function in postmenopausal women: the Women's Health Initiative Memory Study: a randomized controlled trial. JAMA 2003;289(20):2663–72.
[150] Shumaker SA, Legault C, Kuller L, et al. Conjugated equine estrogens and incidence of probable dementia and mild cognitive impairment in postmenopausal women: Women's Health Initiative Memory Study. JAMA 2004;291(24):2947–58.
[151] Espeland MA, Rapp SR, Shumaker SA, et al. Conjugated equine estrogens and global cognitive function in postmenopausal women: Women's Health Initiative Memory Study. JAMA 2004;291(24):2959–68.
[152] Sano M. Moving from treatment to prevention in Alzheimer's disease with vitamin E and estrogen. Psychiatric Times 1999;16:1–4.
[153] McBee WL, Dailey ME, Dugan E, et al. Hormone replacement therapy and other potential treatments for dementias. Endocrinol Metab Clin North Am 1997;26(2):329–45.
[154] Mulnard RA, Cotman CW, Kawas C, et al. Estrogen replacement therapy for treatment of mild to moderate Alzheimer disease: a randomized controlled trial. Alzheimer's Disease Cooperative Study. JAMA 2000;283(8):1007–15.
[155] Henderson VW, Paganini-Hill A, Miller BL, et al. Estrogen for Alzheimer's disease in women: randomized, double-blind, placebo-controlled trial. Neurology 2000;54(2): 295–301.
[156] Roberts RO, Cha RH, Knopman DS, et al. Postmenopausal estrogen therapy and Alzheimer disease: overall negative findings. Alzheimer Dis Assoc Disord 2006;20(3):141–6.
[157] Masters CL, Beyreuther K. Alzheimer's centennial legacy: prospects for rational therapeutic intervention targeting the Abeta amyloid pathway. Brain 2006;129(Pt 11):2823–39.
[158] Selkoe DJ. The genetics and molecular pathology of Alzheimer's disease: roles of amyloid and the presenilins. Neurol Clin 2000;18(4):903–22.
[159] Hussain I, Powell D, Howlett DR, et al. Identification of a novel aspartic protease (Asp 2) as beta-secretase. Mol Cell Neurosci 1999;14(6):419–27.
[160] Sinha S, Anderson JP, Barbour R, et al. Purification and cloning of amyloid precursor protein beta-secretase from human brain. Nature 1999;402(6761):537–40.
[161] Vassar R, Bennett BD, Babu-Khan S, et al. Beta-secretase cleavage of Alzheimer's amyloid precursor protein by the transmembrane aspartic protease BACE. Science 1999;286(5440): 735–41.
[162] Yan R, Bienkowski MJ, Shuck ME, et al. Membrane-anchored aspartyl protease with Alzheimer's disease beta-secretase activity. Nature 1999;402(6761):533–7.
[163] Garino C, Tomita T, Pietrancosta N, et al. Naphthyl and coumarinyl biarylpiperazine derivatives as highly potent human beta-secretase inhibitors. Design, synthesis, and enzymatic BACE-1 and cell assays. J Med Chem 2006;49(14):4275–85.
[164] Siemers ER, Quinn JF, Kaye J, et al. Effects of a gamma-secretase inhibitor in a randomized study of patients with Alzheimer disease. Neurology 2006;66(4):602–4.
[165] Dovey HF, John V, Anderson JP, et al. Functional gamma-secretase inhibitors reduce beta-amyloid peptide levels in brain. J Neurochem 2001;76(1):173–81.
[166] Eriksen JL, Sagi SA, Smith TE, et al. NSAIDs and enantiomers of flurbiprofen target gamma-secretase and lower Abeta 42 in vivo. J Clin Invest 2003;112(3):440–9.
[167] Anderson JJ, Holtz G, Baskin PP, et al. Reductions in beta-amyloid concentrations in vivo by the gamma-secretase inhibitors BMS-289948 and BMS-299897. Biochem Pharmacol 2005;69(4):689–98.
[168] Black S, Wilcock G, Haworth J, et al. Efficacy and safety of MPC-7869 (R-flurbiprofen), a selective ab42-lowering agent, in mild Alzheimer's disease (AD): results of a 12-month phase 2 trial and 1-year follow-on study. Neurology 2006;66(5 Suppl 2):A347.
[169] Schenk D, Barbour R, Dunn W, et al. Immunization with amyloid-beta attenuates Alzheimer-disease-like pathology in the PDAPP mouse. Nature 1999;400(6740):173–7.
[170] Orgogozo JM, Gilman S, Dartigues JF, et al. Subacute meningoencephalitis in a subset of patients with AD after Abeta42 immunization. Neurology 2003;61(1):46–54.

[171] Gilman S, Koller M, Black RS, et al. Clinical effects of Abeta immunization (AN1792) in patients with AD in an interrupted trial. Neurology 2005;64(9):1553–62.
[172] Masliah E, Hansen L, Adame A, et al. Abeta vaccination effects on plaque pathology in the absence of encephalitis in Alzheimer disease. Neurology 2005;64(1):129–31.
[173] Fox NC, Black RS, Gilman S, et al. Effects of Abeta immunization (AN1792) on MRI measures of cerebral volume in Alzheimer disease. Neurology 2005;64(9):1563–72.
[174] Dodel R, Hampel H, Depboylu C, et al. Human antibodies against amyloid beta peptide: a potential treatment for Alzheimer's disease. Ann Neurol 2002;52(2):253–6.
[175] Dodel RC, Du Y, Depboylu C, et al. Intravenous immunoglobulins containing antibodies against beta-amyloid for the treatment of Alzheimer's disease. J Neurol Neurosurg Psychiatry 2004;75(10):1472–4.
[176] Adamiak B, Monthe C, Bender H, et al. Intravenous immunoglobulin (IVIg) maintains cognition over 18 months in patients with Alzheimer's disease (AD). Alzheimers Dement 2006;2(3):S62–3.
[177] Chung JA, Cummings JL. Neurobehavioral and neuropsychiatric symptoms in Alzheimer's disease: characteristics and treatment. Neurol Clin 2000;18(4):829–46.
[178] Henderson DC, Cagliero E, Copeland PM, et al. Glucose metabolism in patients with schizophrenia treated with atypical antipsychotic agents: a frequently sampled intravenous glucose tolerance test and minimal model analysis. Arch Gen Psychiatry 2005;62(1):19–28.
[179] Ballard C, Bannister C, Solis M, et al. The prevalence, associations and symptoms of depression amongst dementia sufferers. J Affect Disord 1996;36(3–4):135–44.
[180] Borson S, Raskind MA. Clinical features and pharmacologic treatment of behavioral symptoms of Alzheimer's disease. Neurology 1997;48(5 Suppl 6):S17–24.
[181] Devanand DP, Jacobs DM, Tang MX, et al. The course of psychopathologic features in mild to moderate Alzheimer disease. Arch Gen Psychiatry 1997;54(3):257–63.
[182] Mega MS, Cummings JL, Fiorello T, et al. The spectrum of behavioral changes in Alzheimer's disease. Neurology 1996;46(1):130–5.
[183] Reisberg B, Borenstein J, Salob SP, et al. Behavioral symptoms in Alzheimer's disease: phenomenology and treatment. J Clin Psychiatry 1987;48(Suppl):9–15.
[184] Cohen-Mansfield J, Deutsch LH. Agitation: subtypes and their mechanisms. Semin Clin Neuropsychiatry 1996;1(4):325–39.
[185] Cummings JL, Mega M, Gray K, et al. The Neuropsychiatric Inventory: comprehensive assessment of psychopathology in dementia. Neurology 1994;44(12):2308–14.
[186] Kaufer DI, Cummings JL, Ketchel P, et al. Validation of the NPI-Q, a brief clinical form of the Neuropsychiatric Inventory. J Neuropsychiatry Clin Neurosci 2000;12(2):233–9.
[187] Devanand DP, Sano M, Tang MX, et al. Depressed mood and the incidence of Alzheimer's disease in the elderly living in the community. Arch Gen Psychiatry 1996;53(2):175–82.
[188] Cooper JK, Mungas D, Verma M, et al. Psychotic symptoms in Alzheimer's disease. Int J Geriatr Psychiatry 1991;6(10):721–6.
[189] Rubin EH, Drevets WC, Burke WJ. The nature of psychotic symptoms in senile dementia of the Alzheimer type. J Geriatr Psychiatry Neurol 1988;1(1):16–20.
[190] Stern Y, Albert M, Brandt J, et al. Utility of extrapyramidal signs and psychosis as predictors of cognitive and functional decline, nursing home admission, and death in Alzheimer's disease: prospective analyses from the Predictors Study. Neurology 1994;44(12):2300–7.
[191] Katz IR, Jeste DV, Mintzer JE, et al. Comparison of risperidone and placebo for psychosis and behavioral disturbances associated with dementia: a randomized, double-blind trial. Risperidone Study Group. J Clin Psychiatry 1999;60(2):107–15.
[192] McManus DQ, Arvanitis LA, Kowalcyk BB. Quetiapine, a novel antipsychotic: experience in elderly patients with psychotic disorders. Seroquel Trial 48 Study Group. J Clin Psychiatry 1999;60(5):292–8.
[193] Street JS, Clark WS, Gannon KS, et al. Olanzapine treatment of psychotic and behavioral symptoms in patients with Alzheimer disease in nursing care facilities: a double-blind,

randomized, placebo-controlled trial. The HGEU Study Group. Arch Gen Psychiatry 2000;57(10):968–76.

[194] Schneider LS, Tariot PN, Dagerman KS, et al. Effectiveness of atypical antipsychotic drugs in patients with Alzheimer's disease. N Engl J Med 2006;355(15):1525–38.

[195] Schneider LS, Dagerman K, Insel PS. Efficacy and adverse effects of atypical antipsychotics for dementia: meta-analysis of randomized, placebo-controlled trials. Am J Geriatr Psychiatry 2006;14(3):191–210.

[196] McAllister TW. Apathy. Semin Clin Neuropsychiatry 2000;5(4):275–82.

[197] Deutsch LH, Bylsma FW, Rovner BW, et al. Psychosis and physical aggression in probable Alzheimer's disease. Am J Psychiatry 1991;148(9):1159–63.

[198] Sultzer DL, Gray KF, Gunay I, et al. A double-blind comparison of trazodone and haloperidol for treatment of agitation in patients with dementia. Am J Geriatr Psychiatry 1997; 5(1):60–9.

[199] Tariot PN, Erb R, Podgorski CA, et al. Efficacy and tolerability of carbamazepine for agitation and aggression in dementia. Am J Psychiatry 1998;155(1):54–61.

[200] Porsteinsson AP, Tariot PN, Erb R, et al. An open trial of valproate for agitation in geriatric neuropsychiatric disorders. Am J Geriatr Psychiatry 1997;5(4):344–51.

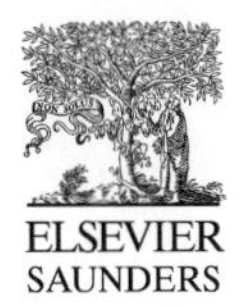

ELSEVIER
SAUNDERS

Neurol Clin 25 (2007) 611–667

NEUROLOGIC
CLINICS

Genetics of Alzheimer's Disease: A Centennial Review

Nilüfer Ertekin-Taner, MD, PhD

Departments of Neurology and Neuroscience, Mayo Clinic Rochester, 200 First Street SW, Rochester, MN 55905, USA

Alzheimer's disease (AD) genetics may be one of the most prolifically published areas in medicine and biology. Nearly 200 reviews on this topic have been published since 1991, when the first report on an autosomal dominant mutation in the amyloid precursor protein gene (*APP*) came out. Three early-onset AD genes with causative mutations (*APP*, presenilin 1 [*PSEN1*] and presenilin 2 [*PSEN2*]) and one late-onset AD susceptibility gene, apolipoprotein E (*APOE*) exist with ample biologic, genetic, and epidemiologic data and, essentially, universal acceptance about their roles in AD. Evidence from family and twin studies suggests a significant genetic component underlying AD that is not explained by the known genetic risk factors. The past 10 years in AD genetics research have led to 10 independent whole-genome linkage and association studies with implications for multiple genomic areas for harboring AD susceptibility genes. To date, about 900 papers have reported associations between variations in more than 350 genes spread over 23 autosomes. One hundred years after the first published article on AD, much is known about the pathophysiology of this disease; however, much more remains to be discovered about its cause. This article summarizes the evidence for the genetic component in AD and the identification of the early-onset familial AD (EOFAD) genes and *APOE*, and examines the current state of knowledge about additional AD susceptibility loci and alleles. The future directions for genetic research in AD as a common and complex condition are also discussed.

Public impact of Alzheimer's disease as a common disorder

AD is the most common adult neurodegenerative disease, with an estimated 10% to 30% prevalence by age 85 or older, and an incidence of

E-mail address: taner.nilufer@mayo.edu

0733-8619/07/$ - see front matter
doi:10.1016/j.ncl.2007.03.009

6% to 8% in the same age group [1]. With about 3 to 4 million affected individuals in the United States, 350,000 new cases per year (range: 200,000–600,000), and average annual cost per patient varying between $10,400 and $34,517 [2,3], AD is an epidemic with major health, social, and economic impacts. In the absence of any interventions to delay its onset, which is the current status, the prevalence of AD is expected to reach 8.64 million (range: 4.37–15.4 million) by the year 2047 [3]. Brookmeyer and colleagues [3] estimated that the 50-year projected prevalence of AD could decrease by 380,000 individuals, if an intervention could delay disease onset by a mere 6 months, corresponding to annual savings of nearly $18 billion after 50 years. Although this study was restricted to the epidemiologic data from four studies in the United States only, with cost estimates from a single region in the United States, the message is clear: the personal, social, and economic impact of AD will continue to expand, given the status quo of management approaches.

Role of environment in Alzheimer's disease

A multitude of environmental factors, concomitant health conditions, and life events have been proposed as associated with the risk for developing AD [1,3–5]. These proposed risk factors can be divided arbitrarily into the following categories: (1) nonmodifiable (eg, age, ethnicity, perinatal conditions, early-life development, and growth); (2) socioeconomically modifiable (eg, socioeconomic conditions, environmental enrichment, cognitive reserve, diet); and (3) medically modifiable (obesity, hyperlipidemia, hypertension, diabetes). Although epidemiologic studies assessing nongenetic risk factors can provide useful insights into the origins of AD, their interpretation and establishment as causative factors rather than mere associations are usually problematic, given the natural lack of an experimental setting, the difficulty in assessing early-life events for a disease of the elderly population (retrospective rather than prospective studies), and the concomitant existence of multiple common conditions (such as hypertension, diabetes, and AD). Exceptions include the Lazarov and colleagues [6] study, which showed that transgenic mice coexpressing two familial AD genes with mutations (APPswe and PS1δE9) and raised in an "enriched environment" had less AD pathology reflected as reduced brain amyloid beta (Aβ) levels, compared with transgenic mice raised in a "standard environment." Of the transgenic mice in the "enriched environment," those that were more physically active had the most significant reductions in brain Aβ levels. The investigators also identified elevated activity of neprilysin, an Aβ-degrading protease, in the environmentally enriched transgenic mice, and differential gene expression, suggesting gene–environment interactions and a possible role of exercise and environmental enrichment for protection against AD. Others determined that environmental enrichment improved cognition in the same transgenic mouse model of AD [7]. Although a discrepancy exists between these studies regarding the effects of environmental enrichment on brain Aβ levels [6,7], a discussion of which is beyond the scope of this article, both studies are important because they provide a paradigm to test the effects of environment and gene–environment interactions in an experimental setting. Despite such advances, exploring the effects of environment on a common, complex condition such as AD remains a challenging task, only surpassed in difficulty by the prospect of modifying environmental factors to decrease disease risk.

Alzheimer's disease has a significant genetic component

Given the public impact of common, complex disorders such as AD and the challenges associated with studying and, more importantly, modifying environmental factors, much focus has been placed on genetic investigations. The rationale for studying genetics of any disease is multifold:

- Uncovering the underlying genetics leads to an understanding about disease pathophysiology.
- Genetic risk factors may be modifiable, unlike many environmental risk factors.
- Molecules encoded by genetic risk factors can be drug targets.
- Genetic risk factors may provide clues into modifiable environmental risk factors.
- Genetic variants and molecules identified through genetic studies can serve as biomarkers to identify at-risk populations for disease prevention.
- Knowledge about genetic risk factors in individuals may allow for personalized medicine in the future.

The first reports to suggest a genetic component for AD were published only 2 to 3 decades ago, about 70 to 80 years after Alzheimer's [8] publication on the very first case of this disease. Early reports focused on the invariable development of AD-like disease in Down syndrome (DS) patients after age 40, the increased risk for disease in family members of AD patients who had disease onset at younger than 65, and the autosomal dominant inheritance pattern in the rare families with early-onset forms of this disease [9]. Systematic analyses geared toward estimation of the genetic component of AD can be grouped into the following categories: (1) familial aggregation, (2) transmission pattern, and (3) twin studies. These studies are discussed.

Familial aggregation studies

Familial aggregation studies have revealed that having a first-degree relative with AD increases one's risk for developing AD significantly. Breitner and colleagues [10] investigated 379 first-degree relatives of 79 probands in a longitudinal study of AD and found that the cumulative incidence of AD among relatives increased strikingly with age, to 49% by age 87, in comparison with an incidence of less than 10% for controls. They did not observe an appreciable difference between the risks to relatives of presenile-onset (AD age of onset <65) and senile-onset AD probands (AD age of onset >65), suggesting the existence of a genetic origin for both early-onset AD (EOAD) and late-onset AD (LOAD). They emphasized that their results should not be interpreted as evidence of autosomal dominant transmission in LOAD, but as a rationale for pursuing genetic studies in LOAD and EOAD. Farrer and colleagues [11] independently assessed 70 families with one or more AD subjects using survival analysis, and found evidence of different transmission patterns for EOAD (defined as mean onset age less than 58 in their study) and LOAD (older than 58). Offspring of AD subjects had an estimated lifetime risk of 53% in EOAD families and 86% in LOAD families. These results supported an autosomal dominant transmission pattern for EOAD, whereas LOAD likely had a more heterogeneous transmission, possibly with both genetic and environmental contributions. Thus, despite the differences in the risk-to-relative estimates, it was evident from these early studies that both EOAD and LOAD had a transmissible component.

More recent longitudinal familial aggregation studies based on much larger data sets supported the earlier findings of familial aggregation and inheritance of AD. As part of the Multi-Institutional Research in Alzheimer Genetic Epidemiology (MIRAGE) project, Lautenschlager and colleagues [12] estimated the risk to 12,971 first-degree relatives of 1,694 AD probands (mean age at onset of 69.8) using survival analysis procedures. They found this risk to be $39.0\% \pm 2.1\%$ by age 96 years, which is approximately twice the estimated cumulative incidence of AD in the general population, establishing the substantial genetic component affecting this disorder. Furthermore, the lifetime risk for LOAD (≥ 65 years) estimated separately was still high, at $38.7 \pm 2.4\%$, though somewhat less than that for EOAD ($39.5 \pm 4.1\%$). Given that the cumulative risk to first-degree relatives in autosomal dominant disorders is expected to be 50%, it was deduced from this study that the lifetime risk among relatives did not support a simple autosomal dominant inheritance pattern of disease, unlike some of the earlier familial aggregation studies, and that AD likely had a more complicated transmission pattern, such as additive, multifactorial, or polygenic inheritance. This study found a lower lifetime risk estimate, compared with other studies [10,11]. The difference was attributed to inflated estimates resulting from missing information, especially in older age groups in other studies. The MIRAGE study, which included about 400 subjects aged older than 90, found a decreased risk for AD in this oldest age group, raising the interesting hypothesis that not only genetic risk factors for AD, but also protective genes, are at play in the healthy, elderly population.

Recent analysis of the MIRAGE data [13] comparing risk to first-degree relatives in the African-American (255 probands) versus the white population (2339 probands) indicated a higher cumulative risk by age 85 for the former (43.7±3.1% versus 26.9±0.8%, $P<.001$). However, risk to the spouses was also found to be higher in the African-American population, indicating that the risk attributable to familial aggregation was similar in the two ethnic groups. Given that the risk to first-degree relatives was higher than that for spouses in all *APOE* strata, this study concluded that a substantial heritable component to AD exists in both African-American and white populations, which is different from *APOE*. Other familial aggregation studies controlling for the *APOE* genotype also found similar evidence supporting the presence of factors other than *APOE* accounting for risk for AD [14–16]. In these studies, the presence of an *APOE* ε4 allele in the proband increased AD susceptibility in the relatives. However, the relatives of patients without an *APOE* ε4 allele also had an increased risk for AD, and the estimated risk to AD relatives was higher than their predicted *APOE* ε4 carrier status, implicating familial factors other than *APOE* as a risk for developing AD.

Transmission pattern studies

Although familial aggregation studies using survival analysis methods provided evidence of a transmissible factor accounting for risk for AD, these approaches did not necessarily distinguish a genetic factor from a transmissible environmental factor. To address this issue and to determine the mode of inheritance of genetic factors, segregation studies were pursued in AD families. Using a segregation analysis of 232 AD families (age at onset of 42–86 years), Farrer and colleagues [17] determined that the model of inheritance with the best fit was autosomal dominant genetic factor plus a multifactorial component. In this study, the models for a single major locus, multifactorial component only, no genetic susceptibility, and autosomal recessive transmission were all rejected. These findings could be explained by the existence of multiple genetic and environmental risk factors for AD and heterogeneity, with some families harboring a major risk gene and others, multifactorial transmissible factors. Segregation analysis of Dutch AD families of EOAD (<65 years) yielded similar results, implicating heterogeneity in EOAD [18]. Rao and colleagues [19] performed segregation analysis on a total of 401 AD families, 68 of which were early-onset (age at onset of AD cutoff = 65). They determined that stratification of the families according to the age of onset always yielded a better model fit, an indication of the etiologic heterogeneity between EOAD and LOAD families. AD in early-onset families was found to have an autosomal dominant transmission pattern. However, all the transmission models tested were rejected in the LOAD families, suggesting the possibility of heterogeneity or a complex genetic mechanism such as oligogenic inheritance. Thus, results from independent segregation analyses provided further support for genetic risk factors for both EOAD and LOAD. They implicated multiple genetic and environmental factors, especially for LOAD, and suggested a role for autosomal dominant transmission for at least some EOAD families.

More recently, Warwick Daw and colleagues [20] used oligogenic segregation analysis to study 75 AD families ascertained through a proband with LOAD and composed of 742 subjects, to estimate the number of trait loci affecting age at onset in LOAD. They accounted for the effects of *APOE* and sex in their study and determined that four or more quantitative trait loci (QTLs) exist, in addition to *APOE*, which contributed to age at onset in LOAD. They estimated that these loci had an effect size equal to or greater than that of *APOE*, which itself accounts for 7% to 9% of the total variance for age at onset. These studies clearly provided evidence for a significant genetic component for AD, with a complex mode of inheritance for LOAD, and provided a clear rationale for the search for novel LOAD genes.

Twin studies

Twin studies, particularly from Scandinavian twin registries, have been instrumental in establishing the genetic component for AD [21–23]. These studies compare the concordance of disease in monozygotic (MZ) twins, who share 100% of their genetic material, and dizygotic (DZ) twins, who, on average, share 50%. For a disease that is entirely caused by genes, the lifetime concordance for MZ twins is expected to approach 100%, allowing for lesser estimates because of diagnostic inaccuracies and the inherent late-onset nature of certain diseases (such as AD). The same estimate for DZ twins would be expected to approach 50%, the same estimate for sibpairs, or slightly more, secondary to possibly increased environmental sharing in DZ twins compared with other sibpairs. Given that MZ and DZ twins are assumed to share similar intrauterine and rearing environments [24], concordance rates significantly higher for MZ than DZ twins can be attributed to the effect of shared genes. The uses and potential pitfalls of twin studies in AD have been reviewed previously [24,25]. In a study of the Finnish Twin Cohort [21], MZ twins (n = 51) had a significantly higher cumulative incidence of AD than did DZ twins (n = 43), whereas the incidence of vascular or mixed dementia between the MZ and DZ twins showed no difference. The MZ twins had higher pairwise disease concordance rates than the DZ twins did, for both AD (18.6% versus 4.7%) and vascular dementia (18.2% versus 6.7%). Bergem and colleagues [22] found a significantly higher pairwise concordance rate for AD in MZ (78%) than in DZ twins (39%), but no difference for vascular dementia (17% of MZ versus 25% of DZ). By using tetrachoric correlations, they estimated the heritability (proportion of total variance caused by genes) for AD to be 60%. The largest AD twin study to date was based on the Swedish Twin Registry that analyzed 392 twin pairs who had clinical diagnoses [23]. The MZ twins' concordance of AD in this study was also higher than that of the DZ twins, confirming the general conclusions of earlier twin studies. In this study, unlike in the earlier twin studies, the investigators adjusted the findings for age and also addressed the issue of sex-difference on genetic factors by using both same-sex and opposite-sex twins. They estimated the age-adjusted heritability of AD to be 58% to 79% (varying based on model used) and concluded that no significant gender difference existed for either the prevalence or heritability of AD after controlling for age. Gatz and colleagues [23] also discussed the discrepancy in the concordance and heritability estimates between the different twin studies and highlighted differences among ascertainment, sample size, follow-up period, diagnostic methods, and age of analysis of subjects. Regardless of the individual parameter estimates obtained from these studies, the ultimate conclusion is unifying and supports a significant genetic component for AD, estimated at 60% to 80%.

Twin studies have also been used to study familial aggregation and the influence of *APOE* on the genetic component of AD. In a study of 94 twin pairs who were either members of the National Academy of Sciences Registry of Aging Twin Veterans (44 pairs) or volunteers (50 pairs), Steffens and colleagues [26] determined that concordance for AD among twins was significantly associated with a higher rate of AD among first-degree relatives (21%), compared with first-degree relatives of discordant twins (9.5%). They also assessed the effect of *APOE* genotype in the twins for development of AD and determined that the presence of *APOE* ε4 genotype in a twin pair was associated with an increased likelihood of AD in first-degree relatives. One family in this study was concordant for AD and without *APOE* ε4, with the highest degree of AD in the first-degree relatives (4/6 relatives), suggesting the instrumental presence of additional AD genes, at least in this family. Given that *APOE* status was not determined or inferred for the AD relatives in this study, and the small number of non-ε4–positive concordant twins, it is not possible to estimate accurately the contribution of genes other than *APOE* toward the development of AD in first-degree relatives of AD twins. Bergem and Lannfelt [27] determined that in a collection of Norwegian twin pairs, the frequency of the *APOE* ε4 allele did not differ between concordant and discordant DZ twin pairs, although the presence of this allele was associated with an earlier age at onset. These findings from twin studies suggest that although *APOE* accounts for risk and earlier age at onset of AD (the two phenotypes are interdependent for late-onset diseases), this gene does not explain all of the genetic risk for AD.

The collective evidence from familial aggregation, segregation, and twin studies for AD suggests a significant genetic component for this disease. The next section discusses the identification of the three known EOFAD genes.

Early-onset Alzheimer's disease genetics

Initial identification of the early-onset familial Alzheimer's disease genes

Amyloid precursor protein

Genetic linkage studies followed by candidate gene analysis or positional cloning have been successful historically in EOFAD and have led to the identification of the three known EOFAD genes. The *APP* gene on chromosome 21 is the first one found to have a mutation that causes EOFAD [28]. It is a good example of how linkage analysis, coupled with candidate gene approach, led to the successful identification of one of the EOFAD genes.

The identification of an association between trisomy 21 (DS) and AD led researchers to focus on chromosome 21 as the possible locus for an AD gene. The first report that discovered the link between DS and AD dates back to the nineteenth century, when Fraser and Mitchell [29] reported "precipitated senility" as a cause of death in DS patients. In studies conducted half a century later, autopsies of DS patients who died after the age of 40 revealed an AD-like histopathology, namely, senile plaques and neurofibrillary tangles [30–32]. During the early 1980s, researchers discovered that the "amyloid protein" isolated from the brains of AD patients had the same biochemical properties and amino acid sequence as that isolated from DS brains [33,34]. Because of the clinical, histopathologic, and biochemical association of DS with AD, and the existence of an extra copy of chromosome 21 in DS, researchers started to focus on chromosome 21 as the possible location for an AD susceptibility gene. In 1987, St. George-Hyslop and colleagues [35] found a linkage to a locus on chromosome 21 in extended families with the autosomal dominant form of EOAD. In two related articles, Goldgaber and colleagues [36] and Tanzi and colleagues [37] reported the mapping of the Aβ protein found in the brains of AD and DS patients to a region on chromosome 21 that was near the newly identified AD locus. After several reports that refuted linkage of autosomal dominant EOFAD to Aβ or to chromosome 21 in general [38–40], Goate and colleagues [41] first found evidence of linkage to chromosome 21 in EOFAD families, and then identified a missense mutation in the *APP* gene segregating with AD in some of the families they analyzed [28]. The mutation occurred in exon 17 of the *APP* gene, partially encoding for the Aβ peptide, and led to a valine-to-isoleucine change at amino acid 717 (Val717Ile), corresponding to the transmembrane domain of the protein. It was thus predicted that this first EOFAD mutation (also known as the London mutation) would lead to AD through its effects on Aβ. These predictions were subsequently proven to be accurate through functional analyses (see later discussion). Since then, according to the Alzheimer Disease and Frontotemporal Dementia Mutation Database (http://www.molgen.ua.ac.be/ADMutations), 26 other mutations have been identified within *APP* from 74 EOFAD families. Many of these mutations were functionally assessed for their effects on *APP* processing [42]. These studies provided strong support for the "amyloid hypothesis" discussed in detail in the related section of the article by Eckman elsewhere in this issue. The prevalence and clinical phenotype of the EOFAD *APP* mutations are discussed in subsequent sections.

Presenilins

Linkage analysis and positional cloning studies led to the identification of the second EOFAD gene, *PSEN1* on chromosome 14. In 1992, Schellenberg and colleagues [43] reported the results from a genome search they conducted in non–Volga-German kindreds with EOFAD, whereby they found significant linkage to a locus on chromosome 14. This finding was confirmed by the positive linkage results obtained by other groups to the same region of chromosome 14 in EOFAD families [44–46]. Sherrington and colleagues [47] cloned AD3 in 1995, later known as *PSN1*, by identifying a minimal cosegregating region on the chromosome 14 linkage area and determining the transcripts within this region. They found that one of the transcripts corresponded to a novel gene harboring a mutation that segregated with EOFAD in the families they studied. Subsequent studies described the structure of the *PSEN1* gene and identified new *PSEN1* mutations segregating with EOFAD [48–50]. To date, 157 pathogenic *PSEN1* mutations have been identified in 347 EOFAD families (http://www.molgen.ua.ac.be/ADMutations), making *PSEN1* mutations the most common known genetic cause of EOFAD.

The third EOFAD gene, *PSEN2*, was identified as a result of linkage studies accompanied by homology analysis of the transcripts in the linkage region. In 1995, Levy-Lahad and colleagues [51] reported significant linkage to a region on chromosome 1 in EOFAD kindreds of Volga-German origin, where linkage to chromosomes 14 and 21 had previously been excluded [40,43]. They identified a candidate gene in this region that showed sequence homology to *PSEN1* and that had a segregating mutation resulting in an asparagines-to-isoleucine substitution (Asn141Ile) [52]. Concurrently, Rogaev and colleagues [53] independently identified the same *PSEN2* N141L mutation in the affected probands of Volga-German families. They also identified a second missense mutation in this gene (Met239Val) segregating in an extended EOFAD pedigree of Italian origin. Unlike *PSEN1* mutations, *PSEN2* mutations are a rare cause of EOFAD. With 11 mutations identified from 19 pedigrees, most *PSEN2* mutations are thought to be private to pedigrees (http://www.molgen.ua.ac.be/ADMutations) [50,54,55].

Impact of autosomal dominant mutations for population risk for Alzheimer's disease

Compared with LOAD, EOAD is exceedingly rare. Campion and colleagues [56] defined EOAD as age of onset less than 61, and assessed the population-based prevalence of this disease in Rouen, France. They determined that the prevalence of EOAD was 41.2 per 100,000 people at risk (defined as ages 41 to 60). Their estimations were similar to those obtained from earlier population-based prevalence estimates of EOAD, which ranged between 18.2 and 45.2 per 100,000 inhabitants [57–60]. Campion and colleagues [56] further defined autosomal dominant EOAD (ADEOAD) as having three EOAD cases in three generations, and determined the prevalence of ADEOAD to be 5.3 per 100,000 people at risk. They then performed mutational analysis of the three known EOAD genes in the ADEOAD families they identified in the prevalence study combined with ADEOAD families referred to their laboratory. In their screen of 34 ADEOAD families, *PSEN1* mutations were identified in 56%, *APP* mutations in 15%, and *PSEN2* mutations in none of the families. Other screens of EOAD identified *PSEN1* mutations at a frequency of 18% to 56% [49,61], with different estimates among the studies attributed to the different selection criteria for the EOAD families analyzed. Others identified *APP* variations at a frequency of 13% in EOAD [62,63]. According to the Alzheimer Disease and Frontotemporal Dementia Mutation Database (http://www.molgen.ua.ac.be/ADMutations), of the EOFAD mutations identified, *PSEN1* mutations account for the most (81%), followed by *APP* (14%), with *PSEN2* mutations identified in only a handful of families (6%).

In summary, EOAD accounts for 6% to 7% of all AD [57,64] and EOFAD (or ADEOAD) accounts for 13% of EOAD. Given that mutations in *APP*, *PSEN1*, or *PSEN2* can explain up to 71% of the autosomal dominant transmission pattern in EOFAD, these genes account for about 0.5% of all AD. Although these are essentially negligible figures in terms of population-attributable risk posed by the known EOFAD mutations, their discoveries were, nonetheless, monumental in terms of understanding the pathophysiology of AD discussed briefly later and in detail elsewhere in this issue by Eckman. Importantly, 50% or more of EOAD are not explained by the known EOFAD mutations, indicating that this aggressive form of AD could possibly harbor as-yet-unknown genetic factors. Furthermore, the existence of LOAD families with an apparent autosomal dominant pattern of transmission suggests the presence of other Mendelian mutations with less aggressive phenotypes [64,65]. In a recent whole-genome scan of 12 AD families with an autosomal dominant pattern of inheritance, Giedraitis and colleagues [66] found evidence of a shared 40-cM haplotypic region on chromosome 8p in affected individuals from two families with age at onset of 54 to75. Analyses of single, extended families with autosomal dominant transmission patterns and members with either EOAD or LOAD in multiple generations have shown a linkage to numerous chromosomal regions, some of which have not been identified in prior whole-genome linkage scans of AD [66–68]. Thus, analyses of EOAD families and large LOAD families with Mendelian transmission patterns may emerge as a way to identify other genetic causes of AD. Although the population-based impact of such discoveries is expected to be small, the discoveries can provide new insights to the pathogenesis of AD and be instrumental in the development of drugs, novel quantitative phenotypes, and biomarkers for the prevention and treatment of the more common forms of this devastating condition.

Impact of autosomal dominant mutations for pathophysiology of Alzheimer's disease

Aβ, the major proteinaceous component of senile plaques in AD brains, is processed from APP by the cleavage of two secretases: β-secretase and γ-secretase [69–72]. Processing of APP by α-secretase and γ-secretase precludes the formation of the Aβ peptide and, instead, leads to the production of the shorter, nonfibrillogenic and nonamyloidogenic P3 peptide [73]. The EOFAD mutations identified in the *APP* gene all reside close to the secretase cleavage sites [74]. Analysis of plasma Aβ from affected families and the secreted Aβ from cell lines transfected with mutant forms of *APP* all showed an increase in the production of Aβ42 ± an increase in Aβ40, increased Aβ42/Aβ40 ratios or enhanced Aβ protofibril formation for all functionally assessed *APP* mutations [42,75–79]. Finally, transgenic mice carrying the mutant *APP* were shown to have elevated Aβ, amyloid plaques, and correlative memory deficits, abnormalities that are reminiscent of AD [80]. *PSEN* mutations similarly have been shown to increase the production of Aβ [75]. Moreover, transgenic mice overexpressing a mutant form of the *PSEN1* have been shown to have increased Aβ42(43) in their brains [81], providing further support for the amyloid cascade hypothesis as the mechanism of AD. Knock-out studies have determined that endogenous, wild-type *PSEN1* and *PSEN2* are required for the γ-secretase cleavage of APP [82]. The finding that all of the functionally tested EOFAD mutations affect Aβ metabolism that is reflected in the plasma or fibroblasts studied from EOFAD patients, presymptomatic mutation-carriers, and transgenic mice, and the evidence that *PSEN*s are a key component of the γ-secretase complex, suggest a common pathologic pathway for AD, involving Aβ [42,75–83].

Thus, although exceedingly rare, the identification of the autosomal dominant mutations in the three known EOFAD genes and the subsequent functional studies led to the development of the amyloid cascade hypothesis. Although the exact steps involved in the cascade of events in this pathophysiologic mechanism are as yet unknown and debatable, this mechanism has clearly set the stage for the ongoing drug discovery efforts for AD [84–86].

Late-onset Alzheimer's disease genetics

Initial identification of apolipoprotein E as a late-onset Alzheimer's disease susceptibility gene

The failure of multiple research groups to replicate the initial linkage reports to chromosome 21 [35] in various independent collections of AD families led to the hypothesis that AD may be a heterogeneous disorder [39,40,87]. In 1991, Pericak-Vance and colleagues [88] reported the results of a genome search they conducted in EOAD and LOAD families, whereby they found linkage to chromosome 21 in their EOAD families, and a novel locus on chromosome 19. The novel locus seemed to have an especially strong effect in the LOAD families (defined as age at onset older than 60). Given the previous association between an *APOC2* allele and AD reported by Schellenberg and colleagues [89], this gene on chromosome 19 initially emerged as a candidate for LOAD.

Concurrently, a group studying the change of lipids in AD brains by using an antibody to apolipoprotein E, a protein having a special relevance to nervous tissue, unexpectedly found that apolipoprotein E immunoreactivity was associated with amyloid in senile plaques and cerebral vessels, and in neurofibrillary tangles [90]. Because the gene for *APOE* mapped to the same locus as that identified in the Pericak-Vance and colleagues [88] linkage study, researchers started investigating the genetic and biologic association of apolipoprotein E with AD. In 1993, Strittmatter and colleagues [91] showed in an in vitro assay that apolipoprotein E binds Aβ with high avidity and that *APOE* ε4, a particular allelic form of *APOE*, is found at a higher frequency in LOAD, when compared with unrelated, age-matched controls. Subsequently, Corder and colleagues [92] demonstrated a dose-dependent increase in risk and a decrease in age at onset for LOAD, in *APOE* ε4 carriers. This study, which assessed 42 LOAD families, found a hazard ratio of 2.84 for carriers of a single *APOE* ε4 allele and 8.07 for those with the *APOE* ε4/ε4 genotype.

Since then, multiple, large, population- or clinic-based studies established the effect of *APOE* ε4 as a genetic risk factor for LOAD [93–99]. Table 1 gives a list of studies arbitrarily defined as having a large number of participants and performed on either population-based samples or multicenter collections. This table is not meant to depict the exhaustive list of all studies testing for an association between AD risk and *APOE*. Clearly, a large number of such studies are in the literature, because a simple search on PubMed (www.pubmed.org) using the keywords "*APOE*, association, Alzheimer, risk" yields an impressive 647 articles to date (January 18, 2007). Instead, Table 1 shows a collection of the studies with the largest sample sizes, which led to the establishment of *APOE* as a susceptibility gene for AD. Several conclusions can immediately be drawn from this list.

- *APOE* ε4 allele increases risk for AD in a dose-dependent manner.
- The risk conferred by *APOE* ε4 in predominantly or entirely Caucasian populations is unequivocal, with largely overlapping odds ratios (ORs) and confidence intervals.
- Studies in the African-American and Hispanic populations yield conflicting results.

Using these studies as a starting point, the population impact of *APOE*, possible ethnicity differences, and the role of *APOE* in the diagnosis of AD and as a premorbid predictor for its development are discussed in the following sections.

Impact of apolipoprotein E for population risk for Alzheimer's disease

In a population-based prospective study of the predominantly Caucasian Framingham cohort, Myers and colleagues [93] determined that the cumulative incidence of AD increased in a dose-dependent fashion, whereby 55% of the *APOE* ε4/ε4 group developed AD by age 80, compared with 27% of the *APOE* ε3/ε4 and 9% of the *APOE* ε3/ε3 groups by age 85. Despite the small number of *APOE* ε4/ε4 individuals (n = 16), this study clearly demonstrated that, unlike the autosomal dominant EOFAD mutations, *APOE* ε4 is a susceptibility, not a deterministic, factor for the development of AD. Furthermore, because only 10% of the individuals with one or more copies of *APOE* ε4 developed AD (positive predictive value 0.1), with specificity 0.81 and sensitivity 0.49, *APOE* ε4 is unlikely to be useful for the diagnosis of AD. Similar dose-dependent increases in the incidence or prevalence of AD were determined in other population-based prospective cohorts [96,97] or case-control studies [94,95,98].

Farrer and colleagues [94] performed a meta-analysis of 40 different clinic, population, or autopsy-based studies and assessed the effects of sex, age, and ethnicity on *APOE* association with AD. They reported results from population-based and clinic-based Caucasian samples separately (Table 1 depicts their population-based results only), which showed largely overlapping ORs for the *APOE* genotypes in these two different study groups. This study showed an age-dependent effect for the risk conferred by *APOE* ε4, such that this allele was associated with risk for AD across all age groups between 40 and 90 years, but the effect was strongest for ages 60 to 75, with a decline after age 70. Similar age-specific effects were also detected by others [95,98,99]. This age specificity, with declines in the risky effect of *APOE* ε4 in the older age groups, could have several causes:

- *APOE* ε4 may decrease age at onset of AD and lead to a more aggressive form of disease and a shorter survival.
- Genetic and nongenetic factors may render certain individuals relatively invulnerable to AD, and promote longevity.
- Genetic and nongenetic factors may interact with *APOE* ε4 in an age-dependent manner.

The results from studies in non-Caucasian populations were not as consistent for the association between AD and *APOE* [94,97,99]. The meta-analysis study by Farrer and colleagues [94] determined that the *APOE* ε3/ε4 association is nonsignificant, and the *APOE* ε4/ε4 genotype had lower, though overlapping, OR estimates in the African-American population, compared with the Caucasian population from that study. Farrer and colleagues [94] emphasized the presence of heterogeneity between these two ethnic groups,

Table 1
Studies of Apo E association in Alzheimer's disease series

Study (ref)	Study type	Ethnicity/ source	*APOE* 3:4 odds ratio (95% CI)	*APOE* 4:4 odds ratio (95% CI)	Number of subjects
Myers et al, 1996 [93]	Population based cohort	Predominantly Caucasian (Italian-American; Framingham, MA, USA)	3.7 (1.9–7.5)	30.06 (10.7–84.4)	68 AD, 962 controls
Farrer et al, 1997 [94]	Meta-analysis (population based)	Caucasian	2.7 (2.2–3.2)	12.5 (8.8–17.7)	4858 (total)
Bickeboller et al, 1997 [95]	Population based case control	Caucasian (France)	2.2 (1.5–3.5)	11.2 (4.0–31.6)	417 AD, 1030 controls
Slooter et al, 1998 [96]	Population based cohort	Caucasian (Rotterdam, Netherlands)	1.8 (1.0–3.1)	6.2 (1.4–28.2)	97 AD, 997 controls
Tang et al, 1998 [97]	Population-based cohort	Caucasian (New York City, NY, USA)	2.5 (1.1–6.4)[a]	—	23 AD, 214 contols
Breitner et al, 1999[b] [98]	Population based case control	Predominantly Caucasian (Cache County, UT, USA)	4.77 (2.71–8.40)[c]	8.52 (3.24–22.39)	230 AD, 698 controls
Farrer et al, 1997 [94]	Meta-analysis (population/ clinic-based)	African-American	1.1 (0.7–1.8)	5.7 (2.3–14.1)	235 AD, 240 controls

Tang et al, 1998 [97]	Population based cohort	African-American (New York City, NY, USA)	1.0 (0.6–1.6)[a]	—	53 AD, 128 controls
Graff-Radford et al, 2002 [99]	Clinic-based, multicenter case-control	African-American	2.6 (1.8–3.7)	10.5 (5.1–21.8)	338 AD, 301 controls
Evans et al, 2003 [100]	Population-based cohort	African-American (Chicago, IL, USA)	1.02 (0.39–2.68)[a]	—	362 (total)
Murrell et al, 2006 [101]	Population-based cohort	African-American (Indianapolis, IN, USA)	2.32 (1.41–3.82)	7.19 (3.00–17.29)	162 AD, 318 controls
Farrer et al, 1997 [94]	Meta-analysis (population/clinic based)	Hispanic	2.2 (1.3–3.4)	2.2 (0.7–6.7)	261 AD, 267 controls
Tang et al, 1998 [97]	Population-based cohort	Hispanic (New York City, NY, USA)	1.1 (0.7–1.6)[a]	—	145 AD, 516 controls
Farrer et al, 1997 [94]	Meta-analysis (population/clinic based)	Japanese	5.6 (3.9–6.0)	33.1 (13.6–80.5)	336 AD, 1977 controls

APOE ε3/ε4 and ε4/ε4 odds ratios are depicted in reference to the ε3/ε3 genotypes except as follows:

[a] Subjects with one or more *APOE* ε4 allele versus *APOE* ε3/ε3 genotype.

[b] Reference group is subjects with *APOE* ε2/ε2, ε2/ε3, and ε3/ε3 genotypes.

[c] Subjects with one *APOE* ε4 allele versus *APOE* ε3/ε3 genotype.

in terms of *APOE*. Tang and colleagues [97] found that the presence of an *APOE* ε4 allele did not pose a significant risk to the African-Americans or Hispanics in their longitudinal cohort from New York City. The African-Americans, Hispanics, and Caucasians in their study had a similar cumulative risk for AD in the presence of *APOE* ε4, whereas in its absence, the cumulative risks to the African-Americans and Hispanics were four and two times higher, respectively, even after adjusting for education and family history of AD. The investigators concluded that these results provided evidence for the presence of other genetic and nongenetic risk factors for AD in these two ethnic groups. Another longitudinal study, on an African-American cohort from Chicago, found similar nonsignificance for an *APOE* ε4 association with AD [100], whereas a longitudinal cohort from Indianapolis [101] and a multicenter case-control study from the southeastern United States [99] determined significant *APOE* ε4 risk for AD, in clear contrast. A recent review discusses these opposing results in the African-American population, and the potential reasons for this discrepancy in this literature [102]. The *APOE* ε4 allele frequencies are higher in controls from those studies that failed to show a significant association [97,100], compared with those that did [99,101], suggesting different underlying population structures. Indeed, the *APOE* ε4 allele control frequencies from the nonsignificant studies are similar to those seen in the Yoruban African population from Nigeria [103], where AD association with *APOE* is also lacking. The incidence of AD is also lower in the Yoruban African population [103], in comparison to the African-American populations from studies both confirming and refuting *APOE*–AD association [97,100–102]. Thus, the lack of association, despite high incidence rates, in the cohorts from Chicago and New York suggest (1) the presence of factors that prevent the development of AD in the controls from these cohorts with the *APOE* ε4 allele; (2) the presence of risk factors other than *APOE*, which lead to the development of AD in non-*APOE* ε4 carriers; (3) the presence of gene x gene, gene x environment interactions specific to, or more prominent in, certain populations; (4) the presence of a population admixture that led to false-negative results; (5) a combination of one or more of these possibilities.

The association studies in Hispanics have similarly been equivocal [94,97]. More recent studies have demonstrated significant *APOE* association and age-at-onset effect in Caribbean Hispanics with familial (but not sporadic) LOAD [104,105], suggesting the role of additional genes and other gene × *APOE* effects in this population. The discrepancies between the *APOE* ε4 frequencies and AD associations among Hispanic populations of different source and geography also imply the effects of genetic, and possibly environmental, heterogeneity in this ethnic group [106].

These findings highlight several important issues regarding AD and genetic studies of complex diseases in general:

Large studies from multiple centers are required to dissect complex genetics.

These studies need to control for potential population substructure arising from genetic heterogeneity.

Multiple genetic and nongenetic factors likely account for risk for, and protection from, AD. Analysis of various ethnic groups, using their genetic and environmental differences, may prove to be highly useful in the detection of these factors.

The population-attributable risk for AD or dementia caused by the *APOE* ε4 allele was estimated to be between 20% to 70% [96,98]. These estimates provide further evidence for the existence of additional genetic factors underlying the risk for AD.

Role of apolipoprotein E for the diagnosis of Alzheimer's disease and as a premorbid marker

Clinicopathologic series where the role of *APOE* in diagnosing AD was estimated did not support a rationale for its genotyping in the clinical setting [107–109]. Mayeux and colleagues [107] assessed the accuracy of clinical diagnosis alone, *APOE* genotyping alone, and their combination, in a clinicopathologic series of 2188 patients from 26 AD centers, 1833 of whom had clinical and 1770 of whom had pathologic diagnosis of AD, with 418 patients who had a pathologic diagnosis of other causes of dementia. The sensitivity and specificity of clinical diagnosis alone were 93% and 55%, respectively, whereas *APOE* genotyping alone had 65% and 68% sensitivity and specificity, respectively. The addition of *APOE* genotyping to the clinical diagnosis of AD decreased the sensitivity to 61%, but increased the specificity to 84%, thus reducing the false-positive rate. Tsuang and colleagues [108] found similar results in a community-based longitudinal series of 132 patients who had cognitive complaints and subsequent autopsy. The sensitivity and specificity of clinical diagnosis alone were 84% and 50%, respectively, in this study, whereas those for *APOE* alone were 59% and 71%, respectively. In the presence of a clinical diagnosis of AD, *APOE* decreased sensitivity to 49% and increased specificity to 84%. In the absence of a clinical diagnosis of AD, *APOE* increased sensitivity to 94% and decreased specificity to 37%, indicating a high false-positive rate of diagnosing AD in individuals with an *APOE* ε4 allele but no pathologic evidence of AD. Although *APOE* genotyping increased the specificity (decreased false-positive rate) when a clinical diagnosis of AD was made, this association is not absolute; some individuals lack the *APOE* ε4 allele and have pathologically confirmed AD, and some have *APOE* ε4 and cognitive impairment but non-AD pathology. Thus, *APOE* genotyping is not advocated as part of the diagnostic work-up for AD [105].

Given the importance of early detection for development of AD from prodromal cognitive impairment states, multiple studies focused on the use of *APOE* genotyping as a predictor for the development of AD. Most population- or clinic-based longitudinal prospective studies that used mild cognitive impairment (MCI) or other clinical criteria for predementia cognitive impairment found *APOE* ε4 to be a significant predictor for the development of AD [110–113]. In two longitudinal studies assessing cognitive testing, *APOE* ε4 was found to be a predictor for the development of AD when used independently, but not in combination with cognitive assessment [114,115], which is in contrast to the findings of Petersen and colleagues [110], whereby *APOE* ε4 was a strong predictor for conversion from MCI to AD, even in the presence of cognitive testing. This discrepancy may arise from the definition of cognitive state in the starting populations in these studies. Cervilla and colleagues [114] assessed conversion from a cognitively normal state, and Lee and colleagues [115] studied subjects with questionable dementia. Both of these populations are likely more heterogeneous than the MCI subjects studied by Petersen and colleagues [110]. In conclusion, although *APOE* ε4 appears to be an important predictor of conversion to AD, especially from well-defined cognitive impairment states, its use in the clinical setting is not substantiated. Nonetheless, future studies of other potential premorbid biomarkers of AD need to include this genetic factor for increased accuracy.

Whole-genome linkage and association studies

Study characteristics

The extensive data from prior twin, segregation, family aggregation, EOFAD autosomal dominant families, and *APOE* association studies discussed earlier have led to the conclusion that AD has a substantial genetic component not explained by the known EOFAD mutations or *APOE*. This conclusion, along with the development of high-throughput techniques for genotyping an ever-expanding number of markers (microsatellites and single nucleotide polymorphisms [SNPs]), statistical methodologies geared toward identification of genetic loci in the absence of known Mendelian patterns of inheritance, and collective efforts to obtain collections of LOAD families, relative pairs, and case-control series led to the pursuit of a number of whole-genome linkage and association studies in the literature [116–136]. A summary of the key characteristics of these studies is presented in Table 2. As seen here, the three groups of studies are essentially as follows: "A" denotes those whole-genome linkage studies on AD families or sibpairs (see Refs. [116,120,125,126,128,131,134,135]). These studies are independent, in that they were either performed entirely on ethnically distinct data sets of Caribbean Hispanic [125,131], Amish [134], or Swedish [135] subjects, or, even if they did have overlapping data (National Institute of Mental Health [NIMH] or National Institute on Aging [NIA] data sets), they also had considerable nonoverlapping data [116,120,126,128]. The initial linkage analysis by Pericak-Vance and colleagues [116] performed on a total of 54 LOAD families may be a subset of their subsequent work on a significantly larger data set [120] based on the similar sources of the study subjects, although the extent of overlap is not mentioned explicitly in their latter publication. Nonetheless, the results from their initial study are presented separately here (Tables 3–8) because this whole-genome linkage analysis was the first conducted in LOAD and also because it led to the identification of the chromosome 12 locus, subsequently replicated in other studies [125,126,129]. Although the extent of overlap is not clearly evident among the three predominantly United States-sample–based studies using the NIMH and NIA data sets [120,126,128], Blacker and colleagues [128] tried to address this issue by reporting results from both their entire data set, and the subset of subjects nonoverlapping with the first [119] and second stages [126] of the Washington University study. Their results from the nonoverlapping (non-Kehoe) subset are depicted here.

The second type of study, denoted by "B," identifies whole-genome association studies conducted on case-control series [118,122,129]. These three studies are entirely independent and assess subjects within the United States [118], Finland [122], or from an inbred Arab community [129]. Their results are shown in Tables 3–8. Studies in group "C" are performed on data sets that have complete, or major, overlaps with other published genome scans (see Refs. [121,123,124,127,130,132,133]). Group C studies reassess these data sets either by using alternative analytic strategies, such as conditional linkage analysis [121], ordered subsets analyses [130], or linkage analysis with covariates [127,132,133]; or by using alternative phenotypes such as age at onset [124] or defined subsets within the data such as LOAD with psychosis [123]. The summary results from these alternative approaches are depicted in the text rather than in Tables 3–8. Finally, the first stage of the Washington University genome scan, which is a subset of their subsequent study [126] and the Pericak-Vance and colleagues [117] study from 1998, which appears to be the same study as Ref. [116], are denoted as a separate category, "D." Their results are not discussed separately.

As seen in Table 2, most of the studies are based on AD families or sibpairs with age at onset older than 60 (see Refs. [116–120,122,123, 126,127,129,133,135]). Most studies with both late and early/mixed age-at-onset data sets showed separate results for these different age groups (see Refs. [125,128,131,132]). Where applicable, the age subsets for the results are shown in Tables 3–8. Many of the studies performed subset analyses based on *APOE* genotypes (see Refs. [116,123,125,126,135]), although their definitions of E4+ (*APOE* ε4+) or E4− subsets varied between the studies. Again, results for the various *APOE* subsets are shown in Tables 3–8.

Results of whole-genome linkage and association studies

Tables 3–8 summarize the results of the whole-genome linkage (group A from Table 2) and association (group B from Table 2) studies in the

Table 2
Characteristics of the whole-genome linkage and association studies in Alzheimer's disease

Study ref.	Authors	Study type	Sample source	Sample type	Age at onset	Sample size	Analytic approach	Number of markers	Marker density	Subset analysis
[116]	Pericak-Vance et al, 1997	A	US (NIA, Duke, UCLA, MGH)	Multiplex families	≥60	16 families (52 ADs versus 83 controls)	ARP, ASP, LOD	280 microsatellites	10–15 cM	E4+ (all ADs with ≥1 E4 = 27 families) versus E4– (≥1 AD member without E4 = 27 families)[a]
[116]	Pericak-Vance et al, 1997	A				38 families (89 ADs versus 216 controls)				
[117]	Pericak-Vance et al, 1998[b]	D	US (NIA, Duke, UCLA, MGH)	Multiplex families	>60	16 families (52 ADs versus 83 controls)	ARP, ASP, LOD	280 microsatellites	10–15 cM	
[117]	Pericak-Vance et al, 1998[b]	D				38 families (89 ADs versus 216 controls)				

[118]	Zubenko et al, 1998	B	US (Belmont, Pittsburgh)	Case control	> 60	100 AD cases (autopsied) versus 100 controls (50 autopsied, 50 90+)	Chi-square	391 microsatellites	10 cM	
[119]	Kehoe et al, 1999	D	US (NIMH)	Sibpairs	≥ 65	292 sibpairs (230 families)	ASP	237 microsatellites	16.3 cM	
[120]	Pericak-Vance et al, 2000[c]	A	US (NIMH, NIA, Duke, UCLA, Vanderbilt)	Families	> 60	466 families (1051 ADs versus 591 controls; 199 families autopsied)	ARP, ASP	326 microsatellite	10 cM	Autopsied (N = 199) versus not (N = 267)
[121]	Curtis et al, 2001[d]	C	US (NIMH)	Families	most ≥ 65	241 families	Conditional nonparametric linkage	237 microsatellites	16.3 cM	
[122]	Hiltunen et al, 2001	B	Finland	Case control	> 60	47 ADs versus 51 controls	Chi-square	366 microsatellites	10 cM	
[123]	Bacanu et al, 2002[e]	C	US (NIMH)	Families[f]	≥ 65	65 families (42 with E4+)	ARP (LOAD +psychosis)	237 microsatellites	16.3 cM	E4+ (≥ 2 members with E4+)

(*continued on next page*)

Table 2 (*continued*)

Study ref.	Authors	Study type	Sample source	Sample type	Age at onset	Sample size	Analytic approach	Number of markers	Marker density	Subset analysis
[124]	Li et al, 2002[g,h]	C	US (NIMH, NIA, Duke, UCLA, Vanderbilt)	Families	≥49	449 families (1121 ADs versus 746 controls)	QTL (AAO)	323 microsatellites	10 cM	
[125]	Mayeux et al, 2002[i]	A	Caribbean Hispanics	Families	mixed (>65 and ≤65)	79 families (320 subjects)	ARP	35 markers (Ch 12)	3.4 cM	Late-onset (≥65) versus early/mixed-onset (<65); E4+ (≥75% of ADs with ≥1 E4) versus E4− (<75% of ADs with ≥1 E4)
[126]	Myers et al, 2002[j]	A	US (NIMH, NIA) UK	Sibpairs	≥65	451 sibpairs (174 new from Ref. [119])	ASP	328 microsatellites (91 additional to Ref. [119])	5 cM (select regions)	E4+ (each sib with ≥1 E4 = 280 ASP) versus E4− (all E4−/E4− = 76 ASP)
[127]	Olson et al, 2002[e]	C	US (NIMH)	Sibpairs	≥60	272 sibpairs	ASP with covariates (age, *APOE*)	(see footnote k)	(see footnote k)	

[128]	Blacker et al, 2003[d]	A	US (NIMH)	Families	≥ 50	437 families (994 AD versus 445 controls; 238 non-Kehoe families)	ARP, LOD	381 microsatellites	9 cM	Late-onset (≥ 65) versus early/mixed-onset (< 65)
[129]	Farrer et al, 2003[l]	B	Inbred Arab community	Case-control	≥ 60	5 ADs versus 5 controls	Chi-square	375 microsatellites	10 cM	
[129]	Farrer et al, 2003[l]	B				100 ADs versus 110 controls				
[130]	Scott et al, 2003[m]	C	US (NIMH, NIA, Duke, UCLA, Vanderbilt)	Families	≥ 49	437 multiplex families (1014 ADs versus 238 controls)	Ordered subsets analysis	336 microsatellites	10 cM	
[131]	Lee et al, 2004	A	Caribbean Hispanics	Families	Mixed (> 65 and ≤ 65)	96 families (490 subjects; 237 ADs versus 157 controls, others unknown); 104 families (2nd stage, 521 subjects)	ASP, ARP, affected only dominant model	340 microsatellites	10.2 cM	Late-onset (≥ 65) versus early/mixed-onset (< 65)

(*continued on next page*)

Table 2 (*continued*)

Study ref.	Authors	Study type	Sample source	Sample type	Age at onset	Sample size	Analytic approach	Number of markers	Marker density	Subset analysis
[131]	Lee et al, 2004	A				104 families (521 subjects)		Additional markers on Ch 10, 18, 12		
[132]	Avramopoulos et al, 2005[n]	C	US (NIMH)	Families	>50	148 families (348 ADs versus 153 controls)	ASP with covariates (delusions, hallucinations)	381 microsatellites	9 cM	Late-onset (>65) versus early-onset (<65)
[133]	Holmans et al, 2005[o]	C	US (NIMH, NIA) UK	Sibpairs	≥ 65	453 sibpairs (600–789 subjects, depending on covariate)	ASP with covariates (mean AAO, difference AAO, mean ROD, difference ROD)	328 microsatellites (91 additional to Ref. 120)	5 cM (select regions)	
[134]	Hahs et al, 2006	A	US (Amish)	Extended families	≥ 58	5 families (115 subjects; 40 AD, 9 MCI, 66 controls)	LOD	407 microsatellites	7 cM	

[135]	Sillen et al, 2006	A	Sweden	Multiplex and sibpair families	≥65	71 families (188 subjects)	ARP	365 microsatellites	9 cM	E4+ = all ADs with ≥1 E4 versus E4− = ≥1 AD without any E4 (in E4− families, the E4+ individuals were excluded from analysis)

Study types: A, Linkage analysis of families, relative pairs, independent studies; B, Association analysis of case-controls, independent studies; C, Linkage analysis of families, using alternative analytic methods on largely overlapping data sets with previously published results; D, First-stage linkage results or results on subsets of other data sets.

Abbreviations: AAO, age at onset; ARP, affected relative pair; ASP, affected sibpair; Ch, chromosome; LOD, logarithm of the odds (parametric linkage); MGH, Massachusetts General Hospital; NIA, National Institute on Aging; NIMH, National Institute of Mental Health; ROD, rate of decline; UCLA, University of California at Los Angeles.

[a] E4 = *APOE* ε4.

[b] Appears to be same study as Ref. [116].

[c] Sample overlaps with Refs. [116,117]; 80% overlap with Ref. [126].

[d] Sample overlaps significantly with Ref. [119].

[e] Subset of Ref. [119].

[f] Families with ≥2 members with LOAD and psychosis and ≥2 members with *APOE* ε4+.

[g] Only results for AD are used herein.

[h] Sample overlaps with other NIMH data, major overlaps with Refs. [116,117,120].

[i] Subset of Ref. [131].

[j] Follow-up study of 120; 80% sample overlap with Ref. 121.

[k] Likely same markers as Ref. [119], but not mentioned explicitly in text.

[l] Ch 12 results are not follow-up from stage I, but based on previous studies.

[m] Subset of Ref. [120].

[n] Sample overlaps with other NIMH data.

[o] Same data set as Ref. [126].

Table 3
Results of the whole-genome linkage and association studies in Alzheimer's disease chromosomes 1 to 4

Chromosome	1			2			3			4		
Study ref.	Marker	Locus	Result	Marker	Locus	Result	Marker	Locus	Result	Marker	Locus	Result
Pericak-Vance et al, 1997[a] [116]										D4S1629	4q32.1	> 1.0
Pericak-Vance et al, 2000[b] [120]										D4S1629	4q32.1	1.32
Myers et al, 2002[c] [126]	D1S1675	1p13.2	1.7 (E4+)									
Blacker et al, 2003[d] [128]	D1S1597	1p36.21	1.3 (late)				D3S2387	3p26.3	2.9 (early/ mixed)	D4S1629	4q32.1	1.1 (total)
	D1S551	1p31.1	1.7 (early/ mixed)				D3S4542	3p14.1	1.5 (total)	D4S1652	4q35.2	1.1 (late)
Mayeux et al, 2002 (Ch12), Lee et al, 2004[e] [125,131]	D1S551	1p31.1	1.12 (late)	D2S1777	2p12	1.51 (all)	D3S2418	3q28	1.07 (total)	D4S2366	4p16.1	1.59 (all)
				D2S1353	2q24.1	1.59 (late)				D4S2382	4p14	1.26 (late)
				D2S2944	2q34	1.31 (all and late)				D4S3335	4q35.1	1.25 (late)

Hahs et al, 2006[b] [134]	D1S1665	1p31.1	1.07	D2S2978	2q31.3	1.94	DS31766	3p14.2	1.78	D4S2632	4p15.1	1.33
	D1S1631	1p21.1	1.83	D2S1363	2q36.3	1.17	D3S3045	3q13.12	1	D4S2394	4q28.2	2.12
							D3S1763	3q26.1	1.69	D4S1548	4q31.3	3.01
							D3S2398	3q28	2.16	D4S2417	4q34.3	1.21
Sillen et al, 2006[c] [135]										D4S406	4q25	2 (E4+)
Zubenko et al, 1998[f] [118]	D1S518	1q31.1	0.003									
	D1S547	1q43	0.001									
Hiltunen et al, 2001[f] (results for Ch 13 from Ref. [136]) [122]	D1S552	1p36.13	0.006	D2S405	2p23.2	0.009	D3S1602	3q27.2–27.3	0.007	D4S1627	4p13	0.004
	D1S1679	1q23.3	0.015									
Farrer et al, 2003[f] [129]				D2S310	2p24.1	0.005						

Abbreviation: Ch, chromosome.

[a] Two-point (38 families, except Ch 12 = 54 families; Ch 19 results are significant but caused by *APOE* and therefore not shown in this article).

[b] Two-point.

[c] Multipoint.

[d] Multipoint (non-Kehoe data set).

[e] Ch 10, 12, 18 second-stage multipoint linkage, others single-stage two-point.

[f] Chi-square *P*.

Table 4
Results of the whole-genome linkage and association studies in Alzheimer's disease chromosomes 5 to 8

Chromosome	5			6			7			8		
Study ref.	Marker	Locus	Result	Marker	Locus	Result	Marker	Locus	Result	Marker	Locus	Result
Pericak-Vance et al, 1997 [116]				D6S1004 D6S1019	6q15 6p21.2	> 1.5 > 1.0						
Pericak-Vance et al, 2000 [120]	D5S1470	5p13.3	2.23 (autopsy)	D6S1027	6q27	1.20 (autopsy)	D7S2847	7q31.31	2.18 (autopsy)			
Myers et al, 2002 [126]	D5S1470	5p13.3	1.0/1.6 (all, E4+)	D6S1017 D6S1018	6p21.1 p12.3	1.3 (E4+)						
Blacker et al, 2003 [128]				D6S1027	6q27	2.7 (total)						
Mayeux et al, 2002 (Ch 12), Lee et al, 2004 [125,131]	D5S2488	5p15.33	1.76 (late)	GAAT3A06 D6S1280	6p22.3 6p12.3	1.65 (all) 1.58 (late = all)				D8S1136	8q13.1	1.08 (late)
Hahs et al, 2006 [134]	D5S1725	5q14.3	1.47	D6S1040	6q23.1	1.94	D7S2204 D7S3070	7q21.11 7q36.1	1.14 1.74			
Sillen et al, 2006 [135]	D5S498	5q35.2	2.4									
Zubenko et al, 1998 [118]												
Hiltunen et al, 2001 [122]	D5S807	5p15.2	0.001	D6S1017	6p21.1	0.003				GAAT1A4	8q22.2	0.028
Farrer et al, 2003 [129]												

Abbreviation: Ch, chromosome.

literature. Different analytic approaches have been used between and within the studies. Where a given study has more than one analytic approach, findings from the approach yielding the most significant result are depicted. Likewise, when subset analyses exist, the results of the subset with the most significant result are used, and these are depicted in the table. For multistage genome scans, the results from the second stage or follow-up study are used, where available. When both two-point and multipoint linkage results are available, the latter result is shown. Logarithm of the odds (LOD) scores (parametric or nonparametric linkage results) above 1.0 or *P* values below 0.05 are shown, unless the study investigators determined a more significant cutoff in their paper. When two or more "interesting" results exist on a single chromosome separated by an arbitrary distance cutoff of greater than 15 cM, each one is reported separately. Otherwise, the most significant result is reported. When a multipoint linkage curve spans more than15 cM with one or more peaks separated only by sharp "dips" (as opposed to a plateau of "no suggestive linkage," with LOD scores consistently less than one in between), the highest multipoint result is reported. Otherwise, each multipoint result is reported separately. For locations of the multipoint LOD score results, unless given explicitly, the nearest marker location is used.

Fig. 1 is a compilation of all chromosomes where more than one suggestive or significant result exists in more than one study from Tables 3–8. The plain karyotype figures (not showing the study results) are taken from the Ensemble website (http://www.ensembl.org/info/software/website/installation/build.html) [137]. The chromosomal locations for the markers are as per the March 2006 human genome assembly on the UCSC Genome Browser (http://genome.ucsc.edu/) [138].

Despite the differences in the study subjects, study designs, and analytic approaches among the various studies, inspection of Tables 3–8 and Fig. 1 reveals a number of chromosomal regions where evidence for linkage or association exists, based on a number of studies. For chromosome 19, all but two studies [129,131] showed significant or suggestive evidence of linkage or association. One of these studies was performed on the specific ethnic group of an inbred Arab community, where *APOE* frequency is low in controls and in AD cases [129]. The other study was on a collection of Caribbean-Hispanic families, where an association but no significant linkage was evident [131]. These results strongly suggest the existence of genetic risk factors for AD other than *APOE*, especially in ethnic groups of non-European or non-North American origin. Furthermore, in three studies, one or more locus yields greater significance for linkage or association, compared with the *APOE* locus on chromosome 19 [122,126,134]. Hiltunen and colleagues [122] identified loci on chromosomes 1 to 6, 10, 13, and 18 in their study of a Finnish case-control series in which evidence for association was greater than that for *APOE*. They reported simulated *P* values. Myers and colleagues [126] found the strongest evidence of linkage on chromosome 10q, with a LOD score of 3.9 in their whole data set, compared with 1.3

Table 5
Results of the whole-genome linkage and association studies in Alzheimer's disease chromosomes 9 to 12

Chromosome	9			10			11			12		
Study ref.	Marker	Locus	Result	Marker	Locus	Result	Marker	Locus	Result	Marker	Locus	Result
Pericak-Vance et al, 1997 [116]										D12S1042	12p11.23	3.2 (multi all=3.5; multi E4 − =3.9)
										D12S390	12q13.13	2.3
Pericak-Vance et al, 2000 [120]	D9S741	9p21.3	4.31 (autopsy)	D10S1426	10p11.23	1.22 (autopsy)						
	D9S1818	9q34.2	2.05 (autopsy)									
Myers et al, 2002 [126]	D9S741	9p21.3	1.8 (all)	D10S1211	10q21.3	3.9/3.2 (all/E4+)				LOX-1	12p13.2	1.3/1.4 (whole/E4−)
	D9S176	9q22.33	1.0/1.8 (all/E4+)									
Blacker et al, 2003 [128]				D10S189	10p14	1.2 (early/mixed)	D11S968	11q25	1.1 (total)			
Mayeux et al, 2002 (Ch 12), Lee et al, 2004 [125,131]				D10S190	10q26.11	2.02 (all)				D12S1623	12p13.31	2.01 (late)
										D12S1057	12p12.1	1.63 (late)

Hahs et al, 2006 [134]				D10S2327	10q22.3	2.42	D11S1392	11p13	2.14			
Sillen et al, 2006 [135]												
Zubenko et al, 1998 [118]				D10S1423	10p12.33	0.001				D12S1045	12q24.33	0.03
Hiltunen et al, 2001 [122]				D10S1664	10p13	0.007						
Farrer et al, 2003 [129]	AFM220XF2	9p21.3	2.3 × 10^-7	D10S580	10q22.3	0.001				D12S1722	12q15	1.3×10^-6
				D10S1426	10p11.23	<0.01						

Abbreviation: Ch, chromosome.

Table 6
Results of the whole-genome linkage and association studies in Alzheimer's disease chromosomes 13 to 16

Chromosome	13			14			15			16		
Study ref.	Marker	Locus	Result	Marker	Locus	Result	Marker	Locus	Result	Marker	Locus	Result
Pericak-Vance et al, 1997 [116]												
Pericak-Vance et al, 2000 [120]	D13S787	13q12.12	1.05									
Myers et al, 2002 [126]												
Blacker et al, 2003 [128]	D13S793	13q32.1	1.4 (late)	D14S587	14q22.2	2.9 (early/ mixed)	D15S642	15q26.3	1.2 (early/ mixed)			
Mayeux et al, 2002 (Ch 12), Lee et al, 2004 [125,131]				D14S587	14q22.2	2.0 (total)						
Hahs et al, 2006 [134]				D14S588	14q24.1	1.54						
Sillen et al, 2006 [135]												
Zubenko et al, 1998 [118]												
Hiltunen et al, 2001 [122]	D13S292	13q12.12	0.002	D14S77	14q24.2	0.048	D15S659	15q21.1	0.036	D16S403	16p12.1	0.012
Farrer et al, 2003 [129]												

Abbreviation: Ch, chromosome.

Table 7
Results of the whole-genome linkage and association studies in Alzheimer's disease chromosomes 17 to 20

Chromosome	17			18			19			20		
Study ref.	Marker	Locus	Result	Marker	Locus	Result	Marker	Locus	Result	Marker	Locus	Result
Pericak-Vance et al, 1997 [116]										D20S94	20q13.32	< 1.0
Pericak-Vance et al, 2000 [120]				D18S878	18q22.1	1.02 (autopsy)	D19S246	19q13.33	3.64 (autopsy)			
				D18S1371	18q22.3-23	1.14 (autopsy)	*APOE*	19q13.32	11.85			
Myers et al, 2002 [126]							D19S412	19q13.32	1.3			
Blacker et al, 2003 [128]							D19S178	19q13.31	7.6 (early/ mixed)			
Mayeux et al, 2002 (Ch 12), Lee et al, 2004 [125,131]				D18S1106	18q22.3	3.65 (all)						
Hahs et al, 2006 [134]				D18S858	18q21.31	1.88	D19S586 D19S245 D19S246	19p13.2 19q13.11 19q13.33	2.06 1.41 1.57	D20S477	20p11.21	1.05
Sillen et al, 2006 [135]							D19S902	19q13.32	4.84			
Zubenko et al, 1998 [118]							*APOE*	19q13.32	< 0.0001			
Hiltunen et al, 2001 [122]	D17S1293	17q12	0.025	D18S66 D18S59	18q11.2 18p11.32	0.025 0.009	D19S1034 D19S433	19p13.3 19q12	0.013 0.021	D20S604	20p12.1	0.036
Farrer et al, 2003 [129]												

Abbreviation: Ch, chromosome.

Table 8
Results of the whole-genome linkage and association studies in Alzheimer's disease chromosomes 21 to X

Chromosome	21			22			X		
Study ref.	Marker	Locus	Result	Marker	Locus	Result	Marker	Locus	Result
Pericak-Vance et al, 1997 [116]									
Pericak-Vance et al, 2000 [120]									
Myers et al, 2002 [126]	D21S1909	21q22.11	1.6 (E4−)				DXS8015	Xp11.4	1.2/1.2 (all/E4−)
Blacker et al, 2003 [128]									
Mayeux et al, 2002 (Ch 12), Lee et al, 2004 [125,131]									
Hahs et al, 2006 [134]				D22S425	22q11.22	1.38			
Sillen et al, 2006 [135]									
Zubenko et al, 1998 [118]							DXS1047	Xq25	0.0002
Hiltunen et al, 2001 [122]									
Farrer et al, 2003 [129]									

Abbreviation: Ch, chromosome.

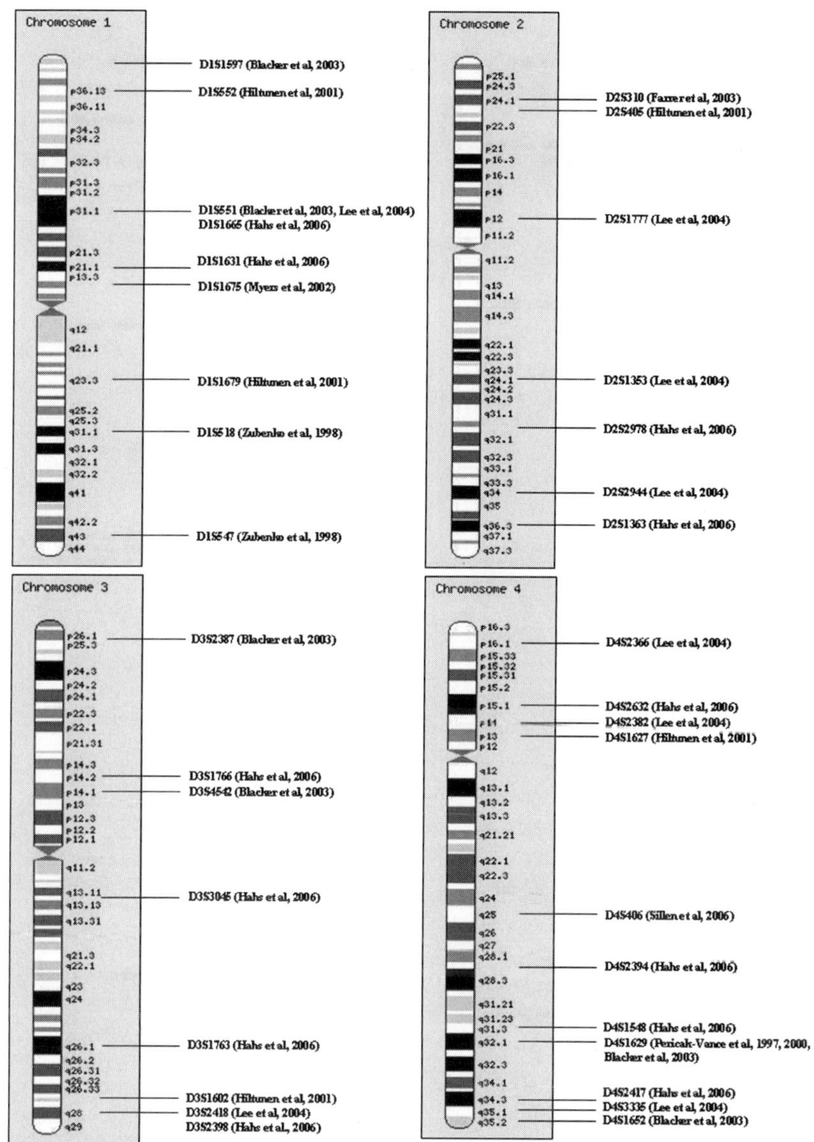

Fig. 1. Chromosomal map summaries of whole-genome linkage and association studies in AD. Chromosomes 16, 17, 21, and 22 are not shown because only a single result from a single study was suggestive or significant for these chromosomes.

for chromosome 19q [126]. Finally, Hahs and colleagues [134], in their study of extended Amish families from the United States, where *APOE* was previously shown not to be an important risk factor for AD, identified both novel (chromosomes 4–7, 11, 18–20) and previously reported (chromosomes

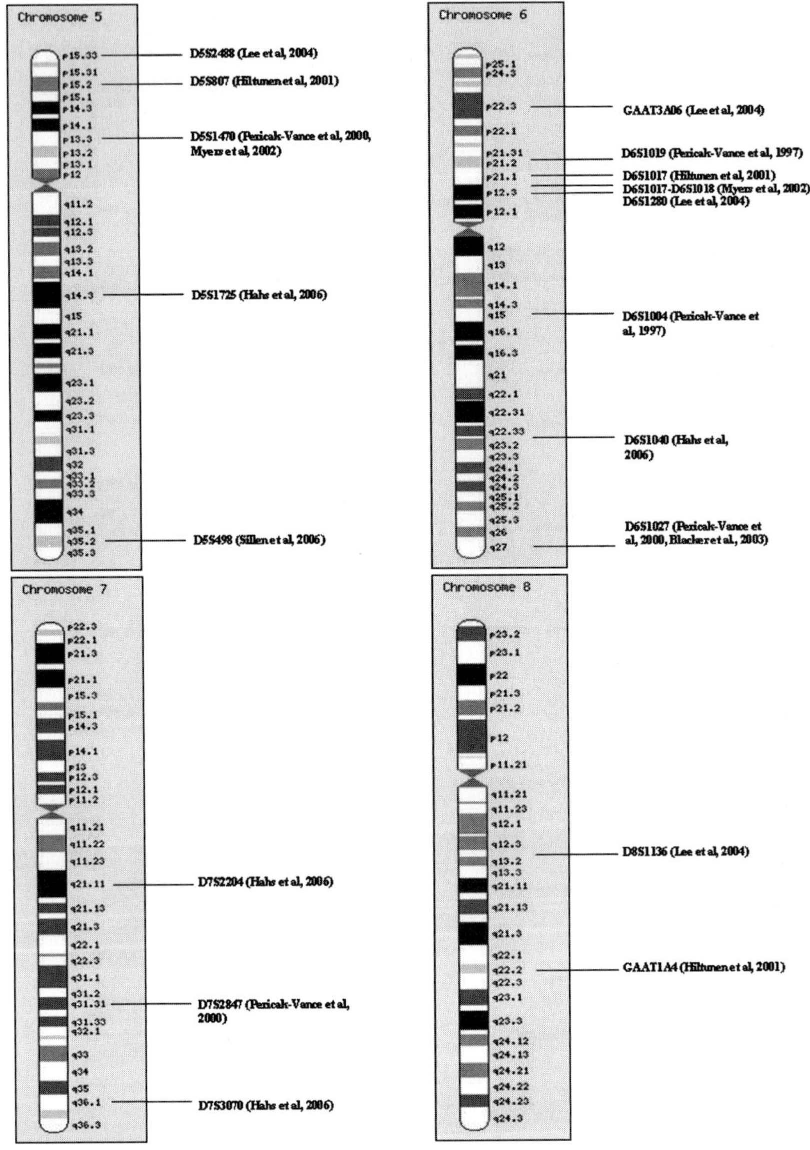

Fig. 1 (*continued*)

4–7, 11, 18–20) regions with evidence for linkage. Thus, evidence is ample from these whole-genome linkage and association studies for the existence of novel LOAD risk loci.

Given the plethora of positive findings, it is important to be able to discern true-positive from false-positive results. Evidence of linkage or

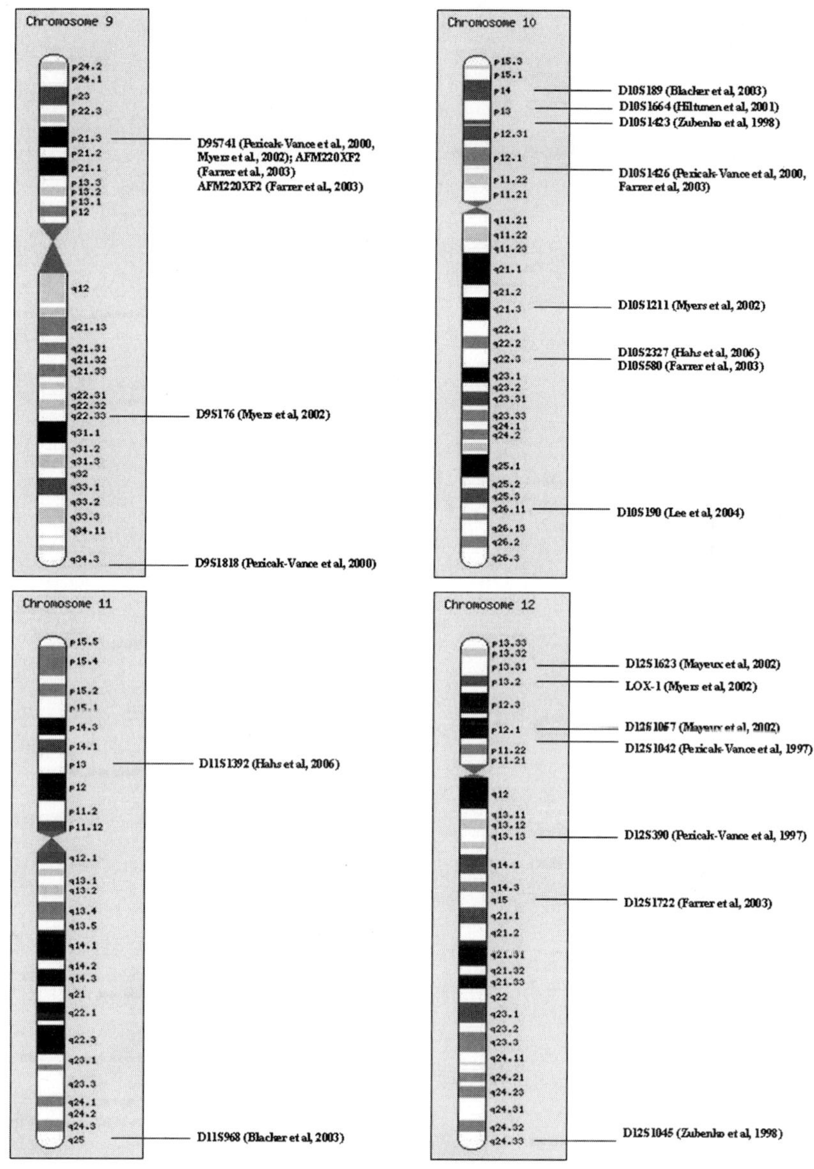

Fig. 1 (*continued*)

association from multiple independent studies is an important indicator for a result as being a true positive. Although studies with overlapping data sets [116,120,126,128] render such a comparison difficult, attempts are being made to approach this analytic difficulty. Blacker and colleagues [128] reported the results of their linkage analyses on overlapping and

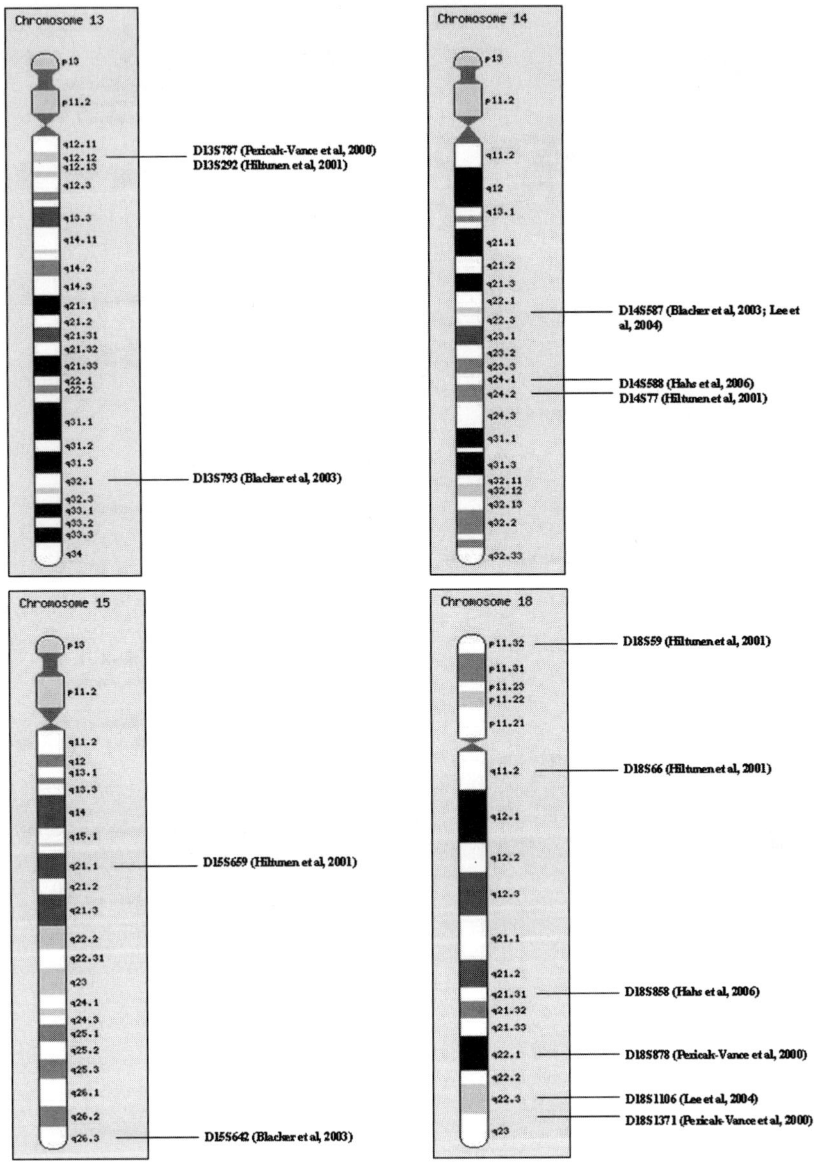

Fig. 1 (*continued*)

nonoverlapping (non-Kehoe) data sets separately, where the latter results can be seen as an independent assessment of the findings of Pericak-Vance and colleagues [116,120] and Myers and colleagues [126]. Despite these confounders, several chromosomal loci emerge as potential risk loci for AD.

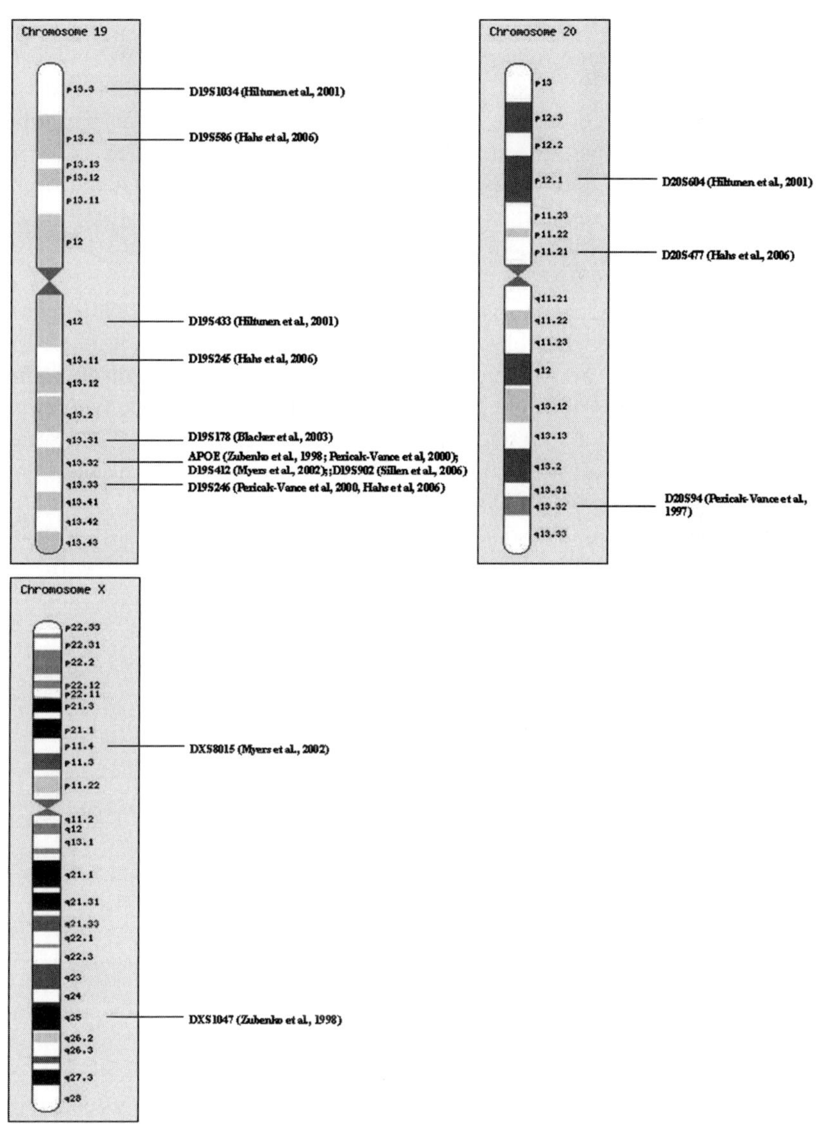

Fig. 1 (*continued*)

Chromosomal loci 1p31.1 [128,131,134], 2p24.1–23.2 [122,129], 3p14.1–2 [128,134], 3q27.2–28 [122,131,134], 4p13–15.1 [122,131,134], 4q31.3–32.1 [116,120,128,134], 4q34.3–35.2 [128,131,134], 13q12.12 [120,122], 14q22.2 [128,131], 14q24.1–2 [122,134], and 18q22.3–23 [120,131] have been implicated in at least two completely independent whole-genome linkage or association studies. Of the chromosomal loci with independent replication, those on chromosomes 6 (see Refs. [120,122,126,128,131]), 9 (see Refs. [120,126,128,129]), 10 (see Refs. [118,120,122,126,129,134]), and 12 [116,125,126] have received the greatest interest because of the large number of confirmatory studies, the strength of these results, and the existence of multiple strong candidate genes in these regions with positive association results from one or more studies.

Chromosome 6

Chromosome 6p21.2–12.3 [116,122,126,131] and 6q27 [120,128] regions have been implicated in whole-genome linkage and association studies. Initially, Pericak-Vance and colleagues [116] identified linkage to chromosome 6p21.2 and 6q15 in a follow-up analysis of 38 LOAD families, where evidence for linkage was also replicated for chromosomes 4, 12, and 20. In their larger subsequent analyses of 466 LOAD families, continued linkage signal was observed for the 6q27 region [120]. The chromosome 6p21.1–12.1 region showed significant association in a whole-genome association study from Finland [122]. Myers and colleagues [126], in a sample with "as much as 80%" overlap with Pericak-Vance and colleagues [120], also detected linkage to the chromosome 6p21.1–12.3 region in their *APOE* ε4+ sample. Their maximum multipoint LOD score is near marker D6S1017, which showed evidence of association in the Finnish association study [122]. Blacker and colleagues [128] confirmed the linkage in the 6p21 and 6q27 regions, which is perhaps not surprising, given their sample overlap with the two prior linkage studies [120,126]. Nonetheless, the D6S1017 marker also yielded a two-point LOD score of 1.2 in their non-Kehoe families, which do not overlap with the Myers and colleagues [126] study. Furthermore, this subset continued to have suggestive multipoint linkage to the 6q27 region. Finally, in a Caribbean-Hispanic series, evidence for linkage was identified to the chromosome 6p22.3 and 12.3 regions [131]. These studies provide independent evidence for the existence of two AD risk regions of interest on chromosome 6 on the p and q arms. A number of candidate genes have been analyzed in these regions, which are depicted graphically on the AlzGene website (http://www.alzforum.org/res/com/gen/alzgene/) [139] and reviewed previously [140,141]. In a recent meta-analysis of the available candidate gene studies compiled by the AlzGene database, tumor necrosis factor emerged as a promising candidate gene. The rs4647198 (–1031) SNP in a transcriptional regulatory site for tumor necrosis factor showed significant association with AD in a meta-analysis of three studies [139].

Chromosome 10

Several chromosome 10 regions were identified as candidate AD risk loci in numerous linkage and association studies (see Refs. [118,120,122,126,128,129,131,134]). Zubenko and colleagues [118] identified significant

AD association with D10S1423 on 10p12.33 in their 10 cM whole-genome scan of 100 AD cases and 100 controls. Chromosome 10p11.23, about 13 cM downstream of this region, showed suggestive linkage in 199 autopsy-confirmed LOAD families studied by Pericak-Vance and colleagues [120]. Two studies implicated the more upstream chromosome 10p region [122,128], whereas Farrer and colleagues [129] confirmed the findings in the 10p11.23 region. The 10p13 region implicated in the Finnish association study [122], 10p14 identified with linkage in early/mixed-onset non-Kehoe LOAD families [128], and the initial association region by Zubenko and colleagues [118] span about 17 cM on the short arm of chromosome 10. Whether this region and the more downstream 10p11.23 region identified independently in a United States–based linkage [120] and an inbred Arab-based association study [129] represent the same locus is not known as yet.

The most significant linkage evidence for chromosome 10 identified 10q21.3 as a potential AD risk region, with a maximum multipoint LOD score of 3.9 at about 82.2 cM, which is significant at the whole-genome level [126]. In this study by Myers and colleagues [126] of 451 affected sibpairs, the *APOE* ε4+ group yielded the strongest linkage signal. In an independent study of 10 extended LOAD families, using plasma Aβ42 levels as a quantitative phenotype, Ertekin-Taner and colleagues [142] found evidence of linkage to the same region on chromosome 10, with greatest evidence of linkage in those 5 extended LOAD families whose AD proband had extremely high plasma Aβ levels. This study was the first one in AD genetics to use a quantitative, biologically relevant phenotype for mapping an AD risk locus. Jointly, these two independent studies provided evidence for a novel AD risk locus on 10q21.3 that acts by way of the Aβ pathway [142,143]. The linkage peak in the Myers and colleagues [126] study covers a broad region (59 cM–103 cM). In a study of Amish pedigrees, Hahs and colleagues [134] found linkage to about 101 cM on 10q22.3. Similarly, Farrer and colleagues [129] found evidence of association in their inbred Arab sample to a number of chromosome 10 markers spanning 81 to 115 cM, with the greatest single marker association at 10q22.3 (97 cM) and four contiguous markers showing association between 105 and 115 cM. Not surprisingly, Blacker and colleagues [128] found linkage in their overlapping NIMH sample at 10q22 and 10q24, but not in the non-Kehoe sample. In another analysis of the same data set using a different set of markers, this group reported significant linkage and association at 115 to 127 cM near the insulin-degrading enzyme (*IDE*) gene [144]. Finally, using age at onset as a quantitative phenotype, Li and colleagues [124] identified linkage to 10q25.3 at 139 cM. These studies provide evidence for the existence of one or more AD risk loci on chromosome 10, some or all of which appear to affect Aβ levels and age at onset. According to the AlzGene website (www.alzgene.org), 69 candidate genes have been studied on chromosome 10 [139]. Some of these candidate gene studies are discussed briefly.

Chromosome 12

The first evidence of linkage to chromosome 12 came from Pericak-Vance and colleagues [116], who detected the strongest linkage signal with a maximum multipoint LOD score of 3.5 at 12p11.23 in their 54 LOAD families. The evidence for linkage was strongest in a subset of *APOE* ε4– families defined as those families with at least one patient who lacked the *APOE* ε4 allele. This group subsequently genotyped additional markers and reanalyzed the same data set, using different subgroups, by their *APOE* genotypes and underlying pathology [145]. Their analyses of all affected sibpairs confirmed the initial linkage findings about 12p11.23, although they identified a second, smaller peak about 18 cM more downstream at 12q13.13. When the analyses were weighted by *APOE* ε4– individuals, the peak linkage occurred at 12q13.2 and was significantly stronger than the *APOE* ε4+–weighted linkage. Furthermore, subset analyses of the 8 families with Lewy body pathology yielded stronger linkage than that in the remaining 46 families. The families with Lewy body pathology had linkage to the 12p region, whereas the other families linked to the 12q region. These results suggest the presence of one or more loci around the 30cM region encompassing the linkage peaks in the various subgroups at 12p and 12q. Myers and colleagues [126] found a suggestive linkage to chromosome 12 at 12p13.2, also with stronger results in the *APOE* ε4– subset. Finally, Rogaeva and colleagues [146] found the strongest evidence of linkage near marker D12S96 at 12q13.13, although their linkage region extended to 12p13.2, spanning about 42 cM region (according to the marker locations from the Marshfield map). An independent analysis of Caribbean-Hispanic LOAD families [125] found evidence of linkage at the 12p13.31 region and the more downstream 12p12.1 regions, close to the Myers and colleagues [126] and Pericak-Vance and colleagues [116] linkage regions, respectively. The evidence of linkage in this study was also stronger in the *APOE* ε4– subset. Two independent association studies also found significant results on chromosome 12 [118,129]; however, the loci identified in these reports were about 15 cM [129] to 93 cM [118] distal to the nearest linkage region.

Thus, similar to the findings on chromosomes 10 and 6, multiple potential LOAD risk regions have been identified on chromosome 12. More than 20 candidate genes have been analyzed on this chromosome, of which α2-macroglobulin mapping to 12p13.31 and low-density lipoprotein-like protein at 12q13.3 have received the greatest interest because of their potential involvement in the Aβ clearance pathway [147]. Both genes are excellent functional and positional candidates; however, their role as Aβ-susceptibility genes has not been established unequivocally because of inconsistent results from association studies [148]. Recently, LOAD association has been detected for glyceraldehyde-3 phosphate dehydrogenase variants in multiple series [149,150].

Chromosome 9

Although chromosome 9 has received interest because of the evidence of linkage or association from several studies [120,126,128,129], data sets assessed by three of these studies overlap [120,126,128] and they, therefore, cannot be considered providers of independent evidence of linkage. Chromosome 9 is therefore considered last in this section. In a whole-genome scan of 466 LOAD families, Pericak-Vance and colleagues [120] identified a region on chromosome 9p to have strong evidence for linkage with a multipoint LOD score of 2.97. The evidence was even stronger in the autopsy-confirmed subset of 199 families with a multipoint LOD score (4.31) even higher than that found in the *APOE* region on chromosome 19 (3.42). The autopsy-confirmed subset also had another downstream region on chromosome 9q with evidence of linkage. In the substantially overlapping data set analyzed by Myers and colleagues [126], evidence for linkage was identified to regions on 9p and 9q. The 9p linkage coincides with that in the Pericak-Vance and colleagues [120] study, although the 9q linkage findings for the two studies are about 46 cM apart. Blacker and colleagues [128] also identified two suggestive linkage peaks on 9p21.1 and 9q22.2 in their overall data set; however, they could not detect a suggestive signal in their nonoverlapping, non-Kehoe families. Finally, Farrer and colleagues [129], in an association analysis of an independent series of Arab case-controls, determined four markers on chromosome 9 spanning 32 to 47 cM (9p22.2–21.2) with significant LOAD association. Their most significant marker (AFM220XF2, $P = 2.3 \times 10^{-7}$) resides in a region coinciding with two other linkage signals [120,126] from overlapping data sets.

Several functional and positional candidate genes reside on chromosome 9, including death-associated protein kinase (*DAPK1*) [151], ATP binding cassette A1-2 transporters (*ABCA1-2*) [152,153], very low density lipoprotein receptor (*VLDLR*) [154], and ubiquilin 1 (*UBQLN1*) [155], with roles in apoptosis [151], lipid metabolism [152–154], and protein degradation [155]. Recent meta-analyses of genetic association studies on LOAD from the AlzGene database determined that variants in *DAPK1* showed significant association in a meta-analyses of three to six independent series [139] and also significantly altered expression of this gene [151].

Alternative analytic methods to detect risk loci for late-onset Alzheimer's disease

In addition to the nine whole-genome linkage or association analyses in predominantly nonoverlapping samples (See Refs. [116,118,120,122, 125,126,128,129,131,134,135]), seven linkage studies are presented here that used alternative analytic strategies to reassess the data in overlapping data sets (see Refs. [121,123,124,127,130,132,133]). The authors briefly discuss the approaches and results of these studies because they potentially bring new understanding and evidence to the LOAD risk loci. Curtis and colleagues [121] reanalyzed the NIMH families, which have significant overlap with the genome-wide scans by Kehoe and colleagues [119] and Myers and colleagues [126], using *APOE* genotypes as liability classes, thus introducing a novel method for simultaneous analysis of any loci conditional on a known risk locus. They were able to confirm the 10q21.3 linkage at D10S1211 and 12p13.2-1 at D12S358. Scott and colleagues [130] used the "ordered subsets analysis," developed by Hauser and colleagues [156], to identify subsets of families ordered by their age at onset; this study yielded stronger evidence of linkage to certain loci, compared with the analyses using the whole data set. This approach was applied to 437 families with complete age-at-onset information, from the original set of 466 families in the Pericak-Vance and colleagues [120] whole-genome screen. Two novel loci were detected at chromosomes 2q34 in EOAD (50–60 years) and 15q22 in very late-onset AD ($\geq$79 years), in addition to increasing the previously detected linkage signal at 9p from 3.0 to 4.6 (n = 334 families, 60–75 years). The chromosome 2q34 locus also showed evidence of linkage in Caribbean Hispanics [131], along with two other regions encompassing 2q34 detected in Amish families [134]. The 15q region is at least 17 cM away from the nearest risk region identified in another study [122].

Several groups included a number of variables as covariates in linkage analyses [127,132,133]. Olson and colleagues [127] studied 272 sibpairs from the NIMH Genetics Initiative with complete covariate information on age at onset, current age, and *APOE* genotype to determine the effects of these covariates on linkage. They were able to obtain stronger evidence of linkage to regions on chromosomes 5, 6, 9, and 21, previously identified in genome scans using the NIMH data [120,126]. In addition, they detected signals at chromosomes 14 and 20 in regions not previously identified by inclusion of covariates. The most significant evidence came from chromosomes 20p and 21p near the *APP* region, where linkage was strongest in the oldest age group lacking the *APOE* ε4 allele. The significant epistasis between these two regions suggested a biologic link. Avramopoulos and colleagues [132] found linkage to the chromosome 14q24 region near the *PSEN1* locus using the presence of psychotic features as a covariate in a subset of the NIMH sibpairs. Their strongest linkage was detected in earlier-onset AD families without comorbid hallucinations. Two other studies identified 14q24 as a risk region [122,134]. Recent meta-analyses of an intronic SNP in *PSEN1* was found to have a significant association with AD in 34 different studies. Given that a substantial number of these studies were conducted in LOAD case-control series, these results suggest a potential involvement of this established EOAD gene for LOAD as well [139]. Bacanu and colleagues [123] analyzed the subset of the NIMH families with psychotic symptoms and *APOE* ε4 allele and determined a linkage to chromosomes 2p, 6q, and 21q. These regions do not overlap with those from the Avramopoulos and colleagues [132] study. Although both studies showed linkage to 2p in LOAD with psychotic features, their locations are about 40 cM apart. Holmans and colleagues [133] analyzed the effects of multiple covariates, including age at onset, rate of decline, and *APOE*, on the linkage of LOAD series with major overlap with the Myers and colleagues [126] study. Their most significant finding was on chromosome 21 in the NIMH data set, where linkage was strongest in the sibpairs with high age at onset, thus confirming the results of Olson and colleagues [127]. Their approach led to improved linkage findings in several other chromosomal loci.

Quantitative trait analyses in LOAD were first performed by Ertekin-Taner and colleagues [142] using plasma Aβ levels as the phenotype, whereby evidence of linkage to chromosome 10 was determined in a locus overlapping that from the Myers and colleagues [126] study. Li and colleagues [124] used age at onset as a quantitative phenotype in AD and Parkinson's disease (PD) families. Their strongest evidence for linkage in AD families came from chromosome 10q at a locus greater than 50 cM downstream that of the Myers and colleagues [126] and Ertekin-Taner and colleagues [142] linkage.

These linkage studies, with alternative analytic approaches, have several important uses. They can

- Lead to identification of novel loci by reducing heterogeneity and increasing power
- Help confirm prior findings
- Identify the subset of individuals where effect of the risk locus is strongest, thus potentially help guide future mapping/association studies
- Bring some potential understanding to the pathophysiologic effects of the risk locus (eg, decreases age at onset, acts by way of the amyloid pathway, and so forth).

Candidate gene studies

To date, 968 association studies on 398 AD candidate genes have been done, according to the AlzGene database updated on February 8, 2007 (http://www.alzforum.org/res/com/gen/alzgene/) [139]. It is neither possible nor effectively informative to provide a thorough review of these studies. Instead, this section focuses on some general pitfalls and guidelines in the association studies for complex diseases, and highlights a few AD candidate genes as examples. The lack of a universally accepted genetic risk factor or factors for LOAD besides *APOE*, despite the substantial genetic component underlying this disorder and the large number of genes studied, is testimony, in part, to the complexity of the genetic underpinnings of AD and the inadequacy of some of the approaches used. Several reviews have highlighted potential reasons for the failure to identify the "next *APOE*" gene for AD [140,157–159]. These include (1) initial false-positive results followed by lack of replication; (2) lack of power because of small sample size (false-negatives); (3) lack of informative markers; (4) genetic heterogeneity (different sets of genes underlying the same AD phenotype); and (5) clinical heterogeneity (multiple clinical subtypes with different sets of susceptibility genes).

Although initial false-positive associations could account for some of the lack of replication in LOAD association studies, it is unlikely to account for all cases of failure to replicate. Lohmueller and colleagues [160] assessed 301 published studies on 25 single variant associations and determined a highly substantial excess of studies with significant replication of the original association results. They determined that, of the 301 follow-up studies to an original significant association, 59, 26, and 10 studies showed significant associations with *P* less than .05, less than 0.01, and less than 0.001, respectively. These numbers were significantly higher than the numbers of significant association studies expected by chance alone (15, 3, and <1, respectively). Ioannidis and colleagues [161] systematically assessed by meta-analysis 370 published studies on 36 genetic associations. Both studies concluded that the initial estimate of genetic effect size from the original positive association study tended to be inflated [160,161], with modest true effect sizes with ORs of 0.5 to 2.0, in most cases. Therefore, many association studies assessed by these investigators and also from the LOAD literature are sorely underpowered to detect true, but modest, effects. Two groups systematically analyzed AD association studies published within a given period of time [140,159]. Bertram and Tanzi [140] assessed 105 (38 positive, 67 negative) AD association studies published in 2003, whereas Blomqvist and colleagues [159] analyzed 138 (86 positive, 52 negative) articles published between January 2004 to April 2005. Both studies excluded reports on *APOE*. They both observed insufficient sample sizes. Blomqvist and colleagues [159] found that 59% of the studies (82/138) had less than 500 subjects, whereas Bertram and Tanzi [140] determined that about 20% of the studies had less than 200 individuals. Because sample sizes on the order of 1000 to 10,000 are often required to achieve power sufficient to detect the expected modest effect sizes for most complex disease susceptibility genes, many of the AD association studies are underpowered. A small sample size is not only problematic for the lack of power for follow-up studies, but also an important determinant for an initial false-positive association. An initial sample size of less than 150 was significantly less likely to be replicated, compared with larger studies, suggesting a higher false-positive rate for initial studies of smaller size [161].

Association of a disease with a genetic variant does not imply causation and may simply be caused by linkage dysequilibrium between the tested marker and an untested susceptibility variant. Furthermore, more than one susceptibility variant can be present in a single gene, acting in an additive or multiplicative fashion. These issues complicate association studies and could potentially lead to false-negative results caused by (1) a different extent of linkage dysequilibrium between the tested marker and the untested susceptibility variant among different populations or (2) incomplete assessment of the true susceptibility conferred by a genic region. To address these issues, choosing potentially functional variants (eg, missense SNPs, insertions/deletions, and variants in highly conserved regions) and assessing multiple variants and haplotypes have been advocated [140,162]. The two recent surveys of AD association studies have revealed that most (>60%) have been performed on a single variant [140,159] and less than 20% pursued haplotype analysis [140].

Genetic heterogeneity because of ethnic or environmental differences leading to false-negative results, and false-positive results secondary to population substructure, have been raised as potential problems affecting association studies [162], although their true impact on AD genetics is yet to be determined. Finally, the use of biologically relevant, quantitative phenotypes has been proposed as a means of overcoming potential clinical heterogeneity because such quantitative traits may (1) be a less heterogeneous and more direct correlate for the genetic variation or variations; (2) be less prone to the imprecisions of a clinical phenotype; (3) be amenable to inclusion of subjects with preclinical disease; and (4) allow for downstream functional testing of putative susceptibility variants [157,159,162]. More recently, the use of quantitative traits such as Aβ levels, mini-mental state examination scores, cerebrospinal fluid (CSF) tau levels, age at onset, pathologic disease burden, and CSF cholesterol levels [163–167] have emerged as novel approaches for studying candidate AD genes.

Despite the pitfalls and shortcomings of association studies of AD, a recent meta-analysis of 127 polymorphisms in 69 AD candidate genes identified 20 polymorphisms in 13 genes (other than *APOE* and related genes) with significant results [139]. The effects of these variants were modest, with average ORs of 0.82 to 1.25. Additionally, several recent reports on AD candidate genes have applied many of the suggested guidelines for complex disease association studies and found significant results [163–166,168–171]. Although the role of these genes for AD remains to be established with further confirmatory studies, and despite the presence of negative results, these findings are encouraging.

Chromosome 10 has been an area of great interest in AD because of the convergence of multiple linkage and association signals and the presence of multiple excellent positional and functional candidate genes. The authors thus give examples of several AD candidate gene association studies from this chromosome, highlighting study designs and briefly summarizing the conclusions.

Ertekin-Taner and colleagues [163] analyzed alpha-T-catenin (*VR22*) as a candidate gene on chromosome 10 because of its location and indirect interaction with *PSEN1* by way of β-catenin. They identified two intronic SNPs that showed an association with plasma Aβ42 levels in two independent sets of families, showed that these SNPs accounted for their plasma Aβ linkage on chromosome 10, and bounded the association within the large *VR22* gene by analyzing an additional 49 SNPs within and around this gene, none of which showed as strong an association. The strengths of this study were the use of a quantitative phenotype, multiple variants, internal replication, bounding of the association within a gene, and assessment of linkage conditional on association. Subsequently, three affirmative [172–174] and four negative [168,170,175,176] association studies were published on this genic region.

In 2003, Prince and colleagues [166] identified a haplotype block spanning *IDE*, which showed a significant association with AD or its quantitative traits (mini-mental state examination scores, CSF tau levels, age at onset) in an analysis of five independent case-control series. The strengths of this study were the use of multiple variants, haplotype analysis, multiple independent series from different populations, and clinical and quantitative phenotypes. Assessing the same haplotypes in two case-control and one family series, Ertekin-Taner and colleagues [164] found evidence of an association with AD and plasma Aβ42 levels, with directions of effect similar to those from the Prince and colleagues [166] study. Sixteen additional association studies exist on the *IDE* gene, with five confirmatory reports, all of which are summarized on the AlzGene website [139].

Li and colleagues [169] screened 22,000 genes by an expression assay and identified 52 genes with significant expression difference between ADs and controls, 4 of which resided on chromosome 10. They assessed these candidate genes in their AD and PD series and determined variants in glutathione S-transferase omega-1 and -2 genes (*GSTO1*, *GSTO2*) to be associated significantly with age at onset of AD and PD. They subsequently determined that this association contributed significantly to their linkage results on chromosome 10 [177]. The main strength of this study is the selection of candidate genes based on a functional screen, in addition to the use of multiple markers, multiple series, quantitative phenotypes, and assessing the effect of association on linkage. Of the four follow-up studies on *GSTO1–2*, two show a positive trend [139].

In their exploratory series, Grupe and colleagues [168] genotyped about 1400 gene-based SNPs in the chromosome 10q region to identify 69 with significant association. Of these, one SNP in *LOC439999* showed significant association in four of their six case-control series. The strengths of this study were the use of a high-throughput screening strategy to survey many genes in a nonhypothesis-driven fashion and the presence of internal replication using more than 1000 cases and controls. Their association did not account for the linkage on chromosome 10. Only two negative follow-up studies exist for this association to date [139]. Using a similar screening approach, with 1206 chromosome 10 SNPs in a Japanese case-control series with no *APOE* ε4 allele, Kuwano and colleagues [170] identified six SNPs in a two-stage association study, three of which resided in the dynamin-binding protein gene (*DNMBP*). The strengths of this study are similar to those of Grupe and colleagues [168]. Kuwano and colleagues [170] also determined decreased expression levels for *DNMBP* in the AD, compared with control, brains, thus providing some functional correlate for this gene.

Finally, although not on chromosome 10, recent findings on neuronal sortilin-related receptor (*SORL1*) on chromosome 11 are discussed briefly [171] to highlight the study approach and challenges of complex disease association studies. Rogaeva and colleagues [171] assessed SNPs in several genes from the vacuolar protein sorting family and identified *SORL1* as a candidate for further analyses. Using a two-stage approach with a total of six series from different ethnic groups, with two family-based series in the exploratory set and four combined case-control and family series in the replication set, they assessed *SORL1* variants in more than 1500 cases and controls. In addition, they analyzed three more independent series of 1405 ADs and 2124 controls. The investigators found a significant association with *SORL1* variants in multiple independent data sets, although no single variant had significant association across all data sets. Considerable functional data demonstrated reduced expression of *SORL1* in subjects who were carriers of a *SORL1* risk haplotype. Finally, the investigators showed experimental results depicting the role of *SORL1* in differential sorting of the APP holoprotein. The strengths of this study are the use of many independent series of family and case-control types, with multiple different ethnic groups, the hypothesis-driven assessment of candidate genes in a specific pathway, the multiple single-SNP and haplotype variants assessed, and the presence of expression data in support of the association findings.

Summary

Alzheimer's disease is one of the most challenging disorders of the century because of its personal and public impact. Discovering the underlying genetics of this common, complex disorder harbors the hope for its early detection, prevention, and treatment. With the identification of exceedingly rare, early-onset, autosomal dominant, familial Alzheimer's disease gene mutations over the past 2 decades, substantial progress has been made in understanding the disease pathophysiology. The most common, late-onset form of Alzheimer's disease has a substantial genetic component that remains unexplained, despite the identification of the susceptibility allele *APOE* ε4. Evidence from whole-genome linkage, association, and candidate gene studies strongly implicate multiple different genetic loci responsible for susceptibility to Alzheimer's disease. The ever-growing number of variants in the human genome with systematic cataloguing efforts, development of high-throughput genotyping and phenotyping assays, generation of well-characterized and large study series, and advent of novel analytic strategies will provide the tools essential for studying Alzheimer's disease genetics. Although significant progress is as yet lacking in this area, recent studies hold promise for illuminating important genetic aspects of this multifaceted disorder.

References

[1] Mayeux R. Epidemiology of neurodegeneration. Annu Rev Neurosci 2003;26:81–104.

[2] Rice DP, Fillit HM, Max W, et al. Prevalence, costs, and treatment of Alzheimer's disease and related dementia: a managed care perspective. Am J Manag Care 2001;7(8):809–18.

[3] Brookmeyer R, Gray S, Kawas C. Projections of Alzheimer's disease in the United States and the public health impact of delaying disease onset. Am J Public Health 1998;88(9): 1337–42.
[4] Borenstein AR, Copenhaver CI, Mortimer JA. Early-life risk factors for Alzheimer disease. Alzheimer Dis Assoc Disord 2006;20(1):63–72.
[5] Whalley LJ, Dick FD, McNeill G. A life-course approach to the aetiology of late-onset dementias. Lancet Neurol 2006;5(1):87–96.
[6] Lazarov O, Robinson J, Tang YP, et al. Environmental enrichment reduces Abeta levels and amyloid deposition in transgenic mice. Cell 2005;120(5):701–13.
[7] Jankowsky JL, Melnikova T, Fadale DJ, et al. Environmental enrichment mitigates cognitive deficits in a mouse model of Alzheimer's disease. J Neurosci 2005;25(21):5217–24.
[8] Alzheimer A. A new disease of the cortex (Ger). Allgemeine Zeitschrift für Psychiatrie und psychisch-gerichtliche Medizin 1907;64:146–8.
[9] Harris R. Genetics of Alzheimer's disease. Br Med J (Clin Res Ed) 1982;284(6322):1065–6.
[10] Breitner JC, Silverman JM, Mohs RC, et al. Familial aggregation in Alzheimer's disease: comparison of risk among relatives of early-and late-onset cases, and among male and female relatives in successive generations. Neurology 1988;38(2):207–12.
[11] Farrer LA, Myers RH, Cupples LA, et al. Transmission and age-at-onset patterns in familial Alzheimer's disease: evidence for heterogeneity. Neurology 1990;40(3 Pt 1):395–403.
[12] Lautenschlager NT, Cupples LA, Rao VS, et al. Risk of dementia among relatives of Alzheimer's disease patients in the MIRAGE study: what is in store for the oldest old? Neurology 1996;46(3):641–50.
[13] Green RC, Cupples LA, Go R, et al. Risk of dementia among white and African American relatives of patients with Alzheimer disease. JAMA 2002;287(3):329–36.
[14] Farrer LA, Cupples LA, van Duijn CM, et al. Apolipoprotein E genotype in patients with Alzheimer's disease: implications for the risk of dementia among relatives. Ann Neurol 1995;38(5):797–808.
[15] Martinez M, Campion D, Brice A, et al. Apolipoprotein E epsilon4 allele and familial aggregation of Alzheimer disease. Arch Neurol 1998;55(6):810–6.
[16] Devi G, Ottman R, Tang M, et al. Influence of APOE genotype on familial aggregation of AD in an urban population. Neurology 1999;53(4):789–94.
[17] Farrer LA, Myers RH, Connor L, et al. Segregation analysis reveals evidence of a major gene for Alzheimer disease. Am J Hum Genet 1991;48(6):1026–33.
[18] van Duijn CM, Farrer LA, Cupples LA, et al. Genetic transmission of Alzheimer's disease among families in a Dutch population based study. J Med Genet 1993;30(8):640–6.
[19] Rao VS, van Duijn CM, Connor-Lacke L, et al. Multiple etiologies for Alzheimer disease are revealed by segregation analysis. Am J Hum Genet 1994;55(5):991–1000.
[20] Warwick Daw E, Payami H, Nemens EJ, et al. The number of trait loci in late-onset Alzheimer disease. Am J Hum Genet 2000;66(1):196–204.
[21] Raiha I, Kaprio J, Koskenvuo M, et al. Alzheimer's disease in Finnish twins. Lancet 1996; 347(9001):573–8.
[22] Bergem AL, Engedal K, Kringlen E. The role of heredity in late-onset Alzheimer disease and vascular dementia. A twin study. Arch Gen Psychiatry 1997;54(3):264–70.
[23] Gatz M, Reynolds CA, Fratiglioni L, et al. Role of genes and environments for explaining Alzheimer disease. Arch Gen Psychiatry 2006;63(2):168–74.
[24] Breitner JC, Gatz M, Bergem AL, et al. Use of twin cohorts for research in Alzheimer's disease. Neurology 1993;43(2):261–7.
[25] Raiha I, Kaprio J, Koskenvuo M, et al. Alzheimer's disease in twins. Biomed Pharmacother 1997;51(3):101–4.
[26] Steffens DC, Plassman BL, Helms MJ, et al. APOE and AD concordance in twin pairs as predictors of AD in first-degree relatives. Neurology 2000;54(3):593–8.
[27] Bergem AL, Lannfelt L. Apolipoprotein E type epsilon4 allele, heritability and age at onset in twins with Alzheimer disease and vascular dementia. Clin Genet 1997;52(5):408–13.

[28] Goate A, Chartier-Harlin MC, Mullan M, et al. Segregation of a missense mutation in the amyloid precursor protein gene with familial Alzheimer's disease. Nature 1991;349(6311): 704–6.

[29] Fraser J, Mitchell A. Kalmuc idiocy: report of a case with autopsy, with notes on sixty-two cases. J Ment Sci 1876;22:161–79.

[30] Struwe F. Histopathologische Untersuchungen uber Entstehung und Wesen der senilen Plaques. Z Neurol Psychiatrie 1929;122:291–307.

[31] Jervis G. Early senile dementia in mongoloid idiocy. Am J Psychiatry 1948;105:102–6.

[32] Pary RJ, Rajendran G, Stonecipher A. Overview of Alzheimer's disease in Down syndrome. In: Prasher VP, editor. Down syndrome and Alzheimer's disease biological correlates. Oxen, UK: Radcliffe Publishing; 2006. p. 2–13.

[33] Glenner GG, Wong CW. Alzheimer's disease and Down's syndrome: sharing of a unique cerebrovascular amyloid fibril protein. Biochem Biophys Res Commun 1984;122(3): 1131–5.

[34] Masters CL, Simms G, Weinman NA, et al. Amyloid plaque core protein in Alzheimer disease and Down syndrome. Proc Natl Acad Sci U S A 1985;82(12):4245–9.

[35] St George-Hyslop PH, Tanzi RE, Polinsky RJ, et al. The genetic defect causing familial Alzheimer's disease maps on chromosome 21. Science 1987;235(4791):885–90.

[36] Goldgaber D, Lerman MI, McBride OW, et al. Characterization and chromosomal localization of a cDNA encoding brain amyloid of Alzheimer's disease. Science 1987;235(4791): 877–80.

[37] Tanzi RE, Gusella JF, Watkins PC, et al. Amyloid beta protein gene: cDNA, mRNA distribution, and genetic linkage near the Alzheimer locus. Science 1987;235(4791): 880–4.

[38] Tanzi RE, St George-Hyslop PH, Haines JL, et al. The genetic defect in familial Alzheimer's disease is not tightly linked to the amyloid beta-protein gene. Nature 1987; 329(6135):156–7.

[39] Van Broeckhoven C, Genthe AM, Vandenberghe A, et al. Failure of familial Alzheimer's disease to segregate with the A4-amyloid gene in several European families. Nature 1987; 329(6135):153–5.

[40] Schellenberg GD, Bird TD, Wijsman EM, et al. Absence of linkage of chromosome 21q21 markers to familial Alzheimer's disease. Science 1988;241(4872):1507–10.

[41] Goate AM, Haynes AR, Owen MJ, et al. Predisposing locus for Alzheimer's disease on chromosome 21. Lancet 1989;1(8634):352–5.

[42] Theuns J, Marjaux E, Vandenbulcke M, et al. Alzheimer dementia caused by a novel mutation located in the APP C-terminal intracytosolic fragment. Hum Mutat 2006;27(9): 888–96.

[43] Schellenberg GD, Bird TD, Wijsman EM, et al. Genetic linkage evidence for a familial Alzheimer's disease locus on chromosome 14. Science 1992;258(5082):668–71.

[44] Mullan M, Houlden H, Windelspecht M, et al. A locus for familial early-onset Alzheimer's disease on the long arm of chromosome 14, proximal to the alpha 1-antichymotrypsin gene. Nat Genet 1992;2(4):340–2.

[45] St George-Hyslop P, Haines J, Rogaev E, et al. Genetic evidence for a novel familial Alzheimer's disease locus on chromosome 14. Nat Genet 1992;2(4):330–4.

[46] Van Broeckhoven C, Backhovens H, Cruts M, et al. Mapping of a gene predisposing to early-onset Alzheimer's disease to chromosome 14q24.3. Nat Genet 1992;2(4):335–9.

[47] Sherrington R, Rogaev EI, Liang Y, et al. Cloning of a gene bearing missense mutations in early-onset familial Alzheimer's disease. Nature 1995;375(6534):754–60.

[48] Alzheimer's Disease Collaborative Group. The structure of the presenilin 1 (S182) gene and identification of six novel mutations in early onset AD families. Nat Genet 1995;11(2): 219–22.

[49] Hutton M, Busfield F, Wragg M, et al. Complete analysis of the presenilin 1 gene in early onset Alzheimer's disease. Neuroreport 1996;7(3):801–5.

[50] Cruts M, Van Broeckhoven C. Presenilin mutations in Alzheimer's disease. Hum Mutat 1998;11(3):183–90.
[51] Levy-Lahad E, Wijsman EM, Nemens E, et al. A familial Alzheimer's disease locus on chromosome 1. Science 1995;269(5226):970–3.
[52] Levy-Lahad E, Wasco W, Poorkaj P, et al. Candidate gene for the chromosome 1 familial Alzheimer's disease locus. Science 1995;269(5226):973–7.
[53] Rogaev EI, Sherrington R, Rogaeva EA, et al. Familial Alzheimer's disease in kindreds with missense mutations in a gene on chromosome 1 related to the Alzheimer's disease type 3 gene. Nature 1995;376:775–8.
[54] Sherrington R, Froelich S, Sorbi S, et al. Alzheimer's disease associated with mutations in presenilin 2 is rare and variably penetrant. Hum Mol Genet 1996;5(7):985–8.
[55] Finckh U, Kuschel C, Anagnostouli M, et al. Novel mutations and repeated findings of mutations in familial Alzheimer disease. Neurogenetics 2005;6(2):85–9.
[56] Campion D, Dumanchin C, Hannequin D, et al. Early-onset autosomal dominant Alzheimer disease: prevalence, genetic heterogeneity, and mutation spectrum. Am J Hum Genet 1999;65(3):664–70.
[57] Schoenberg BS, Anderson DW, Haerer AF. Severe dementia. Prevalence and clinical features in a biracial US population. Arch Neurol 1985;42(8):740–3.
[58] Sulkava R, Wikstrom J, Aromaa A, et al. Prevalence of severe dementia in Finland. Neurology 1985;35(7):1025–9.
[59] Kokmen E, Beard CM, Offord KP, et al. Prevalence of medically diagnosed dementia in a defined United States population: Rochester, Minnesota, January 1, 1975. Neurology 1989;39(6):773–6.
[60] Croes EA, Dermaut B, van Der Cammen TJ, et al. Genetic testing should not be advocated as a diagnostic tool in familial forms of dementia. Am J Hum Genet 2000;67(4): 1033–5.
[61] Cruts M, van Duijn CM, Backhovens H, et al. Estimation of the genetic contribution of presenilin-1 and -2 mutations in a population-based study of presenile Alzheimer disease. Hum Mol Genet 1998;7(1):43–51.
[62] Janssen JC, Beck JA, Campbell TA, et al. Early onset familial Alzheimer's disease: mutation frequency in 31 families. Neurology 2003;60(2):235–9.
[63] Nussbaum RL, Ellis CE. Alzheimer's disease and Parkinson's disease. N Engl J Med 2003; 348(14):1356–64.
[64] Sleegers K, Roks G, Theuns J, et al. Familial clustering and genetic risk for dementia in a genetically isolated Dutch population. Brain 2004;127(Pt 7):1641–9.
[65] Jimenez-Escrig A, Gomez-Tortosa E, Baron M, et al. A multigenerational pedigree of late-onset Alzheimer's disease implies new genetic causes. Brain 2005;128(Pt 7):1707–15.
[66] Giedraitis V, Hedlund M, Skoglund L, et al. New Alzheimer's disease locus on chromosome 8. J Med Genet 2006;43(12):931–5.
[67] Ashley-Koch AE, Shao Y, Rimmler JB, et al. An autosomal genomic screen for dementia in an extended Amish family. Neurosci Lett 2005;379(3):199–204.
[68] Rademakers R, Cruts M, Sleegers K, et al. Linkage and association studies identify a novel locus for Alzheimer disease at 7q36 in a Dutch population-based sample. Am J Hum Genet 2005;77(4):643–52.
[69] Sinha S, Anderson JP, Barbour R, et al. Purification and cloning of amyloid precursor protein beta-secretase from human brain. Nature 1999;402(6761):537–40.
[70] Vassar R, Bennett BD, Babu-Khan S, et al. Beta-secretase cleavage of Alzheimer's amyloid precursor protein by the transmembrane aspartic protease BACE. Science 1999;286(5440): 735–41.
[71] Yan R, Bienkowski MJ, Shuck ME, et al. Membrane-anchored aspartyl protease with Alzheimer's disease beta-secretase activity. Nature 1999;402(402):533–7.
[72] Vassar R, Citron M. Abeta-generating enzymes: recent advances in beta- and gamma-secretase research. Neuron 2000;27(3):419–22.

[73] Lammich S, Kojro E, Postina R, et al. Constitutive and regulated alpha-secretase cleavage of Alzheimer's amyloid precursor protein by a disintegrin metalloprotease. Proc Natl Acad Sci U S A 1999;96(7):3922–7.

[74] Hardy J. Amyloid, the presenilins and Alzheimer's disease. Trends Neurosci 1997;20(4): 154–9.

[75] Scheuner D, Eckman C, Jensen M, et al. Secreted amyloid beta-protein similar to that in the senile plaques of Alzheimer's disease is increased in vivo by the presenilin 1 and 2 and *APP* mutations linked to familial Alzheimer's disease. Nat Med 1996;2(8):864–70.

[76] Citron M, Oltersdorf T, Haass C, et al. Mutation of the beta-amyloid precursor protein in familial Alzheimer's disease increases beta-protein production. Nature 1992;360(6405): 672–4.

[77] Suzuki N, Cheung TT, Cai XD, et al. An increased percentage of long amyloid beta protein secreted by familial amyloid beta protein precursor (beta APP717) mutants. Science 1994; 264(5163):1336–40.

[78] Borchelt DR, Thinakaran G, Eckman CB, et al. Familial Alzheimer's disease-linked presenilin 1 variants elevate Abeta1–42/1–40 ratio in vitro and in vivo. Neuron 1996;17(5): 1005–13.

[79] Eckman CB, Mehta ND, Crook R, et al. A new pathogenic mutation in the *APP* gene (I716V) increases the relative proportion of A beta 42(43). Hum Mol Genet 1997;6(12): 2087–9.

[80] Hsiao K, Chapman P, Nilsen S, et al. Correlative memory deficits, Abeta elevation, and amyloid plaques in transgenic mice. Science 1996;274(5284):99–102.

[81] Duff K, Eckman C, Zehr C, et al. Increased amyloid-beta42(43) in brains of mice expressing mutant presenilin1. Nature 1996;383(6602):710–3.

[82] Zhang Z, Nadeau P, Song W, et al. Presenilins are required for gamma-secretase cleavage of beta-APP and transmembrane cleavage of Notch-1. Nat Cell Biol 2000;2(7):463–5.

[83] Golde TE, Younkin SG. Presenilins as therapeutic targets for the treatment of Alzheimer's disease. Trends Mol Med 2001;7(6):264–9.

[84] Lansbury PT, Lashuel HA. A century-old debate on protein aggregation and neurodegeneration enters the clinic. Nature 2006;443(7113):774–9.

[85] Klafki HW, Staufenbiel M, Kornhuber J, et al. Therapeutic approaches to Alzheimer's disease. Brain 2006;129(Pt 11):2840–55.

[86] Masters CL, Beyreuther K. Alzheimer's centennial legacy: prospects for rational therapeutic intervention targeting the Abeta amyloid pathway. Brain 2006;129(Pt 11):2823–39.

[87] Pericak-Vance MA, Yamaoka LH, Haynes CS, et al. Genetic linkage studies in Alzheimer's disease families. Exp Neurol 1988;102(3):271–9.

[88] Pericak-Vance MA, Bebout JL, Gaskell PC, et al. Linkage studies in familial Alzheimer disease: evidence for chromosome 19 linkage. Am J Hum Genet 1991;48(6):1034–50.

[89] Schellenberg GD, Deeb SS, Boehnke M, et al. Association of an apolipoprotein CII allele with familial dementia of the Alzheimer type. J Neurogenet 1987;4(2–3):97–108.

[90] Namba Y, Tomonaga M, Kawasaki H, et al. Apolipoprotein E immunoreactivity in cerebral amyloid deposits and neurofibrillary tangles in Alzheimer's disease and kuru plaque amyloid in Creutzfeldt-Jakob disease. Brain Res 1991;541(1):163–6.

[91] Strittmatter WJ, Saunders AM, Schmechel D, et al. Apolipoprotein E: high-avidity binding to beta-amyloid and increased frequency of type 4 allele in late-onset familial Alzheimer disease. Proc Natl Acad Sci U S A 1993;90(5):1977–81.

[92] Corder EH, Saunders AM, Strittmatter WJ, et al. Gene dose of apolipoprotein E type 4 allele and the risk of Alzheimer's disease in late onset families. Science 1993;261(5123):921–3.

[93] Myers RH, Schaefer EJ, Wilson PW, et al. Apolipoprotein E epsilon4 association with dementia in a population-based study: the Framingham study. Neurology 1996;46(3):673–7.

[94] Farrer LA, Cupples LA, Haines JL, et al. Effects of age, sex, and ethnicity on the association between apolipoprotein E genotype and Alzheimer disease. A meta-analysis. APOE and Alzheimer Disease Meta Analysis Consortium. JAMA 1997;278(16):1349–56.

[95] Bickeboller H, Campion D, Brice A, et al. Apolipoprotein E and Alzheimer disease: genotype-specific risks by age and sex. Am J Hum Genet 1997;60(2):439–46.
[96] Slooter AJ, Cruts M, Kalmijn S, et al. Risk estimates of dementia by apolipoprotein E genotypes from a population-based incidence study: the Rotterdam Study. Arch Neurol 1998; 55(7):964–8.
[97] Tang MX, Stern Y, Marder K, et al. The APOE-epsilon4 allele and the risk of Alzheimer disease among African Americans, whites, and Hispanics. JAMA 1998;279(10):751–5.
[98] Breitner JC, Wyse BW, Anthony JC, et al. APOE-epsilon4 count predicts age when prevalence of AD increases, then declines: the Cache County Study. Neurology 1999;53(2): 321–31.
[99] Graff-Radford NR, Green RC, Go RC, et al. Association between apolipoprotein E genotype and Alzheimer disease in African American subjects. Arch Neurol 2002;59(4):594–600.
[100] Evans DA, Bennett DA, Wilson RS, et al. Incidence of Alzheimer disease in a biracial urban community: relation to apolipoprotein E allele status. Arch Neurol 2003;60(2):185–9.
[101] Murrell JR, Price B, Lane KA, et al. Association of apolipoprotein E genotype and Alzheimer disease in African Americans. Arch Neurol 2006;63(3):431–4.
[102] Hendrie HC, Murrell J, Gao S, et al. International studies in dementia with particular emphasis on populations of African origin. Alzheimer Dis Assoc Disord 2006;20(3 Suppl 2): S42–6.
[103] Gureje O, Ogunniyi A, Baiyewu O, et al. APOE epsilon4 is not associated with Alzheimer's disease in elderly Nigerians. Ann Neurol 2006;59(1):182–5.
[104] Romas SN, Santana V, Williamson J, et al. Familial Alzheimer disease among Caribbean Hispanics: a reexamination of its association with APOE. Arch Neurol 2002;59(1):87–91.
[105] Olarte L, Schupf N, Lee JH, et al. Apolipoprotein E epsilon4 and age at onset of sporadic and familial Alzheimer disease in Caribbean Hispanics. Arch Neurol 2006;63(11):1586–90.
[106] Arboleda GH, Yunis JJ, Pardo R, et al. Apolipoprotein E genotyping in a sample of Colombian patients with Alzheimer's disease. Neurosci Lett 2001;305(2):135–8.
[107] Mayeux R, Saunders AM, Shea S, et al. Utility of the apolipoprotein E genotype in the diagnosis of Alzheimer's disease. Alzheimer's Disease Centers Consortium on apolipoprotein E and Alzheimer's disease. N Engl J Med 1998;338(8):506–11.
[108] Tsuang D, Larson EB, Bowen J, et al. The utility of apolipoprotein E genotyping in the diagnosis of Alzheimer disease in a community-based case series. Arch Neurol 1999;56(12): 1489–95.
[109] Waldemar G, Dubois B, Emre M, et al. Recommendations for the diagnosis and management of Alzheimer's disease and other disorders associated with dementia: EFNS guideline. Eur J Neurol 2007;14(1):E1–26.
[110] Petersen RC, Smith GE, Ivnik RJ, et al. Apolipoprotein E status as a predictor of the development of Alzheimer's disease in memory-impaired individuals. JAMA 1995;273(16): 1274–8.
[111] Hsiung GY, Sadovnick AD, Feldman H. Apolipoprotein E epsilon4 genotype as a risk factor for cognitive decline and dementia: data from the Canadian Study of Health and Aging. CMAJ 2004;171(8):863–7.
[112] Devanand DP, Pelton GH, Zamora D, et al. Predictive utility of apolipoprotein E genotype for Alzheimer disease in outpatients with mild cognitive impairment. Arch Neurol 2005; 62(6):975–80.
[113] Tschanz JT, Welsh-Bohmer KA, Lyketsos CG, et al. Conversion to dementia from mild cognitive disorder: the Cache County Study. Neurology 2006;67(2):229–34.
[114] Cervilla J, Prince M, Joels S, et al. Premorbid cognitive testing predicts the onset of dementia and Alzheimer's disease better than and independently of APOE genotype. J Neurol Neurosurg Psychiatry 2004;75(8):1100–6.
[115] Lee DY, Youn JC, Choo IH, et al. Combination of clinical and neuropsychologic information as a better predictor of the progression to Alzheimer disease in questionable dementia individuals. Am J Geriatr Psychiatry 2006;14(2):130–8.

[116] Pericak-Vance MA, Bass MP, Yamaoka LH, et al. Complete genomic screen in late-onset familial Alzheimer disease. Evidence for a new locus on chromosome 12. JAMA 1997; 278(15):1237–41.

[117] Pericak-Vance MA, Bass ML, Yamaoka LH, et al. Complete genomic screen in late-onset familial Alzheimer's disease. Neurobiol Aging 1998;19(Suppl 1):S39–42.

[118] Zubenko GS, Hughes HB, Stiffler JS, et al. A genome survey for novel Alzheimer disease risk loci: results at 10-cM resolution. Genomics 1998;50(2):121–8.

[119] Kehoe P, Wavrant-De Vrieze F, Crook R, et al. A full genome scan for late onset Alzheimer's disease. Hum Mol Genet 1999;8(2):237–45.

[120] Pericak-Vance MA, Grubber J, Bailey LR, et al. Identification of novel genes in late-onset Alzheimer's disease. Exp Gerontol 2000;35(9–10):1343–52.

[121] Curtis D, North BV, Sham PC. A novel method of two-locus linkage analysis applied to a genome scan for late onset Alzheimer's disease. Ann Hum Genet 2001;65(Pt 5):473–81.

[122] Hiltunen M, Mannermaa A, Thompson D, et al. Genome-wide linkage disequilibrium mapping of late-onset Alzheimer's disease in Finland. Neurology 2001;57(9):1663–8.

[123] Bacanu SA, Devlin B, Chowdari KV, et al. Linkage analysis of Alzheimer disease with psychosis. Neurology 2002;59(1):118–20.

[124] Li YJ, Scott WK, Hedges DJ, et al. Age at onset in two common neurodegenerative diseases is genetically controlled. Am J Hum Genet 2002;70(4):985–93.

[125] Mayeux R, Lee JH, Romas SN, et al. Chromosome-12 mapping of late-onset Alzheimer disease among Caribbean Hispanics. Am J Hum Genet 2002;70(1):237–43.

[126] Myers A, Wavrant De-Vrieze F, Holmans P, et al. Full genome screen for Alzheimer disease: stage II analysis. Am J Med Genet 2002;114(2):235–44.

[127] Olson JM, Goddard KA, Dudek DM. A second locus for very-late-onset Alzheimer disease: a genome scan reveals linkage to 20p and epistasis between 20p and the amyloid precursor protein region. Am J Hum Genet 2002;71(1):154–61.

[128] Blacker D, Bertram L, Saunders AJ, et al. Results of a high-resolution genome screen of 437 Alzheimer's disease families. Hum Mol Genet 2003;12(1):23–32.

[129] Farrer LA, Bowirrat A, Friedland RP, et al. Identification of multiple loci for Alzheimer disease in a consanguineous Israeli-Arab community. Hum Mol Genet 2003;12(4):415–22.

[130] Scott WK, Hauser ER, Schmechel DE, et al. Ordered-subsets linkage analysis detects novel Alzheimer disease loci on chromosomes 2q34 and 15q22. Am J Hum Genet 2003;73(5): 1041–51.

[131] Lee JH, Mayeux R, Mayo D, et al. Fine mapping of 10q and 18q for familial Alzheimer's disease in Caribbean Hispanics. Mol Psychiatry 2004;9(11):1042–51.

[132] Avramopoulos D, Fallin MD, Bassett SS. Linkage to chromosome 14q in Alzheimer's disease (AD) patients without psychotic symptoms. Am J Med Genet B Neuropsychiatr Genet 2005;132(1):9–13.

[133] Holmans P, Hamshere M, Hollingworth P, et al. Genome screen for loci influencing age at onset and rate of decline in late onset Alzheimer's disease. Am J Med Genet B Neuropsychiatr Genet 2005;135(1):24–32.

[134] Hahs DW, McCauley JL, Crunk AE, et al. A genome-wide linkage analysis of dementia in the Amish. Am J Med Genet B Neuropsychiatr Genet 2006;141(2):160–6.

[135] Sillen A, Forsell C, Lilius L, et al. Genome scan on Swedish Alzheimer's disease families. Mol Psychiatry 2006;11(2):182–6.

[136] Hiltunen M, Mannermaa A, Koivisto AM, et al. Linkage disequilibrium in the 13q12 region in Finnish late onset Alzheimer's disease patients. Eur J Hum Genet 1999;7(6):652–8.

[137] Hubbard TJ, Aken BL, Beal K, et al. Ensembl 2007. Nucleic Acids Res 2007;35(Database issue):D610–7.

[138] Kent WJ, Sugnet CW, Furey TS, et al. The human genome browser at UCSC. Genome Res 2002;12(6):996–1006.

[139] Bertram L, McQueen MB, Mullin K, et al. Systematic meta-analyses of Alzheimer disease genetic association studies: the AlzGene database. Nat Genet 2007;39(1):17–23.

[140] Bertram L, Tanzi RE. Alzheimer's disease: one disorder, too many genes? Hum Mol Genet 2004;13(Spec No 1):R135–41.
[141] Kamboh MI. Molecular genetics of late-onset Alzheimer's disease. Ann Hum Genet 2004; 68(Pt 4):381–404.
[142] Ertekin-Taner N, Graff-Radford N, Younkin LH, et al. Linkage of plasma Aß42 to a quantitative locus on chromosome 10 in late-onset Alzheimer's disease pedigrees. Science 2000; 290(5500):2303–4.
[143] Myers A, Holmans P, Marshall H, et al. Susceptibility locus for Alzheimer's disease on chromosome 10. Science 2000;290(5500):2304–5.
[144] Bertram L, Blacker D, Mullin K, et al. Evidence for genetic linkage of Alzheimer's disease to chromosome 10q. Science 2000;290(5500):2302–3.
[145] Scott WK, Grubber JM, Conneally PM, et al. Fine mapping of the chromosome 12 late-onset Alzheimer disease locus: potential genetic and phenotypic heterogeneity. Am J Hum Genet 2000;66(3):922–32.
[146] Rogaeva E, Premkumar S, Song Y, et al. Evidence for an Alzheimer disease susceptibility locus on chromosome 12 and for further locus heterogeneity. JAMA 1998;280(7):614–8.
[147] Kovacs DM. Alpha2-macroglobulin in late-onset Alzheimer's disease. Exp Gerontol 2000; 35(4):473–9.
[148] D'Introno A, Solfrizzi V, Colacicco AM, et al. Current knowledge of chromosome 12 susceptibility genes for late-onset Alzheimer's disease. Neurobiol Aging 2006;27(11):1537–53.
[149] Li Y, Nowotny P, Holmans P, et al. Association of late-onset Alzheimer's disease with genetic variation in multiple members of the GAPD gene family. Proc Natl Acad Sci U S A 2004;101(44):15688–93.
[150] Lin PI, Martin ER, Bronson PG, et al. Exploring the association of glyceraldehyde-3-phosphate dehydrogenase gene and Alzheimer disease. Neurology 2006;67(1):64–8.
[151] Li Y, Grupe A, Rowland C, et al. DAPK1 variants are associated with Alzheimer's disease and allele-specific expression. Hum Mol Genet 2006;15(17):2560–8.
[152] Katzov H, Chalmers K, Palmgren J, et al. Genetic variants of ABCA1 modify Alzheimer disease risk and quantitative traits related to beta-amyloid metabolism. Hum Mutat 2004;23(4):358–67.
[153] Mace S, Cousin E, Ricard S, et al. ABCA2 is a strong genetic risk factor for early-onset Alzheimer's disease. Neurobiol Dis 2005;18(1):119–25.
[154] Okuizumi K, Onodera O, Namba Y, et al. Genetic association of the very low density lipoprotein (VLDL) receptor gene with sporadic Alzheimer's disease. Nat Genet 1995;11(2): 207–9.
[155] Bertram L, Hiltunen M, Parkinson M, et al. Family-based association between Alzheimer's disease and variants in UBQLN1. N Engl J Med 2005;352(9):884–94.
[156] Hauser ER, Watanabe RM, Duren WL, et al. Ordered subset analysis in genetic linkage mapping of complex traits. Genet Epidemiol 2004;27(1):53–63.
[157] Emahazion T, Feuk L, Jobs M, et al. SNP association studies in Alzheimer's disease highlight problems for complex disease analysis. Trends Genet 2001;17(7):407–13.
[158] Finckh U. The future of genetic association studies in Alzheimer disease. J Neural Transm 2003;110(3):253–66.
[159] Blomqvist ME, Reynolds C, Katzov H, et al. Towards compendia of negative genetic association studies: an example for Alzheimer disease. Hum Genet 2006;119(1–2):29–37.
[160] Lohmueller KE, Pearce CL, Pike M, et al. Meta-analysis of genetic association studies supports a contribution of common variants to susceptibility to common disease. Nat Genet 2003;33(2):177–82.
[161] Ioannidis JP, Ntzani EE, Trikalinos TA, et al. Replication validity of genetic association studies. Nat Genet 2001;29(3):306–9.
[162] Newton-Cheh C, Hirschhorn JN. Genetic association studies of complex traits: design and analysis issues. Mutat Res 2005;573(1–2):54–69.

[163] Ertekin-Taner N, Ronald J, Asahara H, et al. Fine mapping of the alpha-T catenin gene to a quantitative trait locus on chromosome 10 in late-onset Alzheimer's disease pedigrees. Hum Mol Genet 2003;12(23):3133–43.
[164] Ertekin-Taner N, Allen M, Fadale D, et al. Genetic variants in a haplotype block spanning IDE are significantly associated with plasma Abeta42 levels and risk for Alzheimer disease. Hum Mutat 2004;23(4):334–42.
[165] Ertekin-Taner N, Ronald J, Feuk L, et al. Elevated amyloid beta protein (Abeta42) and late onset Alzheimer's disease are associated with single nucleotide polymorphisms in the urokinase-type plasminogen activator gene. Hum Mol Genet 2005;14(3):447–60.
[166] Prince JA, Feuk L, Gu HF, et al. Genetic variation in a haplotype block spanning IDE influences Alzheimer disease. Hum Mutat 2003;22(5):363–71.
[167] Wollmer MA, Streffer JR, Tsolaki M, et al. Genetic association of acyl-coenzyme A: cholesterol acyltransferase with cerebrospinal fluid cholesterol levels, brain amyloid load, and risk for Alzheimer's disease. Mol Psychiatry 2003;8(6):635–8.
[168] Grupe A, Li Y, Rowland C, et al. A scan of chromosome 10 identifies a novel locus showing strong association with late-onset Alzheimer disease. Am J Hum Genet 2006;78(1):78–88.
[169] Li YJ, Oliveira SA, Xu P, et al. Glutathione S-transferase omega-1 modifies age-at-onset of Alzheimer disease and Parkinson disease. Hum Mol Genet 2003;12(24):3259–67.
[170] Kuwano R, Miyashita A, Arai H, et al. Dynamin-binding protein gene on chromosome 10q is associated with late-onset Alzheimer's disease. Hum Mol Genet 2006;15(13):2170–82.
[171] Rogaeva E, Meng Y, Lee JH, et al. The neuronal sortilin-related receptor SORL1 is genetically associated with Alzheimer disease. Nat Genet 2007;39(2):168–77.
[172] Martin ER, Bronson PG, Li YJ, et al. Interaction between the alpha-T catenin gene (VR22) and APOE in Alzheimer's disease. J Med Genet 2005;42(10):787–92.
[173] Cellini E, Bagnoli S, Tedde A, et al. Insulin degrading enzyme and alpha-3 catenin polymorphisms in Italian patients with Alzheimer disease. Alzheimer Dis Assoc Disord 2005;19(4): 246–7.
[174] Bertram L, Mullin K, Parkinson M, et al. Is alpha-T catenin (VR22) an Alzheimer's disease risk gene? J Med Genet 2007;44(1):1–4.
[175] Blomqvist ME, Andreasen N, Bogdanovic N, et al. Genetic variation in CTNNA3 encoding alpha-3 catenin and Alzheimer's disease. Neurosci Lett 2004;358(3):220–2.
[176] Busby V, Goossens S, Nowotny P, et al. Alpha-T-catenin is expressed in human brain and interacts with the Wnt signaling pathway but is not responsible for linkage to chromosome 10 in Alzheimer's disease. Neuromolecular Med 2004;5(2):133–46.
[177] Li YJ, Scott WK, Zhang L, et al. Revealing the role of glutathione S-transferase omega in age-at-onset of Alzheimer and Parkinson diseases. Neurobiol Aging 2006;27(8):1087–93.

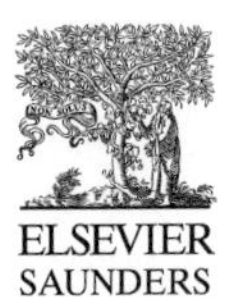

ELSEVIER
SAUNDERS

Neurol Clin 25 (2007) 669–682

NEUROLOGIC
CLINICS

An Update on the Amyloid Hypothesis

Christopher B. Eckman, PhD[a,*],
Elizabeth A. Eckman, PhD[b]

[a]*Department of Neuroscience, Mayo Clinic College of Medicine, Birdsall Building Room 306, 4500 San Pablo Road, Jacksonville, FL 32224, USA*
[b]*Department of Neuroscience, Mayo Clinic College of Medicine, Birdsall Building Room 318a, 4500 San Pablo Road, Jacksonville, FL 32224, USA*

Alzheimer's disease (AD) is a devastating disease, not only for patients but also for their families and loved ones. What typically begins as fairly subtle memory loss progresses relentlessly over a period of approximately 7-10 years, until all higher cognitive functions are eroded and AD patients are robbed of their identity and ability to interact with the outside world. Currently, estimates indicate that more than 27 million individuals are affected by AD worldwide [1]. In the United States alone, more than 4 million individuals have the disease [2]. Unfortunately, without a cure or a means to otherwise prevent this disease or significantly slow its progression, the number of affected individuals in the United States is expected to triple by 2050 due to the aging baby boomer generation [2]. This enormous increase in the number of affected individuals is likely to have dire consequences on the already overburdened health care system in this country.

Based on the statistics alone, the identification of novel therapeutic or preventative agents is of considerable importance. To rationally develop these agents, an understanding of the etiology and pathogenesis of this complex disease is necessary. Over the past century, numerous hypotheses have been proposed, including abnormal phosphorylation of tau, unconventional infectious agents, trace element neurotoxicity, growth factor deficiency, excitatory amino acid insult, altered calcium homeostasis, free radical toxicity, deficits in energy metabolism, and altered protein processing resulting in abnormal β-amyloid peptide (Aβ) accumulation (reviewed in part by

This work was supported by grants from the National Institutes of Neurological Diseases and Stroke (NIH 5R01NS042192 and NIH 5R01NS048554) and by the Mayo Foundation for Medical Education and Research.

* Corresponding author.
E-mail address: eckman@mayo.edu (C.B. Eckman).

doi:10.1016/j.ncl.2007.03.007 ***neurologic.theclinics.com***

Markesbery [3]). Most importantly, any hypothesis describing the etiology and pathogenesis of AD must take into account the neurologic and neuropathologic features of AD as well as the known genetic risk factors, causative mutations, and the heightened risk associated with advanced age.

One such comprehensive hypothesis, that has received significant attention over the past 2 decades (for better or for worse), is the amyloid hypothesis [4–6]. Although many iterations of this hypothesis currently exist, the initial hypothesis stated that the "deposition of amyloid β protein (AβP), the main component of the plaques, is the causative agent of Alzheimer's pathology…" [5]. This article examines the evidence for this hypothesis and its potential limitations, particularly related to the development of novel therapeutic and preventative agents.

Neuropathology of Alzheimer's disease and the identification of beta-amyloid

The first evidence for the amyloid hypothesis came from neuropathologic assessments of brains isolated from AD patients. The earliest examinations published by Alois Alzheimer described the neuropathology in two patients [7–9], and revealed a diffuse atrophy primarily of the cerebral cortex. Staining of the brains isolated from these two patients demonstrated the presence of two types of lesions. The first type, now known as neurofibrillary tangles (NFTs), was observed in the initial patient, and was described as a twisted coil of fibrils derived from degenerating cerebral cortical cells. The second type of lesion, now known as senile plaques, was present in both of the cases to differing degrees. These plaques were found throughout the cerebral cortex and were characterized by a central core surrounded by a more diffuse halo.

We now know that these classical senile plaques are complex, extracellular lesions that are associated with degenerating neuronal processes, have activated microglia intertwined with the central deposit, and are surrounded by reactive astrocytes. These deposits are found throughout the neocortex and hippocampus in patients who have AD [10]. The central deposit in classical senile plaques structurally is similar to the deposits seen in a group of diseases referred to as amyloidoses, wherein there is extracellular deposition of proteins with a beta-pleated sheet conformation (reviewed by Sipe [11,12]). More than 15 different polypeptides have been identified as the primary proteinaceous components of the amyloids that are deposited in various tissues in the clinically diverse amyloidoses.

The central location of the plaque core within this pathology led to the speculation that whatever comprises the core may play a pivotal role in the disease process itself. In a landmark finding in 1984, Glenner and Wong published the purification and sequence of the primary proteinaceous component of amyloid isolated from meningeal vessels obtained from AD brains [13]. By comparing samples from six AD patients and three controls, they identified a unique protein only present in the patients who had AD. Size-exclusion chromatography revealed that the protein had an approximate molecular weight of 4200 daltons, and amino acid analysis and sequencing revealed a novel amino acid sequence now referred to as Aβ.

Alzheimer's disease and Down syndrome: the link to chromosome 21

Previously, it was established that individuals who have Down syndrome who live past age 50 have neuropathologic changes similar to AD patients (reviewed by Mann [14]). In a follow-up to their original finding, Glenner and Wong [15] isolated and analyzed the cerebrovascular amyloid from Down syndrome patients. They established that the amino acid sequence of cerebrovascular amyloid in Down syndrome is identical to that observed in AD patients. Given the similarity of the amyloid deposited in AD and Down syndrome, Glenner and Wong [15] proposed that there was a common pathogenic process involved. Down syndrome results from trisomy of the twenty-first chromosome, which implied that AD pathology could be produced by increased expression of a gene or genes on chromosome 21.

After these initial reports, amino acid sequencing of the amyloid isolated from senile plaques from AD and Down syndrome brains was reported by other groups [16,17]. These reports established that the amino-terminal sequence and amino acid composition of plaque core amyloid was identical to that of cerebrovascular amyloid isolated from AD or Down syndrome brains, except for the presence of ragged NH_2 termini [17].

To isolate the gene encoding Aβ, Kang and colleagues [18] used degenerate primers targeted against amino acids 10-16 of the peptide to screen a complementary DNA library constructed from the brain of a 5-month old fetus. In these experiments, they isolated a clone encoding a 695 amino acid protein that contained the Aβ sequence beginning 99 amino acids from the carboxyl end of the protein. This protein was simultaneously reported by other groups and is now known as β-amyloid protein precursor (βAPP) [19–21]. Southern blot analysis of mouse/human cell hybrids revealed that the gene encoding βAPP is located on the twenty-first chromosome [18]. This data substantiated Glenner and Wong's previous suggestion, that overexpression of a gene or genes on chromosome 21 should be sufficient to cause AD pathology. Subsequent studies by Tamaoka and colleagues showed that Aβ levels were increased significantly in plasma isolated from patients who had Down syndrome when compared with control individuals, indicating that an increased copy number of βAPP does result in increased levels of Aβ in humans [22].

β-amyloid protein precursor metabolism

A basic description of the metabolism of βAPP is necessary to understand how the familial AD (FAD)-linked mutations (discussed later) can influence the accumulation of Aβ. The Aβ peptide sequence is embedded in the βAPP protein, indicating that two separate proteolytic cleavages are required to generate Aβ from its precursor. The N-terminus of Aβ is generated by cleavage of βAPP by β-secretase, producing a 99 amino acid C-terminal fragment (CTF) of βAPP that can be cleaved further by γ-secretase to release Aβ. γ-Secretase generates two major Aβ species, 40 and 42 amino acids in length, termed Aβ40 and Aβ42. βAPP also can be cleaved within the Aβ domain by α-secretase, an action that precludes Aβ generation. The β- and γ-secretase cleavages are discussed further with descriptions of the discovery of the three genes linked to familial early-onset AD and the mechanisms by which they elevate Aβ levels.

Genetics of Alzheimer's disease

Some of the strongest evidence for a critical role for Aβ in AD came from an analysis of the genetic mutations that cause AD. In addition to trisomy 21 causing neuropathology that essentially is identical to that seen in typical late-onset AD, AD can be inherited as a fully penetrant, autosomal dominant trait in certain families [23–24]. In these families, the clinical and neuropathologic presentation of the disease essentially is identical to typical late-onset AD, but the age of onset is earlier, typically in the 50s. Mutations in three distinct genes, on three separate chromosomes, have been identified as the cause of AD in these families: the βAPP gene on chromosome 21 [25–29], the presenilin 1 gene on chromosome 14 [30], and the presenilin 2 gene on chromosome 1 [31]. These genes are reviewed in greater detail in the article by Taner and colleagues elsewhere in this issue. However, some of FAD-linked mutations are highlighted below as they relate to the amyloid hypothesis.

The first mutation shown to cause AD, found in a single family, was a point mutation in the βAPP gene itself. This mutation results in a substitution of the more hydrophobic amino acid, isoleucine, for valine at position 717 (V717I), which is immediately carboxyl to the Aβ sequence [26]. In other families, additional mutations at this position subsequently were identified that result in the substitution of phenylalanine (V717F) [25] or glycine (V717G) [27]. After the identification of mutations at position 717 in the βAPP gene, a double mutation at position 670/671 was identified in a large Swedish family with a mean age of onset of AD of 55 years [28]. The 670/671 double mutation results in a substitution of asparagine and leucine for the lysine and methionine, respectively, immediately preceding the N-terminus of Aβ (K670N/M671L). In context, the identification of causative mutations for AD, not only within the βAPP protein itself but also immediately adjacent to the cleavage sites needed to liberate the Aβ peptide from its precursor protein, provided additional, immediate support for the amyloid hypothesis.

To investigate the hypothesis that the mutations identified in the βAPP gene would alter the amount of Aβ peptide being produced, several groups turned their attention to the analysis of βAPP metabolism and extracellular Aβ accumulation in model systems [32–35]. Analysis of total Aβ concentration in the conditioned medium of transfected cells expressing these FAD-linked mutations indicated that the Swedish mutation caused a several-fold increase in the amount of Aβ accumulated extracellularly [32,33]. Additionally, analysis of the CTFs and secreted forms of βAPP (sAPP) showed elevations in CTFβ and sAPPβ, indicating that the increased Aβ concentration observed with this mutation is likely the result of enhanced β secretase cleavage [36]. Using the same experimental paradigm, no significant differences in total Aβ, CTFs, or sAPPs were observed, however, in cells transfected with the 717 mutations [35].

Pioneering work by Lansbury and colleagues [37–39] showed that the carboxy-terminal length of the Aβ molecule was critical to determining the rate at which Aβ fibrils form. Using synthetic peptides, they showed that Aβ ending at position 42 formed fibrils far more rapidly and at lower concentrations than Aβ ending at position 40. As the deposition of Aβ in the form of amyloid fibrils represents an invariant feature of AD, Younkin and colleagues [33] proposed that the 717 mutations might be acting to selectively increase secretion of Aβ42. In a landmark finding, Younkin's group showed that secreted Aβ42, which normally constitutes only a fraction of total secreted Aβ, is increased significantly in the medium of cells expressing the 717 mutations [35]. Thus, both the Swedish mutation and the 717 mutations increase the concentration of Aβ, in particular Aβ42.

To date, one of the greatest tests of the amyloid hypothesis involved the analysis of mutations that also cause early-onset AD but that do not reside in the βAPP gene or even on chromosome 21. These were the presenilin mutations. (These are covered in detail the article by Taner and colleagues elsewhere in this issue.) Initially, there was no evidence to suggest that these genes were involved with βAPP processing. In fact, they seemed equally as likely to directly influence tau, synapse loss, energy metabolism, or a host of other factors associated with alternate theories regarding the etiology and pathogenesis of AD.

However, studies performed by Younkin and colleagues [40] showed that in cultured medium from primary fibroblasts and plasma isolated from patients who had either presenilin 1 or presenilin 2 mutations, Aβ levels were elevated, in particular Aβ42 levels, similar to the 717 mutations in βAPP. Follow-up studies by several groups examining the influence of these mutations on Aβ levels in either transfected cells or in the brains of animals transgenic for these mutations confirmed these findings.

When the presenilins were discovered as FAD-linked genes in 1995, their functions were unknown and their link to APP metabolism was not clear. Then, in 1997, Selkoe and colleagues [41] showed that APP and presenilin interact in mammalian cells, as evidenced by coimmunoprecipitation experiments. Over the next 5 years, several additional laboratories demonstrated that the presenilins are the catalytic component of the multiprotein complex that is γ-secretase [42–44]. Consequently, the relationship between βAPP, the presenilins, and AD now is clear: Aβ is generated by β-secretase and γ-secretase (presenilin complex) cleavage of the βAPP protein. All of the mutations identified in βAPP, presenilin 1, and presenilin 2 that cause early-onset FAD increase Aβ levels, particularly Aβ42 levels, or otherwise perturb the ratio of Aβ42 to Aβ40 levels [45] in ways likely to foster Aβ aggregation and deposition.

β-amyloid peptide levels increase during aging

Aging clearly is the most significant risk factor associated with AD, and Aβ levels begin to increase in the brains of many people who are cognitively normal between the ages of 40 and 80 [46,47]. According to the study of consecutive autopsy cases by Funato and colleagues [46], insoluble Aβ42 in particular accumulates with age in the cortex and precedes senile plaque formation. Compared with brains from cognitively normal elderly individuals, AD brain had higher levels of soluble and insoluble Aβ42 and Aβ40 and a higher degree of N-terminally truncated or modified Aβ. Similar correlations between Aβ levels and age in individuals who were cognitively normal were reported by Morishima-Kawashima and colleagues [47], with significant increases in Aβ accumulation beginning after age 40. In both studies, insoluble Aβ concentration was related logarithmically to plaque density, and a critical threshold (approximately 100 pmol/g) of insoluble Aβ42 was required for immunocytochemical detection of senile plaques. In the latter study, carriers of the apolipoprotein E ϵ4 allele, a strong risk factor for AD, were found to accumulate Aβ at an earlier age than noncarriers [47].

Increased levels of β-amyloid peptide: causative agent or very good biomarker?

As discussed previously, elevations in Aβ concentration that are likely to enhance aggregation and deposition are linked to the expression of all of the FAD-linked mutations analyzed to date, and in Down syndrome. These elevations can be detected in plasma and in fibroblast-conditioned medium isolated from presymptomatic individuals [36,48] and in transgenic animals before deposition [49,50], suggesting that these changes are early and not simply an epiphenomenon associated with end-stage AD. In addition it seems that Aβ levels increase during aging in humans and in animal models, with age being the highest contributing risk factor for the development of the disease.

The question then remains, do elevations in Aβ play a central, causal role in the pathogenesis of the disease or are they a relatively benign marker of the underlying disease process. Perhaps this question will not be answered until newly developed approaches to lower Ab either fail or show significant improvement in the clinics. However, it can be concluded, based on numerous studies, that elevations in Ab levels are not likely without consequence.

Clinical-neuropathologic correlations in Alzheimer's disease

The extent of correlation between the neuropathologic lesions in AD patients and the severity of their dementia has been an area of considerable debate and continues to be used consistently as an argument against the amyloid hypothesis. As is true with any correlative function, a correlation can be a good indicator of a causal relationship, but close correlation is not definitive proof of causality. For example, a well-correlated change simply can be an inconsequential, reliable biomarker of another process that is causative. With that in mind, some of the earliest studies showed significant correlations between plaque numbers and the extent of dementia [51]. Several other studies, however, reported that the number of NFTs and neuropil threads is a far better indicator of the degree of dementia [52,53]. One of the most comprehensive recent analyses, with respect to the extent of variables examined, was published by Cummings and colleagues [54]. In this study, they found that the number of plaques, NFTs, and dystrophic neurites all correlated significantly with dementia severity and the area occupied by Aβ and tau paired-helical filaments. However, individuals remain who have extensive amyloid deposition and are cognitively normal. For example, in a study by Markesbery's group, significant AD-like pathology (plaques and tangles) was found in the brains of a substantial number of elderly, cognitively normal individuals [55]. These and similar studies led some to argue that the amyloid hypothesis must be wrong. In response, some amyloid theory proponents have adjusted the hypothesis accordingly to accommodate and now argue for preamyloid-like aggregates of Aβ, such as Aβ oligomers, as the causative agent in the disease process. Regardless of the correct hypothesis, the development of AD is a reasonably long process. Therefore, it is not surprising that with nearly one half of the population susceptible to the disease, if they live long enough, individuals can be found who have significant neuropathology and who are cognitively normal. Similar trends are observed in other neurodegenerative diseases, such as Parkinson's disease, where approximately 70% of the dopaminergic neurons in the subtantia nigra are lost before the development of clinical symptoms.

β-amyloid peptide toxicity

If alterations in Aβ are necessary and sufficient to play a causal role in AD pathogenesis, then Aβ should be able to elicit, directly or indirectly, the neuropathologic and cognitive changes observed in patients who have AD. Furthermore, mechanisms must exist that can explain the prevalence of the disease in the aging population and in people carrying causative mutations and known genetic risk factors. Evidence gathered over the past several years builds an increasingly stronger case that the alterations in Aβ observed in the genetic forms of AD are not without consequence and can account for the neuropathology and dementia in AD. This section reviews evidence for the neurotoxicity of abnormal Aβ species. Although neurotoxicity initially was attributed to the fibrillar species of Aβ deposited in plaques, recent data also implicate soluble Aβ oligomers, which may form before plaque deposition and cause neuronal dysfunction that may facilitate many of the downstream pathologic events in AD. Because these soluble oligomers exist in equilibrium with fibrillar Aβ as deposition progresses, the neuronal loss, inflammation, and other pathology seen in the vicinity of plaques may be the result of the oligomers, the plaques, or a combination of the two.

Soluble, synthetic Aβ peptides were shown by Yankner and colleagues [56] to be neurotrophic at low concentration to undifferentiated hippocampal neurons in culture and toxic at higher concentrations to mature neurons. Subsequently, the neurotoxicity of Aβ was shown to be dependent on its aggregation state [57,58]. Stable Aβ aggregates were highly toxic to primary neurons, and partial reversal of aggregation resulted in a loss of toxicity. Similar results were found in in vivo studies, with microinjection of fibrillar, but not soluble, Aβ causing neurotoxicity in the cerebral cortex of aged rhesus monkeys [59]. Neurotoxicity was dependent not only on the aggregation state of Aβ but also on the age and species of the animal model used. Specifically, plaque-equivalent concentrations of fibrillar Aβ resulted in extensive neuronal loss, tau phosphorylation, and microglial activation in the brains of aged monkeys but were not toxic to young adult monkeys or aged rodents. Much higher concentrations of Aβ were required to elicit neurotoxicity in young adult monkeys and in rodents [59–61]. These results may help to explain the vulnerability of the elderly to AD and the difficulty of generating a rodent model that faithfully reproduces all of the neuropathologic features of the disease.

In vitro, fibrils are believed to form via the progression from Aβ monomers to low-molecular-weight oligomers to intermediate species (called protofibrils) that assemble into mature fibrils [62]. The data indicating that Aβ fibrils are neurotoxic and can elicit other AD characteristics, including tau phosphorylation, suggested that disrupting fibrils might be therapeutically beneficial. However, researchers suspected that the disruption of insoluble Aβ fibrils could result in an accumulation of protofibrils and other soluble oligomers. Therefore, experiments were performed to investigate whether these lower-level aggregates apparently were nontoxic, like Aβ monomers, or whether they might elicit neurotoxic effects, like fibrils. Data generated over the past several years demonstrates convincingly that Aβ oligomers neurotoxic, and in many assays they are even more toxic than fibrils [63].

Soluble oligomers range from dimers and trimers to dodecamers, also called Aβ-derived diffusible ligands (ADDLs) [64,65]. The smaller sodium dodecyl sulfate (SDS) stable oligomers are produced by several cell lines and have been detected in human brain and cerebrospinal fluid. Similarly, the larger ADDLs are not merely an artifact of the in vitro assembly of Aβ, as structurally indistinguishable Aβ oligomers are present in soluble extracts of AD brain at average levels 12-fold higher than in control brains [66]. ADDLs, formed in vitro or purified from AD brain, bind specifically to synapses in differentiated hippocampal neuronal cultures [63]. This evidence for specific neuronal attachment, coupled with the fact that ADDLs and lower-molecular-weight Aβ oligomers are shown to be potent inhibitors of long-term potentiation, a model of synaptic plasticity and memory, provides a rational explanation for early memory loss in AD and in animal models of AD [64,67,68].

As discussed previously, a common criticism of the amyloid hypothesis was that in some studies, plaque burden correlated poorly with severity of dementia in AD. The discovery of soluble oligomers as neurotoxic Aβ species led to an examination of the relationship between soluble Aβ concentration and clinical and pathologic severity. A strong correlation between soluble Aβ and markers of disease severity, including synaptic loss, was identified [69,70]. Two additional lines of evidence support the hypothesis that soluble Aβ oligomers are the primary toxic entity in the brain, at least in animal models.

First, impaired synaptic transmission and cognitive function are seen before overt amyloid deposition in mouse models of AD [71–73]. In the widely used APP transgenic mouse model, Tg2576, a partial decline in memory occurs at approximately 6 months, before amyloid deposition. Cognitive function then remains stable over the next 7 to 8 months, even though plaque deposition progresses and becomes significant over this time period. Finally, a further decline in cognitive function is detected at ages greater than 15 months. The initial memory decline at 6 months, followed by the period of stability, was perplexing in terms of the lack of correlation with the course of amyloid plaque deposition in this model. This led Lesné and colleagues [72] to conduct a detailed biochemical analysis of Aβ complexes in the brains of these mice during the time period when the first behavioral deficits are detected. Soluble, extracellular-enriched extracts from the forebrain of 6-month-old Tg2576 contained SDS and urea stable Aβ complexes with molecular weights theoretically corresponding to trimers and multiples thereof, up to a molecular weight of 56 kd. Only the 56-kd (theoretic dodecamer) and 40-kd (theoretic nonamer) species appeared for the first time at 6 months. Both correlated inversely with memory performance, with the 56-kd form (termed Aβ*56) showing the strongest correlation. The levels of the 40- and 56-kd Aβ complexes remained stable on average during the subsequent period of cognitive stability in the mice. To test more directly whether or not Aβ*56 causes cognitive impairment, the complexes were purified from Tg2576 brain extracts and then injected into the lateral ventricle of rats. Aβ*56 caused a transient decrease in spatial memory in rats, supporting the hypothesis that this complex could be responsible for the onset of memory deficits in the Tg2576 mouse model [72]. Whether or not Aβ*56 structurally is identical to the 56-kd ADDLs derived from AD brain [66] is an intriguing question that remains to be determined.

Second, therapeutic interventions, which lower the level of soluble Aβ or disrupt Aβ assembly in animal models, often in the absence of detectable changes in plaque load, ameliorate cognitive deficits [74–79]. This effect is not unique to a single therapeutic approach and has been observed with such divergent strategies as Aβ immunization, acute γ-secretase inhibition, and oligomer neutralization. Recently, Lee and colleagues [77] showed that short-term passive immunization of aged Tg2576 APP transgenic mice with a conformation-specific Aβ antibody that preferentially recognizes dimers, soluble oligomers, and certain amyloid deposits resulted in significant improvements in spatial learning and memory without affecting amyloid burden. These results are similar to those obtained by independent groups using different Aβ antibodies and different transgenic lines [75,76] and support the hypothesis that the neutralization of toxic Aβ species can reverse cognitive deficits in mice. This hypothesis has recently been tested by other investigators [78] using a completely different experimental paradigm but with similar results [78,79]. Cyclohexanehexol stereoisomers, which inhibit Aβ aggregation and favor the disassembly of fibrils, can prevent Aβ oligomer–induced toxicity in cultured primary neurons and hippocampal slices and oligomer-induced memory deficits in rats [79]. When administered orally to TgCRND8 APP transgenic mice from 6 weeks of age (predeposition) to 4 to 6 months (significant amyloid deposition), scyllo-cyclohanehexol showed a dose-dependent improvement in spatial learning accompanied by decreases in amyloid burden and Aβ oligomers [78]. Synaptic loss was ameliorated at 6 months as was accelerated mortality in the treated mice.

Perhaps the most important implication of these studies is that the cognitive impairment in these models is not permanent. To what degree this applies to the human condition is unknown, because the profound neuronal loss in AD is absent in AD mouse models. Nonetheless, reducing soluble Aβ levels or altering a toxic conformation may be a less ambitious goal than clearing plaques. The true test for the amyloid hypothesis of AD, and the specific notion that soluble oligomers mediate Aβ toxicity, awaits the further development of Aβ-targeted therapies and their progression to clinical trial.

References

[1] Wimo A, Jonsson L, Winblad B. An estimate of the worldwide prevalence and direct costs of dementia in 2003. Dement Geriatr Cogn Disord 2006;21(3):175–81.

[2] Hebert LE, Scherr PA, Bienias JL, Bennett DA, Evans DA. Alzheimer disease in the US population: prevalence estimates using the 2000 census. Arch Neurol Aug 2003;60(8):1119–22.
[3] Markesbery WR. Alzheimer's Disease. In: Asbury AK, McKhann GM, McDonald WI, editors. Diseases of the Nervous System: Clinical Neurobiology, Vol I. 2 edition. Philadelphia: W.B. Saunders Company; 1992.
[4] Hardy J, Allsop D. Amyloid deposition as the central event in the aetiology of Alzheimer's disease. Trends Pharmacol Sci Oct 1991;12(10):383–8.
[5] Hardy JA, Higgins GA. Alzheimer's disease: the amyloid cascade hypothesis. Science Apr 10 1992;256(5054):184–5.
[6] Selkoe DJ. The molecular pathology of Alzheimer's disease. Neuron Apr 1991;6(4): 487–98.
[7] Alzheimer A. Uber eine eigenartige, Erkrankung der Hirnrinde. Allg Z Psychiatrie Psychisch-Gerichtl Med 1907;64:146–8.
[8] Alzheimer A. Uber eigenartige Krankheitsfalle des spateren Alters. Zbl Ges Neurol Psych 1911;4:356–85.
[9] Moller HJ, Graeber MB. The case described by Alois Alzheimer in 1911. Historical and conceptual perspectives based on the clinical record and neurohistological sections. Eur Arch Psychiatry Clin Neurosci 1998;248(3):111–22.
[10] Selkoe DJ. Cellular and molecular biology of the beta-amyloid precursor protein and Alzheimer's disease. In: Rosenberg RN, Pruisner SB, DiMauro S, Barchi RL, editors. The Molecular and Genetic Basis of Neurological Disease. 2 edition. Boston: Butterworth-Heinemann; 1997. p. 601–11.
[11] Sipe JD. Amyloidosis. Annu Rev Biochem 1992;61:947–75.
[12] Sipe JD. Amyloidosis. Crit Rev Clin Lab Sci 1994;31(4):325–54.
[13] Glenner GG, Wong CW. Alzheimer's disease: initial report of the purification and characterization of a novel cerebrovascular amyloid protein. Biochem Biophys Res Commun 1984;120(3):885–90.
[14] Mann DM. Alzheimer's disease and Down's syndrome. Histopathology 1988;13(2):125–37.
[15] Glenner GG, Wong CW. Alzheimer's disease and Down's syndrome: sharing of a unique cerebrovascular amyloid fibril protein. Biochem Biophys Res Commun 1984;122(3):1131–5.
[16] Gorevic PD, Goni F, Pons-Estel B, Alvarez F, Peress NS, Frangione B. Isolation and partial characterization of neurofibrillary tangles and amyloid plaque core in Alzheimer's disease: immunohistological studies. J Neuropathol Exp Neurol 1986;45(6):647–64.
[17] Masters CL, Simms G, Weinman NA, Multhaup G, McDonald BL, Beyreuther K. Amyloid plaque core protein in Alzheimer disease and Down syndrome. Proc Natl Acad Sci U S A 1985;82(12):4245–9.
[18] Kang J, Lemaire HG, Unterbeck A, et al. The precursor of Alzheimer's disease amyloid A4 protein resembles a cell-surface receptor. Nature 1987;325(6106):733–6.
[19] Robakis NK, Ramakrishna N, Wolfe G, Wisniewski HM. Molecular cloning and characterization of a cDNA encoding the cerebrovascular and the neuritic plaque amyloid peptides [published erratum appears in Proc Natl Acad Sci U S A 1987 Oct;84(20):7221]. Proc Natl Acad Sci U S A 1987;84(12):4190–4.
[20] Tanzi RE, Gusella JF, Watkins PC, et al. Amyloid beta protein gene: cDNA, mRNA distribution, and genetic linkage near the Alzheimer locus. Science 1987;235(4791):880–4.
[21] Goldgaber D, Lerman MI, McBride OW, Saffiotti U, Gajdusek DC. Characterization and chromosomal localization of a cDNA encoding brain amyloid of Alzheimer's disease. Science 1987;235(4791):877–80.
[22] Tokuda T, Fukushima T, Ikeda S, et al. Plasma levels of amyloid beta proteins Abeta1-40 and Abeta1-42(43) are elevated in Down's syndrome. Ann Neurol 1997;41(2):271–3.
[23] Hardy J. Amyloid, the presenilins and Alzheimer's disease [see comments]. Trends Neurosci 1997;20(4):154–9.
[24] Blacker D, Tanzi RE. The genetics of Alzheimer disease: current status and future prospects. Arch Neurol 1998;55(3):294–6.

[25] Murrell J, Farlow M, Ghetti B, Benson MD. A mutation in the amyloid precursor protein associated with hereditary Alzheimer's disease. Science 1991;254(5028):97–9.
[26] Goate A, Chartier-Harlin MC, Mullan M, et al. Segregation of a missense mutation in the amyloid precursor protein gene with familial Alzheimer's disease [see comments]. Nature 1991;349(6311):704–6.
[27] Chartier-Harlin MC, Crawford F, Houlden H, et al. Early-onset Alzheimer's disease caused by mutations at codon 717 of the beta-amyloid precursor protein gene. Nature 1991; 353(6347):844–6.
[28] Mullan M, Crawford F, Axelman K, et al. A pathogenic mutation for probable Alzheimer's disease in the APP gene at the N-terminus of beta-amyloid. Nat Genet 1992;1(5):345–7.
[29] Eckman CB, Mehta ND, Crook R, et al. A new pathogenic mutation in the APP gene (I716V) increases the relative proportion of A beta 42(43). Hum Mol Genet 1997;6(12): 2087–9.
[30] Sherrington R, Rogaev EI, Liang Y, et al. Cloning of a gene bearing missense mutations in early-onset familial Alzheimer's disease [see comments]. Nature 1995;375(6534):754–60.
[31] Levy-Lahad E, Wasco W, Poorkaj P, et al. Candidate gene for the chromosome 1 familial Alzheimer's disease locus [see comments]. Science 1995;269(5226):973–7.
[32] Citron M, Oltersdorf T, Haass C, et al. Mutation of the beta-amyloid precursor protein in familial Alzheimer's disease increases beta-protein production. Nature 1992;360(6405): 672–4.
[33] Cai XD, Golde TE, Younkin SG. Release of excess amyloid beta protein from a mutant amyloid beta protein precursor [see comments]. Science 1993;259(5094):514–6.
[34] Citron M, Vigo-Pelfrey C, Teplow DB, et al. Excessive production of amyloid beta-protein by peripheral cells of symptomatic and presymptomatic patients carrying the Swedish familial Alzheimer disease mutation. Proc Natl Acad Sci U S A 1994;91(25): 11993–7.
[35] Suzuki N, Cheung TT, Cai XD, et al. An increased percentage of long amyloid beta protein secreted by familial amyloid beta protein precursor (beta APP717) mutants. Science 1994; 264(5163):1336–40.
[36] Felsenstein KM, Hunihan LW, Roberts SB. Altered cleavage and secretion of a recombinant beta-APP bearing the Swedish familial Alzheimer's disease mutation. Nat Genet 1994;6(3): 251–5.
[37] Jarrett JT, Berger EP, Lansbury PT Jr. The C-terminus of the beta protein is critical in amyloidogenesis. Ann N Y Acad Sci 1993;695:144–8.
[38] Jarrett JT, Lansbury PT Jr. Seeding "one-dimensional crystallization" of amyloid: a pathogenic mechanism in Alzheimer's disease and scrapie? Cell 1993;73(6):1055–8.
[39] Jarrett JT, Berger EP, Lansbury PT Jr. The carboxy terminus of the beta amyloid protein is critical for the seeding of amyloid formation: implications for the pathogenesis of Alzheimer's disease. Biochemistry 1993;32(18):4693–7.
[40] Scheuner D, Eckman C, Jensen M, et al. Secreted amyloid beta-protein similar to that in the senile plaques of Alzheimer's disease is increased in vivo by the presenilin 1 and 2 and APP mutations linked to familial Alzheimer's disease. Nat Med 1996;2(8):864–70.
[41] Xia W, Zhang J, Perez R, Koo EH, Selkoe DJ. Interaction between amyloid precursor protein and presenilins in mammalian cells: implications for the pathogenesis of Alzheimer disease. Proc Natl Acad Sci U S A 1997;94(15):8208–13.
[42] De Strooper B. Aph-1, Pen-2, and Nicastrin with Presenilin generate an active gamma-Secretase complex. Neuron Apr 10 2003;38(1):9–12.
[43] Martoglio B, Golde TE. Intramembrane-cleaving aspartic proteases and disease: presenilins, signal peptide peptidase and their homologs. Hum Mol Genet Oct 15 2003;12 Spec No 2: R201–6.
[44] Wolfe MS, Xia W, Ostaszewski BL, Diehl TS, Kimberly WT, Selkoe DJ. Two transmembrane aspartates in presenilin-1 required for presenilin endoproteolysis and gamma-secretase activity [see comments]. Nature 1999;398(6727):513–7.

[45] McGowan E, Pickford F, Kim J, et al. Abeta42 is essential for parenchymal and vascular amyloid deposition in mice. Neuron Jul 21 2005;47(2):191–9.

[46] Funato H, Yoshimura M, Kusui K, et al. Quantitation of amyloid beta-protein (A beta) in the cortex during aging and in Alzheimer's disease. Am J Pathol Jun 1998;152(6):1633–40.

[47] Morishima-Kawashima M, Oshima N, Ogata H, et al. Effect of apolipoprotein E allele epsilon4 on the initial phase of amyloid beta-protein accumulation in the human brain. Am J Pathol Dec 2000;157(6):2093–9.

[48] Scheuner D, Eckman C, Jensen M, et al. Secreted amyloid beta-protein similar to that in the senile plaques of Alzheimer's disease is increased in vivo by the presenilin 1 and 2 and APP mutations linked to familial Alzheimer's disease [see comments]. Nat Med 1996;2(8): 864–70.

[49] Borchelt DR, Thinakaran G, Eckman CB, et al. Familial Alzheimer's disease-linked presenilin 1 variants elevate Abeta1-42/1-40 ratio in vitro and in vivo. Neuron 1996;17(5): 1005–13.

[50] Citron M, Westaway D, Xia W, et al. Mutant presenilins of Alzheimer's disease increase production of 42-residue amyloid beta-protein in both transfected cells and transgenic mice. Nat Med Jan 1997;3(1):67–72.

[51] Blessed G, Tomlinson BE, Roth M. The association between quantitative measures of dementia and of senile change in the cerebral grey matter of elderly subjects. Br J Psychiatry Jul 1968;114(512):797–811.

[52] McKee AC, Kosik KS, Kowall NW. Neuritic pathology and dementia in Alzheimer's disease. Ann Neurol 1991;30(2):156–65.

[53] Nagy Z, Esiri MM, Jobst KA, et al. The effects of additional pathology on the cognitive deficit in Alzheimer disease. J Neuropathol Exp Neurol Feb 1997;56(2):165–70.

[54] Cummings BJ, Pike CJ, Shankle R, Cotman CW. Beta-amyloid deposition and other measures of neuropathology predict cognitive status in Alzheimer's disease [see comments]. Neurobiol Aging 1996;17(6):921–33.

[55] Davis DG, Schmitt FA, Wekstein DR, Markesbery WR. Alzheimer neuropathologic alterations in aged cognitively normal subjects. J Neuropathol Exp Neurol Apr 1999;58(4): 376–88.

[56] Yankner BA, Duffy LK, Kirschner DA. Neurotrophic and neurotoxic effects of amyloid beta protein: reversal by tachykinin neuropeptides. Science 1990;250(4978):279–82.

[57] Pike CJ, Burdick D, Walencewicz AJ, Glabe CG, Cotman CW. Neurodegeneration induced by beta-amyloid peptides in vitro: the role of peptide assembly state. J Neurosci Apr 1993; 13(4):1676–87.

[58] Pike CJ, Walencewicz AJ, Glabe CG, Cotman CW. In vitro aging of beta-amyloid protein causes peptide aggregation and neurotoxicity. Brain Res 1991;563(1–2):311–4.

[59] Geula C, Wu CK, Saroff D, Lorenzo A, Yuan M, Yankner BA. Aging renders the brain vulnerable to amyloid beta-protein neurotoxicity [see comments]. Nat Med 1998;4(7):827–31.

[60] Frautschy SA, Baird A, Cole GM. Effects of injected Alzheimer beta-amyloid cores in rat brain. Proc Natl Acad Sci U S A Oct 1 1991;88(19):8362–6.

[61] Kowall NW, Beal MF, Busciglio J, Duffy LK, Yankner BA. An in vivo model for the neurodegenerative effects of beta amyloid and protection by substance P. Proc Natl Acad Sci U S A Aug 15 1991;88(16):7247–51.

[62] Walsh DM, Lomakin A, Benedek GB, Condron MM, Teplow DB. Amyloid beta-protein fibrillogenesis. Detection of a protofibrillar intermediate. J Biol Chem 1997;272(35): 22364–72.

[63] Klein WL, Stine WB Jr, Teplow DB. Small assemblies of unmodified amyloid beta-protein are the proximate neurotoxin in Alzheimer's disease. Neurobiol Aging May–Jun 2004;25(5): 569–80.

[64] Lambert MP, Barlow AK, Chromy BA, et al. Diffusible, nonfibrillar ligands derived from Abeta1-42 are potent central nervous system neurotoxins. Proc Natl Acad Sci U S A 1998;95(11):6448–53.

[65] Walsh DM, Klyubin I, Fadeeva JV, Rowan MJ, Selkoe DJ. Amyloid-beta oligomers: their production, toxicity and therapeutic inhibition. Biochem Soc Trans Aug 2002;30(4):552–7.

[66] Gong Y, Chang L, Viola KL, et al. Alzheimer's disease-affected brain: presence of oligomeric A beta ligands (ADDLs) suggests a molecular basis for reversible memory loss. Proc Natl Acad Sci U S A Sep 2 2003;100(18):10417–22.

[67] Walsh DM, Klyubin I, Fadeeva JV, et al. Naturally secreted oligomers of amyloid beta protein potently inhibit hippocampal long-term potentiation in vivo. Nature Apr 4 2002; 416(6880):535–9.

[68] Wang HW, Pasternak JF, Kuo H, et al. Soluble oligomers of beta amyloid (1-42) inhibit long-term potentiation but not long-term depression in rat dentate gyrus. Brain Res Jan 11 2002;924(2):133–40.

[69] Lue LF, Kuo YM, Roher AE, et al. Soluble amyloid beta peptide concentration as a predictor of synaptic change in Alzheimer's disease. Am J Pathol Sep 1999;155(3):853–62.

[70] McLean CA, Cherny RA, Fraser FW, et al. Soluble pool of Abeta amyloid as a determinant of severity of neurodegeneration in Alzheimer's disease. Ann Neurol Dec 1999;46(6):860–6.

[71] Jacobsen JS, Wu CC, Redwine JM, et al. Early-onset behavioral and synaptic deficits in a mouse model of Alzheimer's disease. Proc Natl Acad Sci U S A Mar 28 2006;103(13): 5161–6.

[72] Lesne S, Koh MT, Kotilinek L, et al. A specific amyloid-beta protein assembly in the brain impairs memory. Nature Mar 16 2006;440(7082):352–7.

[73] Hsia AY, Masliah E, McConlogue L, et al. Plaque-independent disruption of neural circuits in Alzheimer's disease mouse models. Proc Natl Acad Sci U S A Mar 16 1999;96(6):3228–33.

[74] Comery TA, Martone RL, Aschmies S, et al. Acute gamma-secretase inhibition improves contextual fear conditioning in the Tg2576 mouse model of Alzheimer's disease. J Neurosci Sep 28 2005;25(39):8898–902.

[75] Dodart JC, Bales KR, Gannon KS, et al. Immunization reverses memory deficits without reducing brain Abeta burden in Alzheimer's disease model. Nat Neurosci May 2002;5(5): 452–7.

[76] Kotilinek LA, Bacskai B, Westerman M, et al. Reversible memory loss in a mouse transgenic model of Alzheimer's disease. J Neurosci Aug 1 2002;22(15):6331–5.

[77] Lee EB, Leng LZ, Zhang B, et al. Targeting amyloid-beta peptide (Abeta) oligomers by passive immunization with a conformation-selective monoclonal antibody improves learning and memory in Abeta precursor protein (APP) transgenic mice. J Biol Chem Feb 17 2006; 281(7):4292–9.

[78] McLaurin J, Kierstead ME, Brown ME, et al. Cyclohexanehexol inhibitors of Abeta aggregation prevent and reverse Alzheimer phenotype in a mouse model. Nat Med Jul 2006;12(7): 801–8.

[79] Townsend M, Cleary JP, Mehta T, et al. Orally available compound prevents deficits in memory caused by the Alzheimer amyloid-beta oligomers. Ann Neurol Dec 2006;60(6): 668–76.

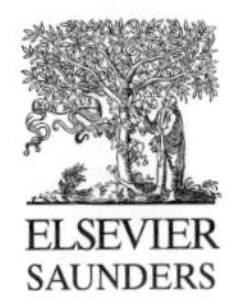

ELSEVIER
SAUNDERS

Neurol Clin 25 (2007) 683–696

NEUROLOGIC
CLINICS

Frontotemporal Lobar Degeneration

Keith A. Josephs, MST, MD

Department of Neurology, Divisions of Behavioral Neurology & Movement Disorders, Mayo Clinic and Mayo Foundation, 200 1st Street S.W., Rochester, MN 55905, USA

Historical perspective

The clinical syndrome associated with frontotemporal lobar degeneration (FTLD) was described first by Arnold Pick in 1892 [1]. It was not until almost 20 years later, however, that the histopathology was described by Alois Alzheimer, in 1911 [2]. He showed an absence of the senile plaques and neurofibrillary tangles that were characteristic of Alzheimer's disease (AD) and rounded inclusions, known today as Pick's bodies, and balloon cells, known today as Pick's cells. Although the term, Pick's disease, first was used to describe lobar atrophy, it now is reserved for one specific type of pathology.

Interest in FTLD waned until the 1980s, when the first diagnostic criteria were proposed by investigators in Lund, Sweden and Manchester, United Kingdom, and the term, frontotemporal dementia (FTD), was used to describe cases of behavioral and language impairment associated with frontal and temporal lobe atrophy [3]. These criteria were refined further by Neary and colleagues in 1998 [4], when the term FTLD was designated to encompass three clinical variants: FTD, characterized by prominent behavioral changes; semantic dementia (SD), characterized by a loss of word meaning; and progressive nonfluent aphasia (PNFA), characterized by agrammatic nonfluent speech. In addition, the term, primary progressive aphasia (PPA), was coined in the United States by Mesulam, in 1982 [5], to describe patients who presented with an isolated language impairment of word usage and comprehension. It now is recognized that there is overlap between PNFA and PPA and between SD and PPA [6]. More recently, there also has been recognition that FTLD can overlap with other well-recognized clinical syndromes, including corticobasal syndrome (CBS) and progressive

KAJ is supported by the NIH Roadmap Multidisciplinary Clinical Research Career Development Award Grant (K12/NICHD)-HD49078 and the Robert H. and Clarice Smith and Abigail Van Buren Alzheimer s Disease Research Program of the Mayo Foundation (Rochester, Minnesota).

E-mail address: josephs.keith@mayo.edu

doi:10.1016/j.ncl.2007.03.005 **_neurologic.theclinics.com_** supranuclear palsy (PSP) [7–10]. The term, Pick complex, was proposed by Kertesz and colleagues to encompass all variants of FTLD, CBS, and PSP [11].

One of the most important developments in the field of FTLD is the recognition that mutations in the tau gene and mutations in the progranulin gene, both located on chromosome 17, cause FTLD. Hutton and colleagues demonstrated that mutations in the microtubule-associated protein tau (MAPT) cause FTLD, with pathologic findings of tau deposition in neurons and glia [12]. Again, Hutton and colleagues demonstrated that mutations in the progranulin gene (*PGRN*) are a cause of FTLD without tau inclusions but with ubiquitin-only immunoreactive inclusions (FTLD-U) [13]. Recently, researchers from the University of Pennsylvania identified the major protein in tau-negative FTLD. This protein, TDP-43, was found in FTLD-U and in cases of motor neuron disease (MND) [14].

Syndromic diagnosis

There are three main clinical variants of FTLD, which are based on consensus statements from an international conference on FTLD [4]. These three syndromes are the behavioral variant of FTD (bvFTD), PNFA, and SD. In addition to these three syndromes, FTLD is linked to CBS, PSP, apraxia of speech (AOS), and MND.

Behavioral variant of frontotemporal dementia

Of all the variants of FTLD, the most common is bvFTD [15], characterized by a significant change in a patient's personality and social behavior and impaired executive function. Patients who have bvFTD usually present with behavioral alterations that are different from their usual personal and social behaviors. These include becoming either more apathetic or more disinhibited. The apathetic patients usually present in a somewhat depressed-like state and lack motivation. These patients also often are hypersomnolent. The disinhibited patients usually present with excessive restlessness, wandering, and socially inappropriate behavior, making, for example, inappropriate conversations in an elevator or in a restaurant with a stranger. Other features of bvFTD include a lack of concern about appearance and a lack of insight into their illness. Increased jocularity, spontaneous giggling or laughter, unusual eating and oral behaviors (for example, gluttony, with cramming food into the mouth and eating nonedible food), hypersexuality, hyper-religiosity, and perseverative and utilization behavior (the need to play with objects that are in visual sight or environment) also can occur. Repetitive behaviors and compulsions may develop later in the disease course, although there are rare occurrences of compulsions being the presenting symptom of bvFTD [16]. For example, one patient who had bvFTD would go to the bathroom to urinate every 5 minutes of each day. Stereotypic behaviors occur in bvFTD, and they take the form of repetitive behaviors, for example rubbing a leg [17]. Paranoia, aggressiveness, selfishness, and lack of empathy can occur. Neuropsychologic testing in patients who have bvFTD may show abnormalities in tests of executive function [18]. Many subjects who have bvFTD may perform normally in neuropsychologic testing, reflecting the insensitivity of test batteries to detect deficits. Language impairment can occur early in the course of the illness in bvFTD but tends to be less prominent than the behavioral features [4]. Parkinsonism occurs in a subset of patients who have bvFTD but tends to be a late feature [19].

Progressive nonfluent aphasia

The second variant of FTLD is PNFA [4]. The characteristic features of PNFA are agrammatism with phonemic paraphasias and anomia, which should be present in isolation during the early stages of the disease. It is common, however, for behavioral abnormalities and executive dysfunction to develop later in the disease course. Patients who have PNFA may have difficulty with comprehension of sentences that syntactically are complex but should have preservation of single-word comprehension. Aphasia can occur in isolation but frequently coexists with AOS (defined later). Agrammatism is defined either as making grammatic errors when speaking, such as the exclusion or incorrect use of articles, propositions, or verbs, or as phonemic paraphasic errors, referring to the transposition of phonemes, which can be prominent particularly when patients are reading, where there can be many phonemic paraphasias, for example, slissors for scissors. Another terminology that overlaps significantly with PNFA is that of PPA, which refers to the presence of isolated language impairment, fluent or nonfluent, for the first 2 years of the disease course [5,20]. One study suggests that a subset of PPA cases has a different pattern of atrophy and may represent a separate syndrome, known as logopenic PPA [21].

Semantic dementia

SD also is referred to as the temporal variant of FTLD [4,22]. In SD there is a progressive loss of word knowledge and meaning, that is, knowledge about objects, facts, and even people. Speech tends to be fluent but may not be meaningful. Comprehension is impaired at the single word level, which differs from PNFA where comprehension is affected at the sentence level. Anomia is prominent; however, the inability to name an object is matched by a patient's inability to give a detailed description of the object. In addition, patients who have SD have a significant visual associative agnosia (impaired object recognition) and, therefore, may not be able to recognize objects that are presented visually [23]. Therefore, word-picture matching tasks are performed poorly. Food preferences and preoccupation with crossword puzzles are common. There is evidence of a surface dyslexia when reading (incorrect pronunciation of orthographically irregular words, for example, yacht is pronounced ya-ch). The majority of cases of SD show temporal lobe atrophy, although on careful inspection the atrophy tends to be asymmetric, more frequently affecting the left than the right temporal lobe [22]. When the right temporal lobe is affected more severely than the left, the presenting features tend to be different from those typically seen in patients who have left-sided atrophy. In the patients who have more right-sided atrophy, prosopagnosia (impaired facial recognition) and geographic disorientation are present, and patients tend to have behavioral abnormalities, including social awkwardness and rudeness.

Corticobasal syndrome

CBS [24] is linked with FTLD, because patients who have CBS can evolve and develop behavioral features, personality changes, and executive dysfunction similar to those observed in bvFTD [9]. This syndrome is characterized by asymmetric cortical (apraxia, cortical sensory loss, or myoclonic jerks) and basal ganglia (bradykinesia, rigidity, tremor, or dystonia) features [24]. Rarely, patients may develop an alien limb phenomenon, in which there are involuntary movements and personification of the limb. Symptoms do not respond to levodopa treatment. CBS may develop in patients who initially had features most characteristic of bvFTD and is even more likely to develop in patients who present initially with PNFA [9]. There also is significant overlap between CBS and PSP. Initially, CBS was believed specific to corticobasal degeneration pathology; however, studies demonstrate that CBS is nonspecific and can occur as a result of any one of several pathologies (discussed later) [25].

Progressive supranuclear palsy

PSP, or Steele-Richardson-Olszewski syndrome, is characterized by early falls, vertical (especially down) gaze, supranuclear palsy, axial greater than appendicular rigidity, and levodopa resistance [26]. Behavior and personality changes are less common and less severe than in CBS. Neuropsychologic testing demonstrates some mild-to-moderate frontal lobe deficiencies. Patients may present with a nonfluent aphasia with prominent AOS and only very late in the disease course show signs characteristic of PSP [27,28]. These patients tend to have PSP pathology. There also are reports of an overlap syndrome between PSP and upper MND [29].

Motor neuron disease

MND is defined as any evidence of pyramidal tract degeneration or anterior horn cell disease. MND can be isolated to the pyramidal tract (upper MND), anterior horn cells (lower MND), or mixed (amyotrophic lateral sclerosis [ALS]). MND infrequently coexists with FTLD. This occurs most frequently with bvFTD and infrequently is reported to coexist with PNFA and SD. Typically in these cases there are findings of lower MND or mixed upper and lower MND [30]. Pathology in these cases almost always shows evidence of lobar degeneration and MND. Not all pathologically confirmed cases show evidence of clinical MND, however [30]. Clinical studies have identified a higher than expected frequency of MND in subjects who have FTLD; conversely, a high frequency of frontal lobe dysfunction on neuropsychologic tests has been observed in subjects who have MND [31,32].

Apraxia of speech

AOS also is referred to as speech apraxia, aphemia, and phonetic disintegration. It is defined as a motor speech disorder with a slow speaking rate, abnormal prosody, and distorted sound substitutions, repetitions, and prolongations, at times accompanied by groping. It is common to lump AOS under the heading of PNFA in neurodegenerative diseases; however, AOS can occur in the absence of aphasia and is considered a separate syndrome by some researchers [27]. Imaging studies have identified specific anatomic correlates of AOS, distinct from those observed in PNFA [27]. Clinicopathologic studies suggest that the presence of AOS is specific to tau biochemistry [27].

Ancillary testing

Routine blood tests

Patients presenting with an FTLD syndrome should undergo routine blood tests. These include a complete blood count, electrolytes including sodium, potassium and chloride, calcium, phosphate thyroid function studies, liver function tests, and renal function tests to rule out systemic illnesses causing a dementia. In very young patients, especially when there is diagnostic uncertainty, more elaborate testing may be required for diagnosis. Some of these tests may include screening for metabolic, genetic, and autoimmune disorders.

Cerebrospinal fluid

Cerebrospinal fluid studies in FTLD are useful to exclude other causes of dementia. In the majority of cases of FTLD, there can be elevated protein; however, the rest of the profile tends to be within normal limits. Oligoclonal bands are not present. Recent studies have investigated the diagnostic usefulness of tau, amyloid beta 42, and neurofilament. Phosphorylated tau protein is reported to be elevated [33] but also reported to be normal [34]. Total tau levels are reported to be low [34] or normal [35]. Some researchers suggest that a combination of cerebrospinal fluid tau and amyloid beta 42 may help differentiate FTLD from AD [36]. Reports aiming to differentiate AD from FTLD by measuring neurofilament proteins have been conducted [35,37] but need to be validated.

Electroencephalogram

An electroencephalogram (EEG) often is performed as part of the clinical evaluation in FTLD. An EEG also is important to rule out other causes of dementia, for example, transient epileptic phenomena. There are, however, no specific EEG findings in FTLD and recently it was shown that there are no EEG abnormalities that are useful in differentiating FTLD from AD [38].

Neuroimaging

Patients show atrophy and hypometabolism of the frontal and temporal cortices, which match the pathologic findings. The occipital lobe almost always is spared, although the parietal lobe can be affected, especially in subjects who present with PNFA or CBS. The presence of frontal and anterior temporal lobe abnormalities on brain imaging is part of the diagnostic criteria for FTLD [4]. There are patients who have FTLD, however, who, even after more than 10 years of illness duration, may show little atrophy [39]. There are characteristic patterns of atrophy that are suggested for each of the syndromic variants of FTLD and their related disorders. Subjects presenting with bvFTD usually show symmetric frontal lobe atrophy (Fig. 1), although asymmetric right-sided atrophy has been reported [40]. Studies using automated image analysis techniques have allowed a more detailed assessment of patterns of atrophy and have shown atrophy in a network of limbic areas that likely are involved in the fine tuning of behavior, including the ventromedial cortex, anterior cingulate cortex, and amygdala [41,42]. It seems to be becoming clearer, however, that subjects who have frontal lobe features suggestive of bvFTD also could have right temporal lobe atrophy. Functional imaging studies show hypometabolism (Fig. 2) or hypoperfusion in the same anatomic regions.

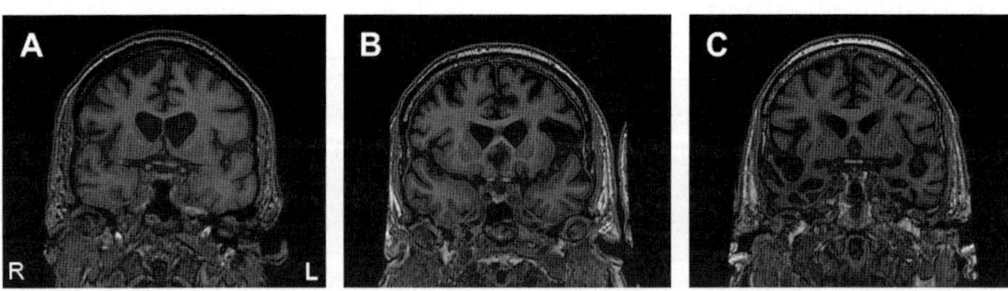

Fig. 1. Coronal T1-weighted MRI scans demonstrating frontal and caudate atrophy in a patient who has behavioral changes and a diagnosis of bvFTD (*A*); left perisylvian atrophy in another patient who has nonfluent speech and a diagnosis of PNFA (*B*); and right greater than left anterior temporal lobe atrophy in a patient who has loss of facial recognition and word meaning and a diagnosis of right temporal variant of SD (*C*).

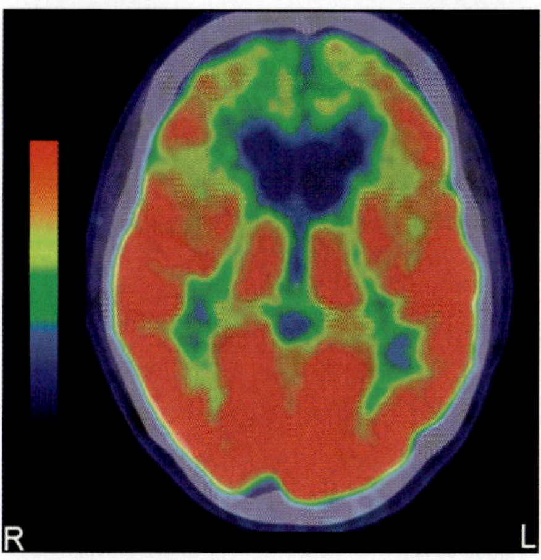

Fig. 2. F18-fluorodeoxyglucose–positive emission tomography scan demonstrating predominant frontal and some temporal lobe hypometabolism in a patient who has personality changes and a diagnosis of bvFTD.

In contrast, patients who have SD show atrophy and hypometabolism predominantly in the left anterior temporal lobe. Patients may present, however, with more right temporal lobe atrophy (see Fig. 1). Practically all left temporal lobe regions can be involved, with particularly severe atrophy in inferior temporal regions, including the fusiform and inferior temporal gyrus, with relative sparing of the superior temporal gyrus [43,44]. Atrophy affects the hippocampus and amygdala significantly [43]. There also often is involvement of the ventromedial and superior frontal lobes, which is consistent with patients who have SD often developing behavioral abnormalities. There also is evidence that as the disease progresses the atrophy can extend from the left anterior temporal lobe to involve more posterior temporal regions, the inferior frontal lobe, and the right anterior temporal lobe [45].

Unlike in SD, patients who have PNFA consistently show left frontal and perisylvian atrophy on MRI (see Fig. 1), with hypoperfusion and hypometabolism demonstrated in the same regions on functional imaging. In those who have become mute, a pattern of atrophy affecting the left perisylvian region and extending into the left basal ganglia has been demonstrated [46].

Imaging studies have been completed in other syndromic variants associated with FTLD. Posterior frontal and superior parietal atrophy is associated with CBS [47,48], whereas those who have PSP show areas of subcortical atrophy affecting the superior cerebellar peduncle and midbrain [48,49]. The anterior-posterior diameter of the midbrain is reduced [50], giving the so-called "face of Mickey mouse" appearance. Patients who have AOS show atrophy of the supplemental motor area and superior posterior frontal lobe [27]. The logopenic variant of PPA was reported to be associated with left posterior temporal and inferior parietal lobule atrophy [51].

Subjects who present with prosopagnosia have shown predominantly right temporal lobe atrophy (see Fig. 1). This pattern of atrophy also can be seen in patients who present with predominant behavior features and in those who have prominent geographic disorientation.

Recent studies suggest that the pathologic subtypes of FTLD also may have characteristic imaging findings. Patients who have FTLD-U (defined later) are shown to have predominant atrophy of the temporal lobes, particularly in posterior gyri, and some involvement of the frontal lobes, whereas patients who have FTLD-MND (defined later) show patterns of atrophy relatively restricted to the frontal lobes [52]. Patients who have Pick's disease show severe involvement of the frontal lobes [53].

Pathology

The gross pathologic findings in FTLD are similar to MRI findings in FTLD. There is atrophy affecting the frontal and temporal lobes (Fig. 3) and in some cases the parietal lobes. The occipital lobes almost always are spared. The frontal, temporal, and parietal lobes all can be affected; however, it is most common to find varying degrees of atrophy in each region, at times correlating with the presenting syndromes. Histologic diagnosis in FTLD, however, is heterogenous [54]. The presence or absence of tau-positive inclusions is used to simplify the classification and to determine if the case is reported as a tauopathy (tau-positive inclusions are the major findings) or a non-tauopathy (tau-positive inclusions are minor or absent). The major diagnostic tauopathies that underlie FTLD are corticobasal degeneration, progressive supranuclear palsy (PSP), and Pick's disease. They all differ by the distribution of the pathology and the morphologic features of the tau-positive inclusions. Corticobasal degeneration originally was believed associated only with the CBS; however, it has been found to underlie many other syndromes, especially PNFA [55]. And although PSP originally

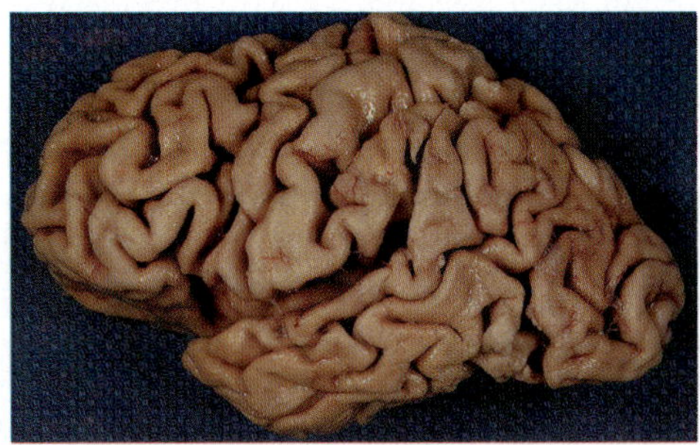

Fig. 3. On gross pathology there is severe frontal lobe atrophy with preserved primary motor and sensory cortex in a patient who had personality changes and executive dysfunction and a diagnosis of bvFTD. (*Courtesy of* Dr. Dennis W. Dickson, Jacksonville, FL.)

was associated with the clinical syndrome of early falls, parkinsonism, and supranuclear gaze palsy, recent evidence has shown that PSP pathology can be found in subjects who have PNFA, especially when AOS also is present [27]. Pick's disease is less common than PSP and corticobasal degeneration in FTLD pathologic studies [7–10].

The two major non-tauopathies include those that have FTLD-U and those that have FTLD-MND. The former, FTLD-U, is the most common pathology that underlies FTLD [56,57]. In addition, FTLD-U is the most common pathology in the SD variant of FTLD [8,58]. There are many different terminologies that have been used to describe this pathology (Box 1) and the presence of intranuclear inclusions in FTLD-U is associated with familial FTLD and may suggest a mutation in the PGRN gene [59]. Similar to the terminologies that define FTLD-U, many terminologies define FTLD-MND (see Box 1). Unlike in FTLD-U where there is no evidence of MND, FTLD-MND is characterized by pathologic findings of MND. When there is clinical evidence of MND, pathologic diagnosis of FTLD-MND is shown to be 100% sensitive [8]. A recent discovery is the identification that a protein, TDP-43, may be the major component of neuronal inclusions in FTLD-U and FTLD-MND; however, this remains to be validated [14]. Two other non-tauopathies worth mentioning are neurofilament inclusion body disease [60] and dementia lacking distinctive histology, which

Box 1. Other pathologic terminologies

FTLD-U

- MND inclusion dementia
- Dementia of MND type
- Dementia with ubiquitin inclusion bodies
- Dementia with inclusions tau and synuclein-negative, ubiquitinated (ITSNU)
- Dementia with ubiquitinated inclusions
- Pick complex with ITSNU
- Dementia with ubiquitinated tau-negative noneosinophilic inclusions

FTLD-MND

- Pick's disease with ALS
- FTD with MND
- MND-type dementia
- Dementia with MND
- Dementia with ALS
- ALS with dementia
- Presenile dementia with MND
- Aphasic dementia and MND

is characterized by neuronal loss and gliosis affecting frontal and temporal cortex but absence of any intraneuronal inclusions [19].

Genetics

A positive family history of dementia occurs in approximately 40% of patients who have FTLD. In the majority of these families, the pattern of inheritance is autosomal dominant. Genetic studies have identified a locus on chromosome 9q and genes on chromosome 3p and 17q. The first gene to be identified and linked to familial FTLD was the MAPT gene (*MAPT*) located on chromosome 17 [12]. Resulting from a consensus conference in 1996, cases linked to tau on chromosome 17q21 were termed, "frontotemporal dementia with parkinsonism linked to chromosome 17 (FTDP-17) [12]." To date, approximately 35 different confirmed mutations in *MAPT* have been identified in more than 100 families. Pathologically, patients who have FTLD and *MAPT* mutations reveal tau-positive inclusions. The second gene to be linked with FTLD is the charged multivesicular body protein, also known as chromatin-modifying protein 2B (*CHMP2B*) [61]. This gene has been linked to a family from the Jutland region of Denmark, and initially believed associated with dementia lacking distinctive histology pathology. Recent re-evaluation of some of the subjects from this family, however, have identified ubiquitin-positive inclusions. Mutations in *CHMP2B*, however, are a rare cause of FTLD and were not identified in 141 familial probands from the United States and United Kingdom [62]. The most recently identified gene that causes FTLD is *PGRN* [13,63]. Mutations in the gene, *PGRN*, are more common than the other two mutations. Mutations in *PGRN* are reported to account for approximately 10% of subjects who have FTLD and 25% of those who have a positive family history of dementia [64]. Pathologic diagnosis in subjects who have a *PGRN* mutation consistently is found to be FTLD-U without any evidence of MND [59,65]. Clinical studies suggest that patients who have *PGRN* mutation have more frequent parkinsonism and language impairment than subjects who do not have the mutation. Imaging and pathologic studies suggest that subjects who have FTLD-U and a *PGRN* mutation have a more severe pattern of atrophy, particularly affecting the frontal and parietal lobes, than FTLD-U subjects who do not have *PGRN* mutations [66]. FTLD-MND has been linked to chromosome 9p in two large families [65,67]. Rarely, FTLD is associated with a muscle disease and Paget's disease of the bone. Mutation in the *valosin-containing protein* (*VCP*) gene, on chromosome 9, is the cause [68].

Treatment

Pharmacologic treatment for FTLD is limited to addressing behavioral dyscontrol. These studies have focused mainly on drugs with serotonergic modulated properties. Treatment trials using serotonin reuptake inhibitors have had, at best, modest effects [69,70].

Although there are no specific pharmacologic treatments for aphasia, many patients may benefit from speech therapy, which aids in their ability to communicate with family and friends. Because speech therapy may be more beneficial for certain aspects of the language impairment, proper syndromic diagnosis and recognition of important signs and symptoms, especially dysarthria, that accompany the aphasia, is important.

Summary

FTLD is a syndromic diagnosis that includes at least three different syndromes: bvFTD, SD, and PNFA. There is significant overlap between FTLD, PSP, CBS, AOS, and MND, suggesting possible common etiopathogenesis. Imaging modalities are helpful in differentiating FTLD from other causes of dementia and usually show a pattern of frontotemporal and parietal abnormalities, depending on which syndrome is the most prominent. Pathology remains the gold standard for definitive diagnosis but is heterogeneous. The most common pathology has been identified as FTLD-U. Recent studies have demonstrated that mutations in the gene, *PGRN*, are associated with FTLD-U pathology. Three additional genes associated with FTLD are *MAPT*, *CHMP2B*, and *VCP*. A genetic loci has been mapped to chromosome 9p in families in which FTLD and MND overlap. Treatment in FTLD is at best modest.

Acknowledgments

The author would like to acknowledge Dr. Jennifer L. Whitwell for critical review and aid with manuscript preparation.

References

[1] Pick A. Uber die Beziehungen der senilen Hirantropie zur aphasie [German]. Prager Medizinishe Wochenscrift 1892;17:165–7.

[2] Alzheimer A. Uber eigenartige Krankheitsfalle des spateren Alters [German]. Zeitscrift fur die Gesamte Neurologie und Psychiatrie 1911;4:356–85.

[3] Brun A. Clinical and neuropathological criteria for frontotemporal dementia. The Lund and Manchester Groups. J Neurol Neurosurg Psychiatr 1994;57:416–8.

[4] Neary D, Snowden JS, Gustafson L, et al. Frontotemporal lobar degeneration: a consensus on clinical diagnostic criteria. Neurology 1998;51:1546–54.

[5] Mesulam MM. Slowly progressive aphasia without generalized dementia. Ann Neurol 1982; 11:592–8.

[6] Adlam AL, Patterson K, Rogers TT, et al. Semantic dementia and fluent primary progressive aphasia: two sides of the same coin? Brain 2006;129:3066–80.

[7] Hodges JR, Davies RR, Xuereb JH, et al. Clinicopathological correlates in frontotemporal dementia. Ann Neurol 2004;56:399–406.

[8] Josephs KA, Petersen RC, Knopman DS, et al. Clinicopathologic analysis of frontotemporal and corticobasal degenerations and PSP. Neurology 2006;66:41–8.

[9] Kertesz A, McMonagle P, Blair M, et al. The evolution and pathology of frontotemporal dementia. Brain 2005;128:1996–2005.
[10] Forman MS, Farmer J, Johnson JK, et al. Frontotemporal dementia: clinicopathological correlations. Ann Neurol 2006;59:952–62.
[11] Kertesz A, Hudson L, Mackenzie IR, et al. The pathology and nosology of primary progressive aphasia. Neurology 1994;44:2065–72.
[12] Hutton M, Lendon CL, Rizzu P, et al. Association of missense and 5′-splice-site mutations in tau with the inherited dementia FTDP-17. Nature 1998;393:702–5.
[13] Baker M, Mackenzie IR, Pickering-Brown SM, et al. Mutations in progranulin cause tau-negative frontotemporal dementia linked to chromosome 17. Nature 2006;442:916–9.
[14] Neumann M, Sampathu DM, Kwong LK, et al. Ubiquitinated TDP-43 in frontotemporal lobar degeneration and amyotrophic lateral sclerosis. Science 2006;314:130–3.
[15] Johnson JK, Diehl J, Mendez MF, et al. Frontotemporal lobar degeneration: demographic characteristics of 353 patients. Arch Neurol 2005;62:925–30.
[16] Mendez MF, Perryman KM, Miller BL, et al. Compulsive behaviors as presenting symptoms of frontotemporal dementia. J Geriatr Psychiatry Neurol 1997;10:154–7.
[17] Mendez MF, Shapira JS, Miller BL. Stereotypical movements and frontotemporal dementia. Mov Disord 2005;20:742–5.
[18] Johanson A, Hagberg B. Psychometric characteristics in patients with frontal lobe degeneration of non-Alzheimer type. Arch Gerontol Geriatr 1989;8:129–37.
[19] Knopman DS, Mastri AR, Frey WH 2nd, et al. Dementia lacking distinctive histologic features: a common non-Alzheimer degenerative dementia. Neurology 1990;40:251–6.
[20] Mesulam MM. Primary progressive aphasia. Ann Neurol 2001;49:425–32.
[21] Gorno-Tempini ML, Dronkers NF, Rankin KP, et al. Cognition and anatomy in three variants of primary progressive aphasia. Ann Neurol 2004;55:335–46.
[22] Thompson SA, Patterson K, Hodges JR. Left/right asymmetry of atrophy in semantic dementia: behavioral-cognitive implications. Neurology 2003;61:1196–203.
[23] Snowden JS. Semantic dementia: a form of circumscribed cerebral atrophy. Behav Neurol 1989;2:167–82.
[24] Boeve BF, Lang AE, Litvan I. Corticobasal degeneration and its relationship to progressive supranuclear palsy and frontotemporal dementia. Ann Neurol 2003;54(Suppl 5):S15–9.
[25] Boeve BF, Maraganore DM, Parisi JE, et al. Pathologic heterogeneity in clinically diagnosed corticobasal degeneration. Neurology 1999;53:795–800.
[26] Litvan I, Agid Y, Calne D, et al. Clinical research criteria for the diagnosis of progressive supranuclear palsy (Steele-Richardson-Olszewski syndrome): report of the NINDS-SPSP international workshop. Neurology 1996;47:1–9.
[27] Josephs KA, Duffy JR, Strand EA, et al. Clinicopathological and imaging correlates of progressive aphasia and apraxia of speech. Brain 2006;129:1385–98.
[28] Josephs KA, Boeve BF, Duffy JR, et al. Atypical progressive supranuclear palsy underlying progressive apraxia of speech and nonfluent aphasia. Neurocase 2005;11:283–96.
[29] Josephs KA, Katsuse O, Beccano-Kelly DA, et al. Atypical progressive supranuclear palsy with corticospinal tract degeneration. J Neuropathol Exp Neurol 2006;65:396–405.
[30] Josephs KA, Parisi JE, Knopman DS, et al. Clinically undetected motor neuron disease in pathologically proven frontotemporal lobar degeneration with motor neuron disease. Arch Neurol 2006;63:506–12.
[31] Lomen-Hoerth C, Anderson T, Miller B. The overlap of amyotrophic lateral sclerosis and frontotemporal dementia. Neurology 2002;59:1077–9.
[32] Lomen-Hoerth C, Murphy J, Langmore S, et al. Are amyotrophic lateral sclerosis patients cognitively normal? Neurology 2003;60:1094–7.
[33] Arai H, Morikawa Y, Higuchi M, et al. Cerebrospinal fluid tau levels in neurodegenerative diseases with distinct tau-related pathology. Biochem Biophys Res Commun 1997;236:262–4.
[34] Grossman M, Farmer J, Leight S, et al. Cerebrospinal fluid profile in frontotemporal dementia and Alzheimer's disease. Ann Neurol 2005;57:721–9.

[35] Sjogren M, Minthon L, Davidsson P, et al. CSF levels of tau, beta-amyloid(1-42) and GAP-43 in frontotemporal dementia, other types of dementia and normal aging. J Neural Transm 2000;107:563–79.
[36] Riemenschneider M, Wagenpfeil S, Diehl J, et al. Tau and Abeta42 protein in CSF of patients with frontotemporal degeneration. Neurology 2002;58:1622–8.
[37] Rosengren LE, Karlsson JE, Sjogren M, et al. Neurofilament protein levels in CSF are increased in dementia. Neurology 1999;52:1090–3.
[38] Chan D, Walters RJ, Sampson EL, et al. EEG abnormalities in frontotemporal lobar degeneration. Neurology 2004;62:1628–30.
[39] Josephs K, Whitwell JL, Jack CR Jr, et al. Frontotemporal lobar degeneration without lobar atrophy. Arch Neurol 2006;63:1632–8.
[40] Fukui T, Kertesz A. Volumetric study of lobar atrophy in Pick complex and Alzheimer's disease. J Neurol Sci 2000;174:111–21.
[41] Boccardi M, Sabattoli F, Laakso MP, et al. Frontotemporal dementia as a neural system disease. Neurobiol Aging 2005;26:37–44.
[42] Rosen HJ, Gorno-Tempini ML, Goldman WP, et al. Patterns of brain atrophy in frontotemporal dementia and semantic dementia. Neurology 2002;58:198–208.
[43] Chan D, Fox NC, Scahill RI, et al. Patterns of temporal lobe atrophy in semantic dementia and Alzheimer's disease [see comment]. Ann Neurol 2001;49:433–42.
[44] Mummery CJ, Patterson K, Price CJ, et al. A voxel-based morphometry study of semantic dementia: relationship between temporal lobe atrophy and semantic memory. Ann Neurol 2000;47:36–45.
[45] Whitwell JL, Anderson VM, Scahill RI, et al. Longitudinal patterns of regional change on volumetric MRI in frontotemporal lobar degeneration. Dement Geriatr Cogn Disord 2004;17:307–10.
[46] Gorno-Tempini ML, Ogar JM, Brambati SM, et al. Anatomical correlates of early mutism in progressive nonfluent aphasia. Neurology 2006;67:1849–51.
[47] Boxer AL, Geschwind MD, Belfor N, et al. Patterns of brain atrophy that differentiate corticobasal degeneration syndrome from progressive supranuclear palsy. Arch Neurol 2006;63:81–6.
[48] Josephs K, Whitwell JL, Dickson D, et al. Voxel-based morphometry in autopsy proven PSP and CBD. Neurobiol Aging 2006; Epub.
[49] Paviour DC, Price SL, Stevens JM, et al. Quantitative MRI measurement of superior cerebellar peduncle in progressive supranuclear palsy. Neurology 2005;64:675–9.
[50] Righini A, Antonini A, De Notaris R, et al. MR imaging of the superior profile of the midbrain: differential diagnosis between progressive supranuclear palsy and Parkinson disease. AJNR Am J Neuroradiol 2004;25:927–32.
[51] Gorno-Tempini ML, Rankin KP, Woolley JD, et al. Cognitive and behavioral profile in a case of right anterior temporal lobe neurodegeneration. Cortex 2004;40:631–44.
[52] Whitwell JL, Jack CR Jr, Senjem ML, et al. Patterns of atrophy in pathologically confirmed FTLD with and without motor neuron degeneration. Neurology 2006;66:102–4.
[53] Whitwell JL, Josephs KA, Rossor MN, et al. Magnetic resonance imaging signatures of tissue pathology in frontotemporal dementia. Arch Neurol 2005;62:1402–8.
[54] McKhann GM, Albert MS, Grossman M, et al. Clinical and pathological diagnosis of frontotemporal dementia: report of the Work Group on Frontotemporal Dementia and Pick's Disease. Arch Neurol 2001;58:1803–9.
[55] McMonagle P, Blair M, Kertesz A. Corticobasal degeneration and progressive aphasia. Neurology 2006;67:1444–51.
[56] Josephs KA, Holton JL, Rossor MN, et al. Frontotemporal lobar degeneration and ubiquitin immunohistochemistry. Neuropathol Appl Neurobiol 2004;30:369–73.
[57] Lipton AM, White CL 3rd, Bigio EH. Frontotemporal lobar degeneration with motor neuron disease-type inclusions predominates in 76 cases of frontotemporal degeneration. Acta Neuropathol (Berl) 2004;108:379–85.

[58] Knibb JA, Xuereb JH, Patterson K, et al. Clinical and pathological characterization of progressive aphasia. Ann Neurol 2006;59:156–65.

[59] Josephs K, Ahmed Z, Katsuse O, et al. Neuropathological features of progranulin gene (PGRN) mutations. 2007, submitted for publication.

[60] Josephs KA, Holton JL, Rossor MN, et al. Neurofilament inclusion body disease: a new proteinopathy? Brain 2003;126:2291–303.

[61] Skibinski G, Parkinson NJ, Brown JM, et al. Mutations in the endosomal ESCRTIII-complex subunit CHMP2B in frontotemporal dementia. Nat Genet 2005;37:806–8.

[62] Cannon A, Baker M, Boeve B, et al. CHMP2B mutations are not a common cause of frontotemporal lobar degeneration. Neurosci Lett 2006;398:83–4.

[63] Cruts M, Gijselinck I, van der Zee J, et al. Null mutations in progranulin cause ubiquitin-positive frontotemporal dementia linked to chromosome 17q21. Nature 2006;442:920–4.

[64] Gass J, Cannon A, Mackenzie IR, et al. Mutations in progranulin are a major cause of ubiquitin-positive frontotemporal lobar degeneration. Hum Mol Genet 2006;15:2988–3001.

[65] Morita M, Al-Chalabi A, Andersen PM, et al. A locus on chromosome 9p confers susceptibility to ALS and frontotemporal dementia. Neurology 2006;66:839–44.

[66] Whitwell JL, Jack CR Jr, Siung M, et al. Voxel based morphometry in progranulin gene (PGRN) mutations. Arch Neurol 2007, in press.

[67] Vance C, Al-Chalabi A, Ruddy D, et al. Familial amyotrophic lateral sclerosis with frontotemporal dementia is linked to a locus on chromosome 9p13.2-21.3. Brain 2006;129:868–76.

[68] Watts GD, Wymer J, Kovach MJ, et al. Inclusion body myopathy associated with Paget disease of bone and frontotemporal dementia is caused by mutant valosin-containing protein. Nat Genet 2004;36:377–81.

[69] Moretti R, Torre P, Antonello RM, et al. Frontotemporal dementia: paroxetine as a possible treatment of behavior symptoms. A randomized, controlled, open 14-month study. Eur Neurol 2003;49:13–9.

[70] Lebert F, Stekke W, Hasenbroekx C, et al. Frontotemporal dementia: a randomised, controlled trial with trazodone. Dement Geriatr Cogn Disord 2004;17:355–9.

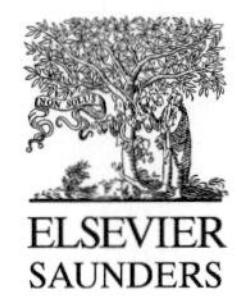

ELSEVIER
SAUNDERS

Neurol Clin 25 (2007) 697–715

NEUROLOGIC
CLINICS

The Genetics of Frontotemporal Dementia

Kristoffer Haugarvoll, MD[a,b,c],
Zbigniew K. Wszolek, MD[b],
Michael Hutton, PhD[a,*]

[a]*Department of Neuroscience, Mayo Clinic College of Medicine, Birdsall Building, 4500 San Pablo Road, Jacksonville, FL 32224, USA*
[b]*Department of Neurology, Mayo Clinic College of Medicine, Cannaday Building, 2E, 4500 San Pablo Road, Jacksonville, FL 32224, USA*
[c]*Department of Neuroscience, NTNU—Norwegian University of Science and Technology MTFS, 7489, Trondheim, Norway*

Last scene of all,
That ends this strange eventful history,
Is second childishness and mere oblivion,
sans teeth, sans eyes, sans taste, sans everything.
From 'As You Like It' by William Shakespeare

Frontotemporal dementia (FTD) (OMIM #60027) is a devastating, midlife- to late-onset disorder characterized by profound alteration in behavior and social conduct. Language impairment, parkinsonism, and amyotrophy also frequently are present . A family history is reported in approximately 35% to 50% of patients. FTD frequently segregates as an autosomal dominant trait. Recently, mutations in the progranulin gene (*PGRN*) (OMIM *138945) were shown to cause FTD. A decade earlier, mutations in the microtubule-associated protein tau gene (*MAPT*) (OMIM +157140) were found to cause FTD. Both these genes are located in close proximity, within 2 megabases (Mb) on chromosome 17q21. Other genes, such as the chromatin-modifying protein 2B gene (*CHMP2B*) (OMIM +609512) and the valosin-containing protein gene (*VCP*) (OMIM 601023), also are implicated in rare autosomal dominant FTD. This article emphasizes the clinical

KH received support from Forsbergs and Aulies legacy. Mayo Clinic Jacksonville is a M. K. Udall Parkinson's Disease Research Center of Excellence (National Institute of Neurological Disorders and Stroke grant P01 NS40256).

* Corresponding author.
E-mail address: hutton.michael@mayo.edu (M. Hutton).

doi:10.1016/j.ncl.2007.03.002 ***neurologic.theclinics.com***

and neuropathologic features of frontotemporal dementia with parkinsonism linked to chromosome 17 (FTDP-17) and the nature of the mutations in *PGRN* and *MAPT*. The work on FTDP-17 over the past 10 years serves as an example of how genetics can be used to understand heterogeneous conditions, such as FTD.

Frontotemporal dementia is a heterogeneous clinical syndrome

Frontotemporal lobar degeneration (FTLD) represents the pathologic correlate to a heterogeneous group of clinical syndromes displaying circumscribed atrophy of the prefrontal and anterior temporal lobes. FTD is the most common syndrome within this group. Two others are primary progressive aphasia and semantic dementia [1,2]. These syndromes display a significant clinical and pathologic overlap. Together, this group of neurodegenerative diseases accounts for 5% to 10% of all patients who have dementia and 10% to 20% of patients who have onset before 65 years [3]. Two other tauopathies, progressive supranuclear palsy (PSP) (OMIM #601104) and corticobasal degeneration (CBD), share clinical features with FTLD and have overlapping neuropathologic findings [4]. FTD is characterized by early disturbance of behavior and personality and language impairment, followed by cognitive decline, eventually leading to dementia. FTD may be associated with parkinsonism [5,6] or Paget disease of bone [7]. In 10% to 15% of cases, clinical features of FTD and motor neuron disease (MND) are present [8–10].

The association of MND with dementia, the dementia being of the frontotemporal type, increasingly is recognized [11]. Moreover, it is reported that patients who have classical MND score poorly on tests of frontal lobe function and, using single photon emission CT (SPECT), have a reduced regional cerebral blood flow in the frontal and anterior temporal regions compared with controls [12,13]. A similar SPECT pattern also is observed with FTD-MND and FTD alone. Talbot and colleagues [13] suggested that "classic MND, FTD-MND and FTD represent a clinical range of a pathological continuum." Evdokimidis and colleagues [14] reported that one third of their MND cohort of 51 patients had frontal lobe dysfunction. Collectively, therefore, there is strong evidence of a frontal lobe involvement in MND and, given the recent linkage to chromosome 9 in families who have MND, FTD-MND, and FTD, it is highly likely that a disease spectrum exists [15–18].

Neuropathology of frontotemporal dementia

Neuropathology in FTD cases reveals bilateral atrophy of the frontal and anterior temporal lobes and degeneration of the striatum [8,19]; microscopic

Table 1
Clinical and pathologic features observed in *PGRN* and *MAPT* mutation carriers

	FTDP-17 (*PGRN*)	FTDP-17 (*MAPT*)
Mean age at onset, years	59 (range, 48–83)	49 (range, 25–76)
Presenting clinical symptom	Personality/behavioral changes, language impairment	Personality/behavioral changes, language impairment, or parkinsonism
Mean disease duration, years	7 (range, 2–17)	7 (range, 2–30)
Additional signs present during the disease course	Cognitive impairment (+++)	Cognitive impairment (+++)
	Parkinsonism (++) Motor neuron dysfunction (+)	Parkinsonism (+++)
Treatments	Levodopa might have temporary effect on parkinsonism (?)	Levodopa might have temporary effect on parkinsonism
Pathology	FTLD with of loss of large cortical neurons Microvacuolation (+++) Gliosis (+) Ub-ir/TDP-43–positive NII and NCI	FTLD with of loss of large cortical neurons Microvacuolation (+) Gliosis (+++) Tau-immunoreactive inclusions in neurons or in neurons and glia

Abbreviations: +, mildly severe; ++, moderately severe; +++, severe.

findings are of two main types (Table 1) [19]. In approximately 50% of FTD cases (microvacuolar type) histopathology is characterized by loss of large cortical neurons and microvacuolation of the neuropil in the superficial cortical layers [8]. Gliosis is minimal and generally there are no distinctive changes (swellings or inclusions) in remaining neurons. The limbic system and striatum are affected mildly. It is becoming increasingly clear that the vast majority of these cases also have varying degrees of cortical ubiquitin-positive neuronal inclusions. A major component of these inclusions recently was shown to be the nuclear protein, TAR DNA-binding protein–43 (TDP-43) [20]. In a proportion of these cases, microvacuolar change is accompanied by histologic features of MND, including anterior horn and bulbar cell loss and ubiquitin/TDP-43–positive inclusions in these regions and in layer 2 of the cortex and the dentate gyrus of the hippocampus [8,11,21,22]. Significantly, recent work shows that some cases of idiopathic amyotrophic lateral sclerosis (ALS) also develops inclusions composed primarily of TDP-43. This provides strong evidence that, as long suspected, this form of FTD and ALS likely is part of the same disease spectrum. Additional studies are required, however, to determine if the mechanism of neurodegeneration requires the accumulation and aggregation of abnormal TDP-43 or if this simply is a marker of a common disease process.

The second form of histopathology (tau-positive type) is observed in a similar proportion of cases and is characterized by loss of large cortical neurons with associated gliosis but minimal microvacuolation. The limbic system and striatum show prominent degeneration in this histopathology type. tTau-positive swollen neurons and, more rarely, spherical inclusions (Pick's bodies) are present [23–25]. Pick's bodies generally contain tau isoforms with three microtubule-binding repeats (3R-tau) [26,27]. More commonly, however, tau-positive FTD cases have features that overlap with CBD and have tau inclusions composed largely of 4R-tau [28].

Although there is clear correspondence between the clinical presentation of FTD/FTLD and the distribution of pathology, these clinical signs do not indicate reliably the molecular and histologic nature of the pathology (eg, tauopathy versus ubiquitin/TDP-43 based) [19,20,24,29]. As a result, FTD and its related syndromes present considerable nosologic problems, and the limitations of these classifications should be recognized; thus, FTD is a clinical term that indicates little about the underlying molecular pathology associated with the disease.

Frontotemporal dementia as a complex trait

FTD is a genetically complex disorder with multiple genetic factors contributing to the disease. A positive family history of dementia is found in up to 50% of patients who have FTD and in the majority of these patients FTD is inherited as an autosomal dominant trait with high penetrance [30–34]. Genetic linkage studies have revealed FTLD loci or genes on the following chromosomes: chromosome 3p [35,36], chromosome 9 [15], chromosome 9p [16–18], and chromosome 17q [6,37–41]. Among them, the most prevalent genes are *PGRN* and *MAPT*, both located on chromosome 17q21 (Fig. 1; see Table 1).

At a consensus conference in Ann Arbor, Michigan, in 1996, the autosomal dominant form of FTLD linked to chromosome 17q21 was identified and the term, FTDP-17, was coined. The initial 13 families known to be linked to this locus in 1996 had variable clinical phenotypes, including cognitive impairment, parkinsonism, amyotrophy, dystonia, and supranuclear gaze palsy [6]. In 1998, mutations in *MAPT* were discovered in some of these

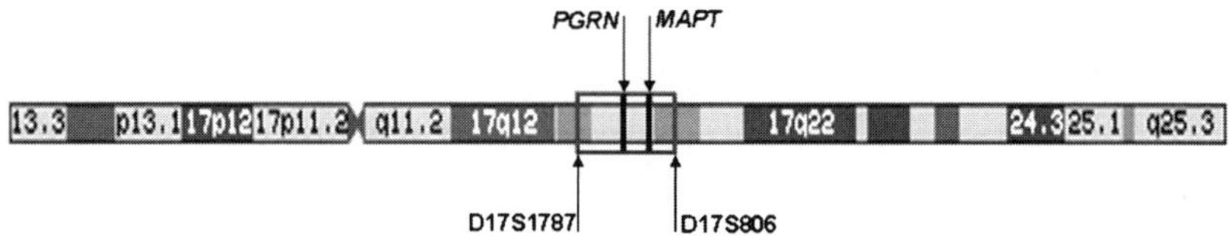

Fig. 1. Chromosome 17 with *PGRN* and *MAPT* gene locations. The 6.1-Mb linkage interval between markers D17S1787–D17S806 on chromosome 17 (q21.2-q21.32) is indicated by the box. The positions of the *PGRN* and *MAPT* genes are indicated.

FTDP-17 families. Thus, this form of disease could be defined genetically as FTDP-17 (*MAPT*). Subsequently, additional families were identified in a worldwide distribution and in different populations. FTDP-17 (*MAPT*) remains, however, a rare disorder with probably fewer than 150 families described so far (personal estimate). More than 30 different confirmed pathogenic mutations in *MAPT* have been identified in these families (FTD mutation database: http://www.molgen.ua.ac.be/FTDMutations) [42].

Over the past decade, six families, including three of the initial FTDP-17 families (Karolinska family, Dutch III, and HDDD2 kindreds) were linked genetically to the chromosome 17q21 locus but without identifiable *MAPT* mutations [38,43–48]. The pathology in patients who had FTD with *MAPT* mutations is characterized by tau-positive inclusions. Autopsy studies of family members, however, from the kindreds linked to chromosome 17q21 but without *tau* mutations revealed no tau pathology. This conundrum finally was resolved in 2006 with the identification of null mutations in *PGRN* that explained the remaining families who had tau-negative FTDP-17 (see Fig. 1) [37,38]. *PGRN* lies within 2Mb of *MAPT* and this finding explained why two such different forms of familial FTD, with tau-positive and ubiquitin/(TDP-43)-positive histopathologies, were linked to the same segment of chromosome 17 [37,38]. At present, there is no obvious mechanistic link between the mutations in *MAPT* and *PGRN* and, as a result, it currently is assumed that their proximity on chromosome 17 simply is coincidence. Despite the fact that *PGRN* was identified recently, the emerging data on prevalence of *PGRN* indicate that it is the form of FTD (FTDP-17 [*PGRN*]) genetically determined most often.

Progranulin

More than 30 nonsense, splice-site, and frameshift mutations have been identified in the *PGRN* gene (Fig. 2) [37,38,49–55]. *PGRN* is located only

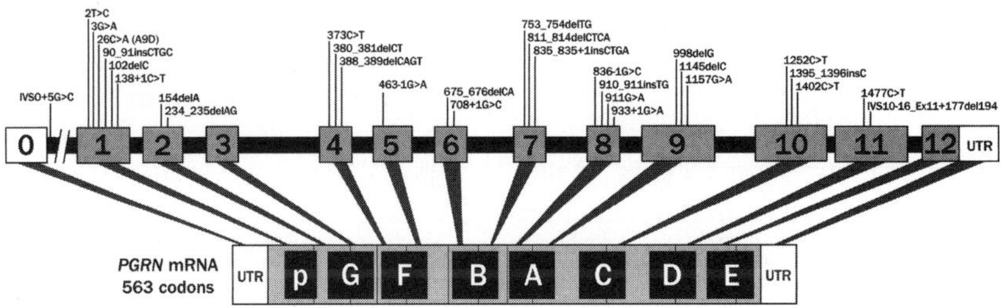

Fig. 2. Schematic representation of the *PGRN* gene (*top*) and the messenger RNA (mRNA) encoding the PGRN protein (*bottom*). Mutations identified in FTDP-17 (*PGRN*) patients by December 2006 are indicated. Individual granulin repeats are highlighted as lettered boxes in the PGRN protein.

approximately 1.7 Mb centromeric of *MAPT* on chromosome 17q21. At this juncture, the most common *PGRN* mutation seems to be 1477C>T. It leads to a premature stop codon (Arg493X) [51,55]. The patients carrying this specific mutation shared an extended haplotype, indicating a common founder [51].

PGRN mutations most likely cause disease by creation of null alleles. The majority of *PGRN* mutations introduce premature termination of codons leading to nonsense-mediated decay of the mutant mRNAs, suggesting that haploinsufficiency is the probable pathogenic mechanism [37,38,51,55]. Therefore, the phenotypes observed in different *PGRN* mutations would not be expected to differ substantially, as they all create nonfunctional mutant allele [37,38].

PGRN encodes the PGRN protein. PGRN is widely expressed and known to play a role in multiple processes linked to tissue remodeling, including development, wound repair, and inflammation, by activating signaling cascades that control cell cycle progression and cell motility [56–58]. Excess PGRN seems to promote tumor formation and, hence, can act as a cell survival signal [59]. Progranulin also can be cleaved proteolytically by an elastase-like activity to form a family of 6 kDa peptides, called granulins. Full-length PGRN and the granulin peptides have opposite activities during wound response, with PGRN stimulating epithelial cell division for wound repair, whereas the granulin peptides stimulate a neutrophil-dependent inflammatory host defense response [57,60]. Despite the increasing literature on the function of PGRN, its role in neuronal function and survival remains uncertain. In the human brain, PGRN is expressed in neurons but significantly also is expressed highly in activated microglia [37], with the result that PGRN expression is increased in many neurodegenerative diseases; again, the function of PGRN in microglia is uncertain but it will be interesting to determine if PGRN regulates a similar repair activity in the brain as in the periphery.

The global frequency of *PGRN* mutations remains to be determined. In the Belgian population, the frequency of *PGRN* mutations is found to be 26% in familial FTD cases. The *PGRN* mutation frequency initially reported is approximately 3.5 times higher than the frequency of *MAPT* mutations as a cause of FTD in the same population [38]. A comprehensive follow-up study identified *PGRN* mutations in 10.5% (39/378) of the Mayo Clinic pathologically proved FTLD series [51]. *PGRN* mutations made up 22.2% of familial cases in this series. Mutations in *PGRN* accounted for approximately 5% of FTD in an unbiased population-based patients subset (n = 167) derived from the Alzheimer's Disease Research Centers [51]. Huey and colleagues [52] identified *PGRN* mutations in 2.4% (2/84) of patients who had FTD from a convenience sample from the United States population.

Despite the predictions made by molecular genetics studies, *PGRN* mutation carriers display heterogeneous clinical presentation. Gass and colleagues [51] reported 38 mutation-positive patients who had mean age of onset of dementia of 59 ± 7 years (range, 48–83 years) and who had a mean disease duration of 7 years (range, 2–17 years) (see Table 1). The clinical presentation of *PGRN* mutation carriers was similar to patients who did not have *PGRN* mutations, FTD being the most frequent clinical diagnosis, followed by primary progressive aphasia. Initially, personality and behavioral changes are most common, followed by language dysfunction. During the course of the illness, the majority of patients developed parkinsonian signs, mainly rigidity and bradykinesia. At times, these symptoms could be strikingly asymmetric, resembling CBD. Impairment of vertical gaze has been observed, however, usually affecting upgaze. Spasticity, exaggerated deep tendon reflexes, and Babinski's signs are common in final stages of the illness [61]. In one patient from the UBC-17 family, tongue muscle atrophy and fasciculations were observed [44]. A liability curve calculation, which included probands, revealed that only 50% of *PGRN* mutation carriers were affected by the age of 60 years, whereas more than 90% were affected by age 70 [51]. This is comparable to the age-dependent risk in another neurodegenerative disease, *LRRK2* parkinsonism, which occasionally can present with cognitive impairment and MND [62].

Two families from Northern Italy linked to chromosome 17q21 (LOD score, 4.173) recently were shown to harbor a 4–base pair deletion in exon 7 of *PGRN* [49]. These two families did not share haplotype background, indicating that they may not have a common ancestor. Even for this specific mutation, highly variable clinical phenotypes were observed, ranging from FTDP-17 to CBD within the same family. Similar findings were seen in a small family in which language disturbance with behavioral alterations was seen in the proband, although a sister presented with an aphasic disorder without behavioral disturbance, despite an identical *PGRN* mutation [61]. The HDDD2 family (discussed previously) presented clinically with prominent changes in behavior and language dysfunction and disease in this family was recently shown to be caused by an Ala9Asp substitution in PGRN [54]. Masellis and colleagues [53] reported a Canadian family of Chinese origin meeting clinical criteria for CBD. A *PGRN* splicing mutation (IVS7+1G>A) was found to cosegregate with disease in this family, and pathology findings were consistent with FTLD-U. There is no known curative treatment of affected *PGRN* carriers and little is known about the effectiveness of symptomatic treatment.

Despite broad clinical phenotypic presentations, including behavioral changes, cognitive impairment, language dysfunction, parkinsonism, dystonia, eye movement impairment, and upper and lower motor neuron dysfunction, neuropathologic studies demonstrate similar abnormalities consistent with FTLD-U. Mackenzie and colleagues [63] reported 13 *PGRN* mutation carriers from six different families who had FTD. The most consistent neuropathologic finding was ubiquitin-immunoreactive (ub-ir) neuronal intranuclear inclusions (NII) in the neocortex and striatum. Additionally, there was moderate to severe superficial laminar spongiosis; chronic degenerative changes; ub-ir neurites; and well-defined neuronal cytoplasmic inclusions (NCI) in the neocortex. Many ub-ir neurites were present in the striatum. NCI of granular appearance were observed in the hippocampus. In contrast, familial FTDL-U cases without *PGRN* mutations had no NII, less severe neocortical and striatal pathology, and more often solid NCI in the hippocampus. This supports the observations from the original reports that ub-ir NCI and NII are found in *PGRN* mutation carriers [37,38]. These ub-ir NCI and NII showed no staining for PGRN [37].

By a remarkable stroke of good fortune, soon after the identification of mutations in PGRN, biochemical analyses demonstrated that truncated and hyperphosphorylated isoforms of TDP-43 are a major component of the ubiquitin-positive inclusions in families who have PGRN mutations and in idiopathic FTD and a proportion of idiopathic ALS cases [20].

This crucial finding re-emphasized a long-recognized clinical and pathologic overlap between ubiquitin-positive FTD and ALS and supported the hypothesis that they are different manifestations of the same neurodegenerative mechanism. TDP-43 is a ubiquitously expressed and highly conserved nuclear protein that can act as a transcription repressor, an activator of exon skipping, or a scaffold for nuclear bodies through interactions with survival motor neuron protein. Under pathologic conditions, TDP-43 has been shown to relocate from the neuronal nucleus to the cytoplasm, a consequence of which may be the loss of TDP-43 nuclear functions [20].

The challenge is to determine the mechanism by which loss of PGRN leads to TDP-43 accumulation and whether or not this is necessary for neurodegeneration in this group of diseases. In this process, the generation of novel mouse models of FTD will be essential. In this way, the genetic discovery of mutations in *PGRN* in FTDP-17 likely will prove as important as the identification of mutations in *MAPT* for determining the pathogenic mechanism in this group of diseases and for the development of therapeutic strategies.

The microtubule-associated protein tau gene

To date, 37 pathogenic mutations have been identified in *MAPT*. The majority of *MAPT* mutations have been found within the microtubule-binding region of *MAPT* or affecting the splicing of exon 10 (Fig. 3). Alternative splicing of exons 2, 3, and 10 produce the six major isoforms that normally are found in the human brain [64]. The alternative splicing of exon 10 produced tau isoforms with either three microtubule-binding repeats (3R-tau) resulting from exclusion of exon 10 or four repeats (4R-tau) resulting from inclusion of exon 10. The deposition of hyperphosphorylated tau in insoluble filaments in the brain is a pathologic hallmark of several neurodegenerative disorders, known collectively as tauopathies [65]. In addition to FTDP-17 (*MAPT*), these include FTD, Pick's disease (OMIM #172700), Alzheimer's disease (AD) (OMIM #104300), argyrophilic grain disease,

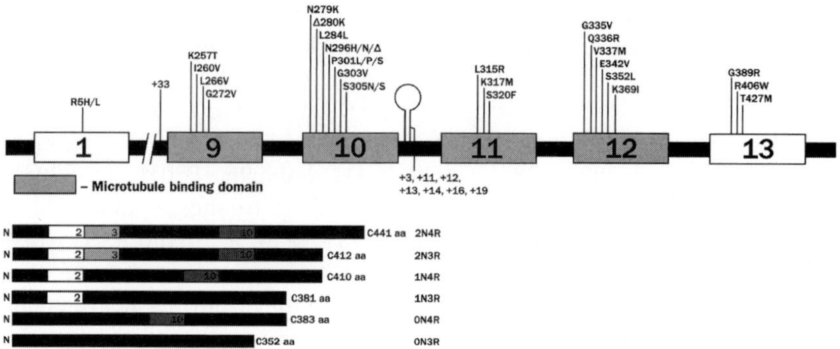

Fig. 3. Schematic representation of the *MAPT* gene (*top*). Mutations identified in FTDP-17 (*MAPT*) are indicated. Tau isoforms (*bottom*). Bars numbered 2, 3, and 10 represent alternatively spliced exons.

PSP, and CBD [42]. It is now believed that several tauopathies are caused by imbalances in the normal 3R-tau:4R-tau ratios. 4R-tau isoforms accumulate in PSP and CBD. Mainly 3R-tau accumulate in Pick's disease, whereas the 3R-tau:4R-tau ratio remains equal in AD [66,67]. The most common tau substitutions associated with FTDP-17 are P301L, N279K, and a splice site mutation (exon10 +16). Together, these three mutations account for approximately 60% of known cases [48]. Two *MAPT* variants (IVS10+29 and A239T) previously were believed to cause disease [68,69]. It now has been shown that these almost certainly are benign *MAPT* variants and that the disease in these patients who have ub-ir pathology is caused by *PGRN* mutations [55].

Two main haplotype clades (H1 and H2) span the entire coding sequence of the *MAPT* gene. The H1 haplotype repeatedly is shown to be associated with PSP [67,70]. In addition, the H1 haplotype is found to form several subhaplotypes, but only one of them (H1c) is associated with PSP. The H1 haplotype also is associated with Parkinson's disease (OMIM #168600) [71]. More recent studies suggest that the H1c subhaplotype may be associated with AD [67]. The molecular mechanism is believed to be an increase in the 4R-tau expression associated with the *MAPT* H1c risk haplotype [72].

MAPT mutations identified in FTDP-17 are believed to cause disease through two main mechanisms:

The first group (missense and deletion mutations) disrupts the binding of tau to microtubules in functional studies [73–75]. The majority of mutations of this type also cause a direct increase in the tendency of tau to aggregate into filaments, in vitro and in vivo [76,77]. Hence, these mutations are predicted to cause an increase in the proportion of unbound tau available for aggregation and increased tendency to form aggregates. The precise mechanism by which the effects of these mutations lead to neurodegeneration and to FTDP-17 is uncertain, however.

The second group of *MAPT* mutations affects the alternative splicing of exon 10. This leads to disruption of 3R-tau:4R-tau ratio [39,41]. Mutations within this group consist of coding changes within exon 10 (N279K, delK280, L284L, N296N/H, delN296, P301L/S, G303V, and S305S/N) and intronic mutations close to the 5′ splice site of exon 10 (at positions +3, +11, +12, +13, +14, +16, and +19) [48].

Tau is a microtubule-binding protein abundant in normal neurons and glia. It commonly is present in axons. Tau binds to and stabilizes microtubules and promotes their formation. Microtubules are cellular structures involved in axonal transport. Therefore, tau most likely regulates the axonal transport processes along the microtubules [42].

The phenotypes seen in *MAPT* mutation carriers include the three cardinal features: behavioral changes (disinhibition, apathy, defective judgment, compulsive behavior, hyper-religiosity, psychosis, alcoholism, verbal and physical aggressiveness, hyperorality and hyperphagia, and neglect of personal hygiene), dementia, and parkinsonism [2]. The average age at onset in FTDP-17(*MAPT*) is 49 years (range, 25–76), this is approximately 10 years younger than in FTDP-17(*PGRN*). The average disease duration is approximately 7 years (range, 2–30 years) (see Table 1) [2].

Personality and behavioral disturbances often are the presenting features in P301L and exon 10+16 mutations. Alternatively, N279K mutation carriers often present with a parkinsonism-plus syndrome (rigidity, bradykinesia, falls, vertical gaze palsy, and poor response to levodopa). The course of the disease is relentlessly progressive and eventually all patients develop significant memory impairment and levodopa-unresponsive parkinsonism, regardless of initial presentation. Resting tremor is seen infrequently. During the course of the illness, however, other clinical signs develop, such as dystonia unrelated to medications, vertical gaze palsy, myoclonus, spasticity, amyotrophy, autonomic dysfunction, and, rarely, seizure disorder difficult to control with standard anticonvulsant therapy. In the final stages of the illness, patients are mute, dysphagic, and urine and stool incontinent, requiring total nursing care.

It still is difficult to perform detailed phenotype/genotype correlations in FTDP-17, because the clinical information is not always available. Nevertheless, two patterns of clinical presentation have emerged: dementia-predominant phenotype and parkinsonism-plus–predominant phenotype.

The dementia-dominant phenotype is more common. It usually is seen in carriers with *MAPT* mutations located on exons 1, 9, and 11 to 13. The parkinsonism-plus–predominant phenotype usually is seen in carriers with *MAPT* mutations located within intron and exon 10, leading to the selective overproduction of 4R-tau isoforms. An association has been found between the H1/H2 genotype and dementia-predominant phenotype and between the H1/H1 genotype and the parkinsonism-plus–predominant phenotype [78].

The pathology in FTDP-17 patients who have *MAPT* mutations (FTDP-17[*MAPT*]) is characterized macroscopically by brain atrophy from 825 to 1290 g. Neuropathologic findings in early stages of the illness are unknown. The cortical atrophy involves frontal and temporal lobes, frequently with a knife-edge appearance [79]. The parietal and occipital lobes are affected less frequently. The subcortical structures in which neuronal loss has been described include caudate nucleus, putamen, globus pallidus, amygdala, hippocampus, and ventral hypothalamus. The substantia nigra and the locus coeruleus show a marked reduction in pigmentation.

Microscopically, the pathologic hallmark of FTDP-17(*MAPT*) is the presence of tau protein deposits in neurons or in both neurons and glial cells. This pathologic variability tends to correlate with *MAPT* mutation and clinical phenotype. *MAPT* mutations in exons 1 and 10 and intron 10 are associated with neuronal and glial tau deposition. This group includes the three most common tau substitutions P301L, N279K, and exon 10 +16 (see Fig. 3). Alternatively, *MAPT* mutations located in exons 9, 11, 12, and 13 usually are associated with neuronal tau inclusions only.

MAPT mutations used to generate transgenic mouse models of tauopathy

The identification of mutations in *MAPT* that cause FTDP-17(*MAPT*) has enabled the generation of transgenic mouse models that develop robust neurofibrillary tangle (NFT) pathology and associated neurodegeneration [80–83]. These models subsequently have been used to explore the role of tau in the pathogenesis of FTDP-17(*MAPT*) and other tauopathies, including AD. In these mouse lines, mutant *MAPT* is overexpressed within the mouse brain. The mutation along with the enhanced level of expression accelerates the formation of MAPT neurofibrillary inclusions to the point where this pathology can be observed within the lifespan of a mouse. The importance of the discovery of *MAPT* mutations to the process of model development cannot be overstated; overexpression of wild-type *MAPT* transgenes has yet to produce a mouse line that recapitulates all stages of NFT formation and associated neurodegeneration.

The mutant *MAPT* transgenic mouse lines that develop robust neurofibrillary pathology, with the structural and biochemical features of human NFT, also show significant neuronal loss in affected brain regions [80–83]. A recent example is the inducible rTg4510 model [82,84], which expresses tau with the P301L substitution [39]. This mouse develops massive neurodegeneration in AD-relevant cortical and limbic structures to the point where global forebrain atrophy is observed and brain weight is reduced significantly. Furthermore, the progression of neurofibrillary pathology and neuronal loss also is correlated with the progression of deficits in spatial reference memory, as assessed by the Morris water maze [82,84]. This and other *MAPT* transgenic mouse models, therefore, show that the development of neurofibrillary pathology and neurodegeneration are linked closely in FTDP-17(*MAPT*) and other tauopathies.

Analysis of the inducible rTg4510 mice, however, demonstrates that the formation of NFT lesions can be dissociated from tau-induced neuronal loss and memory decline [82,84]. In this model, onset of memory deficits (2.5–4 months) precedes the development of significant NFT pathology or neuronal loss (5.5 months). Furthermore, suppressing inducible transgene expression, with doxycycline treatment, after initial NFT formation has occurred (>4 months) did not halt the continuing increase in NFT numbers, with treated and control mice having similar numbers of NFT, in cortex and hippocampus, after 80% transgene suppression for 6 weeks. In contrast, transgene suppression halted the loss of neurons and allowed at least partial recovery of spatial reference memory function. These findings suggest that NFT formation is not directly responsible for neurodegeneration and memory loss in rTg4510; more likely, a toxic intermediate tau species underlies these processes. This parallels the finding that soluble oligomeric amyloid-beta (Aβ) species, rather than insoluble amyloid, drives memory loss in amyloid precursor protein (APP) mice [85,86]. In addition, the results suggest that reversible neuronal dysfunction, as opposed to structural neurodegeneration, explains much of the early memory loss in rTg4510 and suggests that functional (cognitive and motor) deficits in early stage FTDP-17(*MAPT*), AD, and other tauopathies also may be partially reversible.

The mechanism of neuronal cell death in mouse models that develop NFT pathology is uncertain; recent studies in mice expressing mutant *MAPT* transgenes have implicated axonal dysfunction and degeneration as initiators of tau-induced neuronal loss [83,87]. Despite these findings, additional studies are required to determine how tau pathogenesis causes neuronal cell death in these models and in human tauopathy.

Mouse models expressing mutant *MAPT* transgenes also have been used to investigate the relationship between Aβ and *MAPT* in the development of AD. Lewis and colleagues [88] crossed mutant APP and *MAPT* (JNPL3) mice and demonstrated that the double-transgenic TAPP mice developed enhanced limbic neurofibrillary pathology when compared with single transgenic littermates. This suggests that Aβ accumulation is able to accelerate the formation of NFT pathology, consistent with the widely accepted amyloid cascade hypothesis of AD pathogenesis. The enhanced NFT pathology in the TAPP mice, however, also was associated with evidence of neuronal loss in the entorhinal cortex; thus, neurodegeneration was observed only in cortical regions once robust NFT formation was initiated. This result was consistent with the notion that tau dysfunction likely is an important mechanism of neuronal cell death in AD.

Oddo and colleagues [89] extended these studies by generating a triple-transgenic model (3xTg-AD), harboring PS1M146V, APPswe, and *MAPT* (P301L) transgenes. This model accumulates intraneuronal Aβ and subequently forms amyloid plaques and tau lesions in an age-dependent fashion. The stage and extent of the tau pathology in this line have not yet been determined fully; however, that extracellular Aβ deposition precedes tau pathology by several months, suggesting that elevated Aβ enhances tauopathy development in this model. Consistent with this observation, mice expressing only the *MAPT* (P301L) and PS1 transgenes did not develop tau pathology in the absence of APPswe overexpression and Aβ deposition. The 3xTg-AD mice also developed age-dependent synaptic dysfunction, including long-term potentiation (LTP) deficits, and memory deficits that correlate with the accumulation of intraneuronal Aβ [89,90]. As yet, an assessment of neuronal loss in these mice is not reported.

In subsequent studies, Oddo and colleagues [91,92] found that injection of anti-Aβ antibodies, or antibodies specific for oligomeric forms of Aβ, into the brains of 3xTg-AD mice led to the rapid clearance of accumulated Aβ deposition and early tau lesions in the cell body. The removal of Aβ and tau lesions proceeded in a hierarchic, time-dependent manner; clearance of accumulated Aβ occurred before a reduction in the tau pathology. Furthermore, after clearance of the injected Aβ antibody, Aβ pathology re-emerged before the appearance of tau lesions. Later-stage hyperphosphorylated tau (antibody AT8 and AT180 positive) lesions, however, were resistant to clearance by Aβ immunotherapy [91]. These results suggest the existence of reversible and irreversible stages of tau pathology. The nature of this shift from reversible to irreversible pathologic stages is unclear, but one possibility is that tau hyperphosphorylation is associated with aggregation into filaments that renders the lesion resistant to clearance. These data are highly reminiscent of the findings of Santacruz and colleagues [82], who showed that in the rTg4510 inducible model of tauopathy, NFTs were stable and increased in number after *MAPT* (P301L) transgene suppression.

Studies in mice expressing mutant *MAPT* transgenes along with mutant APP have provided clear evidence that Aβ and tau interact in the pathogenesis of AD. Moreover, the results support the hypothesis that Aβ is able to accelerate, if not initiate, the formation of tau neurofibrillary lesions. The close link between NFT formation and neuronal loss observed in multiple *MAPT* transgenic lines and in the TAPP double transgenic mice, however, strongly suggests that in AD the development of pathologic tau species is a major pathway to neurodegeneration. None of these studies could have been performed without the identification of *MAPT* mutations in patients who had FTDP-17.

The chromatin-modifying protein 2B gene

FTD is linked to chromosome 3 (FTD3) in a large Danish family [93]. Affected family members display personality and behavioral changes consistent with FTD. Neuropathologic studies revealed global cortical atrophy with no distinctive histopathologic features. An aberrant splicing mutation in the *CHMP2B* was found to cause disease in this kindred [94]. Several studies using large FTD-patient series failed to detect any *CHMP2B* mutations. Therefore, *CHMP2B* is an uncommon cause of FTD [35,95]. The identification of a similar protein-truncating variant in two unaffected members of an Afrikaner family who had FTD further questions the pathogenicity of mutations in *CHMP2B* [96]. There is a need to identify more families or to perform additional functional work to clarify the role of *CHMP2B* mutations in FTD.

Valosin-containing protein gene

Inclusion body myopathy associated with Paget disease of bone and FTD (IBMPFD) (OMIM #167320) is a rare disorder linked to chromosome 9p21.1-p12 [7]. Watts and colleagues [97] identified six missense mutations in *VCP* as a cause of IBMPDF in families linked to this chromosomal region. *VCP* codes for the protein VCP, which is a member of the AAA-ATPase superfamily, and is associated with several cellular functions, including cell cycle control, membrane fusion, and the ubiquitin-proteasome degradation pathway [97]. The majority of IBMPDF carriers have been identified in North America. This strongly suggests a founder effect.

Other genes and loci

Mutations in the presenilin-1 gene (*PSEN1*) are a known cause of AD. Some *PSEN1* variants, however, were identified in FTD cases. Autopsy of a patient who had the *PSEN1*ins352 mutation demonstrated FTLD-U pathology, but after the discovery of *PGRN*, subsequent genetic analysis revealed the presence of a pathogenic *PGRN* mutation, indicating that the *PSEN1*ins352 mutation may represent a benign variant [50]. Therefore, it is unclear if any *PSEN1* mutation cause FTD, highlighting the need for caution in nominating pathogenic mutations [55].

A patient who had *PGRN* mutation-negative FTD with FTLD-U pathology recently was reported to carry the Lrrk2 G2019S substitution. The G2019S substitution is the most common cause of familial Parkinson's disease known to date. It remains to be seen whether or not this represents a coincidental finding because of reduced penetrance of *LRRK2* parkinsonism or if this may be the result of a pathologic connection between the two neurodegenerative disorders [98].

FTD-MND is linked to two separate loci, both on chromosome 9, located on the long (9q21-22) and short arms (9p13.2-21.3). The responsible genes remain to be identified [15–18].

Summary

Remarkable progress has been made in understanding the genetics of FTD during the past decade. The most important discoveries include the findings that mutations in the *PGRN* and *MAPT* genes are responsible for familial FTD. These two genes, however, are responsible for disease in only a minority of patients who have FTD. Therefore, it is reasonable to assume that additional genes await identification. It is hoped that the exciting molecular genetic discoveries of this past decade will translate into effective treatments of FTD. Progress in functional studies on cell cultures and transgenic animals undoubtedly will help develop therapeutic strategies and foster translational research.

Aknowledgments

The authors thank Jessica Milligan for technical support.

References

[1] Neary D, Snowden JS, Gustafson L, et al. Frontotemporal lobar degeneration: a consensus on clinical diagnostic criteria. Neurology 1998;51(6):1546–54.
[2] Graff-Radford NR, Woodruff BK. Frontotemporal dementia. Semin Neurol 2007;27(1): 48–57.
[3] Ratnavalli E, Brayne C, Dawson K, et al. The prevalence of frontotemporal dementia. Neurology 2002;58(11):1615–21.
[4] Roberson ED. Frontotemporal dementia. Curr Neurol Neurosci Rep 2006;6(6):481–9.
[5] Wszolek ZK, Pfeiffer RF, Bhatt MH, et al. Rapidly progressive autosomal dominant parkinsonism and dementia with pallido-ponto-nigral degeneration. Ann Neurol 1992;32(3): 312–20.
[6] Foster NL, Wilhelmsen K, Sima AA, et al. Frontotemporal dementia and parkinsonism linked to chromosome 17: a consensus conference. Conference participants. Ann Neurol 1997;41(6):706–15.
[7] Kovach MJ, Waggoner B, Leal SM, et al. Clinical delineation and localization to chromosome 9p13.3-p12 of a unique dominant disorder in four families: hereditary inclusion body myopathy, Paget disease of bone, and frontotemporal dementia. Mol Genet Metab 2001;74(4):458–75.
[8] The Lund and Manchester Groups. Clinical and neuropathological criteria for frontotemporal dementia. J Neurol Neurosurg Psychiatry 1994;57(4):416–8.
[9] Neary D, Snowden JS, Mann DM. Classification and description of frontotemporal dementias. Ann N Y Acad Sci 2000;920:46–51.
[10] Neary D, Snowden JS, Mann DM. Cognitive change in motor neurone disease/amyotrophic lateral sclerosis (MND/ALS). J Neurol Sci 2000;180(1–2):15–20.
[11] Neary D, Snowden JS, Mann DM, et al. Frontal lobe dementia and motor neuron disease. J Neurol Neurosurg Psychiatry 1990;53(1):23–32.
[12] Abe K, Fujimura H, Toyooka K, et al. Cognitive function in amyotrophic lateral sclerosis. J Neurol Sci 1997;148(1):95–100.
[13] Talbot PR, Goulding PJ, Lloyd JJ, et al. Inter-relation between "classic" motor neuron disease and frontotemporal dementia: neuropsychological and single photon emission computed tomography study. J Neurol Neurosurg Psychiatry 1995;58(5):541–7.
[14] Evdokimidis I, Constantinidis TS, Gourtzelidis P, et al. Frontal lobe dysfunction in amyotrophic lateral sclerosis. J Neurol Sci 2002;195(1):25–33.
[15] Hosler BA, Siddique T, Sapp PC, et al. Linkage of familial amyotrophic lateral sclerosis with frontotemporal dementia to chromosome 9q21-q22. JAMA 2000;284(13):1664–9.

[16] Morita M, Al-Chalabi A, Andersen PM, et al. A locus on chromosome 9p confers susceptibility to ALS and frontotemporal dementia. Neurology 2006;66(6):839–44.
[17] Valdmanis PN, Dupre N, Bouchard JP, et al. Three families with amyotrophic lateral sclerosis and frontotemporal dementia with evidence of linkage to chromosome 9p. Arch Neurol 2007;64(2):240–5.
[18] Vance C, Al-Chalabi A, Ruddy D, et al. Familial amyotrophic lateral sclerosis with frontotemporal dementia is linked to a locus on chromosome 9p13.2-21.3. Brain 2006;129(Pt 4): 868–76.
[19] Mann DM. Dementia of frontal type and dementias with subcortical gliosis. Brain Pathol 1998;8(2):325–38.
[20] Neumann M, Sampathu DM, Kwong LK, et al. Ubiquitinated TDP-43 in frontotemporal lobar degeneration and amyotrophic lateral sclerosis. Science 2006;314(5796):130–3.
[21] Mackenzie IR, Feldman H. Neuronal intranuclear inclusions distinguish familial FTD-MND type from sporadic cases. Acta Neuropathol (Berl) 2003;105(6):543–8.
[22] Snowden JS, Neary D, Mann DM. Frontotemporal dementia. Br J Psychiatry 2002;180: 140–3.
[23] Dickson DW. Neuropathology of Pick's disease. Neurology 2001;56(11 Suppl 4):S16–20.
[24] Mann DM, McDonagh AM, Snowden J, et al. Molecular classification of the dementias. Lancet 2000;355:626.
[25] McKhann GM, Albert MS, Grossman M, et al. Clinical and pathological diagnosis of frontotemporal dementia: report of the Work Group on Frontotemporal Dementia and Pick's Disease. Arch Neurol 2001;58(11):1803–9.
[26] Buee L, Delacourte A. Comparative biochemistry of tau in progressive supranuclear palsy, corticobasal degeneration, FTDP-17 and Pick's disease. Brain Pathol 1999;9(4): 681–93.
[27] Spillantini MG, Goedert M. Tau protein pathology in neurodegenerative diseases. Trends Neurosci 1998;21(10):428–33.
[28] Forman MS, Farmer J, Johnson JK, et al. Frontotemporal dementia: clinicopathological correlations. Ann Neurol 2006;59(6):952–62.
[29] Dickson DW. Neurodegenerative diseases with cytoskeletal pathology: a biochemical classification. Ann Neurol 1997;42(4):541–4.
[30] Stevens M, van Duijn CM, Kamphorst W, et al. Familial aggregation in frontotemporal dementia. Neurology 1998;50(6):1541–5.
[31] Neary D, Snowden J, Mann D. Frontotemporal dementia. Lancet Neurol 2005;4(11): 771–80.
[32] Chow TW, Miller BL, Hayashi VN, et al. Inheritance of frontotemporal dementia. Arch Neurol 1999;56(7):817–22.
[33] Bird T, Knopman D, VanSwieten J, et al. Epidemiology and genetics of frontotemporal dementia/Pick's disease. Ann Neurol 2003;54(Suppl 5):S29–31.
[34] Rosso SM, Donker Kaat L, Baks T, et al. Frontotemporal dementia in The Netherlands: patient characteristics and prevalence estimates from a population-based study. Brain 2003; 126(Pt 9):2016–22.
[35] Brown J, Ashworth A, Gydesen S, et al. Familial non-specific dementia maps to chromosome 3. Hum Mol Genet 1995;4(9):1625–8.
[36] Gydesen S, Brown JM, Brun A, et al. Chromosome 3 linked frontotemporal dementia (FTD-3). Neurology 2002;59(10):1585–94.
[37] Baker M, Mackenzie IR, Pickering-Brown SM, et al. Mutations in progranulin cause tau-negative frontotemporal dementia linked to chromosome 17. Nature 2006;442(7105): 916–9.
[38] Cruts M, Gijselinck I, van der Zee J, et al. Null mutations in progranulin cause ubiquitin-positive frontotemporal dementia linked to chromosome 17q21. Nature 2006;442(7105):920–4.
[39] Hutton M, Lendon CL, Rizzu P, et al. Association of missense and 5′-splice-site mutations in tau with the inherited dementia FTDP-17. Nature 1998;393(6686):702–5.

[40] Poorkaj P, Bird TD, Wijsman E, et al. Tau is a candidate gene for chromosome 17 frontotemporal dementia. Ann Neurol 1998;43(6):815–25.

[41] Spillantini MG, Murrell JR, Goedert M, et al. Mutation in the tau gene in familial multiple system tauopathy with presenile dementia. Proc Natl Acad Sci U S A 1998;95(13):7737–41.

[42] Rademakers R, Cruts M, van Broeckhoven C. The role of tau (MAPT) in frontotemporal dementia and related tauopathies (http://www.molgen.ua.ac.be/FTDMutations). Hum Mutat 2004;24(4):277–95.

[43] Rademakers R, Cruts M, Dermaut B, et al. Tau negative frontal lobe dementia at 17q21: significant finemapping of the candidate region to a 4.8 cM interval. Mol Psychiatry 2002;7(10): 1064–74.

[44] Mackenzie IR, Baker M, West G, et al. A family with tau-negative frontotemporal dementia and neuronal intranuclear inclusions linked to chromosome 17. Brain 2006;129(Pt 4): 853–67.

[45] Froelich S, Basun H, Forsell C, et al. Mapping of a disease locus for familial rapidly progressive frontotemporal dementia to chromosome 17q12-21. Am J Med Genet 1997;74(4): 380–5.

[46] Lendon CL, Lynch T, Norton J, et al. Hereditary dysphasic disinhibition dementia: a frontotemporal dementia linked to 17q21-22. Neurology 1998;50(6):1546–55.

[47] Rosso SM, Kamphorst W, de Graaf B, et al. Familial frontotemporal dementia with ubiquitin-positive inclusions is linked to chromosome 17q21-22. Brain 2001;124(Pt 10):1948–57.

[48] Wszolek ZK, Tsuboi Y, Ghetti B, et al. Frontotemporal dementia and parkinsonism linked to chromosome 17 (FTDP-17). Orphanet J Rare Dis 2006;1:30–8.

[49] Benussi L, Binetti G, Sina E, et al. A novel deletion in progranulin gene is associated with FTDP-17 and CBS. Neurobiol Aging 2006, in press.

[50] Boeve BF, Baker M, Dickson DW, et al. Frontotemporal dementia and parkinsonism associated with the IVS1+1G->A mutation in progranulin: a clinicopathologic study. Brain 2006;129(Pt 11):3103–14.

[51] Gass J, Cannon A, Mackenzie IR, et al. Mutations in progranulin are a major cause of ubiquitin-positive frontotemporal lobar degeneration. Hum Mol Genet 2006;15(20):2988–3001.

[52] Huey ED, Grafman J, Wassermann EM, et al. Characteristics of frontotemporal dementia patients with a progranulin mutation. Ann Neurol 2006;60(3):374–80.

[53] Masellis M, Momeni P, Meschino W, et al. Novel splicing mutation in the progranulin gene causing familial corticobasal syndrome. Brain 2006;129(Pt 11):3115–23.

[54] Mukherjee O, Pastor P, Cairns NJ, et al. HDDD2 is a familial frontotemporal lobar degeneration with ubiquitin-positive, tau-negative inclusions caused by a missense mutation in the signal peptide of progranulin. Ann Neurol 2006;60(3):314–22.

[55] Pickering-Brown SM, Baker M, Gass J, et al. Mutations in progranulin explain atypical phenotypes with variants in MAPT. Brain 2006;129(Pt 11):3124–6.

[56] He Z, Bateman A. Progranulin (granulin-epithelin precursor, PC-cell-derived growth factor, acrogranin) mediates tissue repair and tumorigenesis. J Mol Med 2003;81(10):600–12.

[57] He Z, Ong CH, Halper J, et al. Progranulin is a mediator of the wound response. Nat Med 2003;9(2):225–9.

[58] Zanocco-Marani T, Bateman A, Romano G, et al. Biological activities and signaling pathways of the granulin/epithelin precursor. Cancer Res 1999;59(20):5331–40.

[59] He Z, Ismail A, Kriazhev L, et al. Progranulin (PC-cell-derived growth factor/acrogranin) regulates invasion and cell survival. Cancer Res 2002;62(19):5590–6.

[60] Zhu J, Nathan C, Jin W, et al. Conversion of proepithelin to epithelins: roles of SLPI and elastase in host defense and wound repair. Cell 2002;111(6):867–78.

[61] Snowden JS, Pickering-Brown SM, Mackenzie IR, et al. Progranulin gene mutations associated with frontotemporal dementia and progressive non-fluent aphasia. Brain 2006; 129(Pt 11):3091–102.

[62] Haugarvoll K, Wszolek ZK. PARK8 LRRK2 parkinsonism. Curr Neurol Neurosci Rep 2006;6(4):287–94.

[63] Mackenzie IR, Baker M, Pickering-Brown S, et al. The neuropathology of frontotemporal lobar degeneration caused by mutations in the progranulin gene. Brain 2006;129(Pt 11): 3081–90.

[64] Goedert M, Spillantini MG, Jakes R, et al. Multiple isoforms of human microtubule-associated protein tau: sequences and localization in neurofibrillary tangles of Alzheimer's disease. Neuron 1989;3(4):519–26.

[65] Spillantini MG, Goedert M, Crowther RA, et al. Familial multiple system tauopathy with presenile dementia: a disease with abundant neuronal and glial tau filaments. Proc Natl Acad Sci U S A 1997;94(8):4113–8.

[66] Wszolek ZK, Tsuboi Y, Farrer M, et al. Hereditary tauopathies and parkinsonism. Adv Neurol 2003;91:153–63.

[67] Pittman AM, Fung HC, de Silva R. Untangling the tau gene association with neurodegenerative disorders. Hum Mol Genet 2006;15(Spec No 2):R188–95.

[68] Stanford PM, Shepherd CE, Halliday GM, et al. Mutations in the tau gene that cause an increase in three repeat tau and frontotemporal dementia. Brain 2003;126(Pt 4):814–26.

[69] Pickering-Brown SM, Richardson AM, Snowden JS, et al. Inherited frontotemporal dementia in nine British families associated with intronic mutations in the tau gene. Brain 2002; 125(Pt 4):732–51.

[70] Baker M, Litvan I, Houlden H, et al. Association of an extended haplotype in the tau gene with progressive supranuclear palsy. Hum Mol Genet 1999;8(4):711–5.

[71] Skipper L, Wilkes K, Toft M, et al. Linkage disequilibrium and association of MAPT H1 in Parkinson disease. Am J Hum Genet 2004;75(4):669–77.

[72] Myers AJ, Pittman AM, Zhao AS, et al. The MAPT H1c risk haplotype is associated with increased expression of tau and especially of 4 repeat containing transcripts. Neurobiol Dis 2007;25(3):561–70.

[73] Dayanandan R, Van Slegtenhorst M, Mack TG, et al. Mutations in tau reduce its microtubule binding properties in intact cells and affect its phosphorylation. FEBS Lett 1999; 446(2–3):228–32.

[74] Hasegawa M, Smith MJ, Goedert M. Tau proteins with FTDP-17 mutations have a reduced ability to promote microtubule assembly. FEBS Lett 1998;437(3):207–10.

[75] Hong M, Zhukareva V, Vogelsberg-Ragaglia V, et al. Mutation-specific functional impairments in distinct tau isoforms of hereditary FTDP-17. Science 1998;282(5395):1914–7.

[76] Nacharaju P, Lewis J, Easson C, et al. Accelerated filament formation from tau protein with specific FTDP-17 missense mutations. FEBS Lett 1999;447(2–3):195–9.

[77] Rizzini C, Goedert M, Hodges JR, et al. Tau gene mutation K257T causes a tauopathy similar to Pick's disease. J Neuropathol Exp Neurol 2000;59(11):990–1001.

[78] Baba Y, Tsuboi Y, Baker MC, et al. The effect of tau genotype on clinical features in FTDP-17. Parkinsonism Relat Disord 2005;11(4):205–8.

[79] Dickson DW. Neurodegeneration: the molecular pathology of dementia and movement disorders. Basel (Switzerland): ISN Neuropath Press; 2003.

[80] Allen B, Ingram E, Takao M, et al. Abundant tau filaments and nonapoptotic neurodegeneration in transgenic mice expressing human P301S tau protein. J Neurosci 2002;22(21): 9340–51.

[81] Lewis J, McGowan E, Rockwood J, et al. Neurofibrillary tangles, amyotrophy and progressive motor disturbance in mice expressing mutant (P301L) tau protein. Nat Genet 2000; 25(4):402–5.

[82] Santacruz K, Lewis J, Spires T, et al. Tau suppression in a neurodegenerative mouse model improves memory function. Science 2005;309(5733):476–81.

[83] Zhang B, Higuchi M, Yoshiyama Y, et al. Retarded axonal transport of R406W mutant tau in transgenic mice with a neurodegenerative tauopathy. J Neurosci 2004;24(19):4657–67.

[84] Ramsden M, Kotilinek L, Forster C, et al. Age-dependent neurofibrillary tangle formation, neuron loss, and memory impairment in a mouse model of human tauopathy (P301L). J Neurosci 2005;25(46):10637–47.

[85] Cleary JP, Walsh DM, Hofmeister JJ, et al. Natural oligomers of the amyloid-beta protein specifically disrupt cognitive function. Nat Neurosci 2005;8(1):79–84.

[86] Walsh DM, Klyubin I, Shankar GM, et al. The role of cell-derived oligomers of Abeta in Alzheimer's disease and avenues for therapeutic intervention. Biochem Soc Trans 2005; 33(Pt 5):1087–90.

[87] Zehr C, Lewis J, McGowan E, et al. Apoptosis in oligodendrocytes is associated with axonal degeneration in P301L tau mice. Neurobiol Dis 2004;15(3):553–62.

[88] Lewis J, Dickson DW, Lin WL, et al. Enhanced neurofibrillary degeneration in transgenic mice expressing mutant tau and APP. Science 2001;293(5534):1487–91.

[89] Oddo S, Caccamo A, Shepherd JD, et al. Triple-transgenic model of Alzheimer's disease with plaques and tangles: intracellular Abeta and synaptic dysfunction. Neuron 2003;39(3): 409–21.

[90] Billings LM, Oddo S, Green KN, et al. Intraneuronal Abeta causes the onset of early Alzheimer's disease-related cognitive deficits in transgenic mice. Neuron 2005;45(5):675–88.

[91] Oddo S, Billings L, Kesslak JP, et al. Abeta immunotherapy leads to clearance of early, but not late, hyperphosphorylated tau aggregates via the proteasome. Neuron 2004;43(3): 321–32.

[92] Oddo S, Caccamo A, Tran L, et al. Temporal profile of amyloid-beta (Abeta) oligomerization in an in vivo model of Alzheimer disease. A link between Abeta and tau pathology. J Biol Chem 2006;281(3):1599–604.

[93] Brown J. Chromosome 3-linked frontotemporal dementia. Cell Mol Life Sci 1998;54(9): 925–7.

[94] Skibinski G, Parkinson NJ, Brown JM, et al. Mutations in the endosomal ESCRTIII-complex subunit CHMP2B in frontotemporal dementia. Nat Genet 2005;37(8):806–8.

[95] Rizzu P, van Mil SE, Anar B, et al. CHMP2B mutations are not a cause of dementia in Dutch patients with familial and sporadic frontotemporal dementia. Am J Med Genet B Neuropsychiatr Genet 2006;141(8):944–6.

[96] Momeni P, Rogaeva E, Van Deerlin V, et al. Genetic variability in CHMP2B and frontotemporal dementia. Neurodegener Dis 2006;3(3):129–33.

[97] Watts GD, Wymer J, Kovach MJ, et al. Inclusion body myopathy associated with Paget disease of bone and frontotemporal dementia is caused by mutant valosin-containing protein. Nat Genet 2004;36(4):377–81.

[98] Dachsel JC, Ross OA, Mata IF, et al. Lrrk2 G2019S substitution in frontotemporal lobar degeneration with ubiquitin-immunoreactive neuronal inclusions. Acta Neuropathol (Berl) 2006, in press.

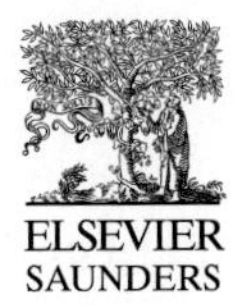

ELSEVIER
SAUNDERS

Neurol Clin 25 (2007) 717–740

NEUROLOGIC
CLINICS

Subcortical Ischemic Vascular Dementia

Helena C. Chui, MD

Department of Neurology, University of Southern California, 1510 San Pablo Street, Suite 618, Los Angeles, CA 90033, USA

This review focuses on subcortical ischemic vascular dementia (SIVD), a proposed subtype of vascular cognitive impairment (VCI). To neurologists, this label conjures up hypertension, diabetes mellitus, small artery disease, lacunar infarctions, white matter changes, subcortical dementia, and dysexecutive syndrome. This article is divided into three main sections: (1) a brief review of the historical syndromes, the conceptual neurobehavioral framework of frontal-subcortical loops, and currently proposed diagnostic criteria; (2) lessons emerging from recent neuroimaging, neuropsychology, and neuropathology studies; and (3) the importance of recognition and treatment of vascular risk factors, in particular hypertension.

Conceptualization: history, frontal-subcortical loops, diagnostic criteria

The wide range of cerebrovascular disease (CVD) and its associated clinical phenotypes have inspired many classification schemes. CVD is divided into large versus small artery disease. Stroke is divided into ischemic versus hemorrhagic subtypes. Multi-infarct dementia (MID) was split into cortical versus subcortical dementia. This article focuses on a proposed subtype known as subcortical vascular dementia (SVD) or SIVD, which is characterized by lacunar infarctions and deep white matter changes. Because lacunar infarctions represent 20% to 30% of symptomatic strokes, SIVD is considered an important subtype of VCI.

History

Three historical syndromes would fall under the current rubric of SIVD: (1) lacunar state, (2) thalamic or strategic infarction dementia, and (3) subcortical arteriosclerotic encephalopathy (Binswanger's syndrome).

This work was supported by NIH Grant P01 AG12435 "The Aging Brain: Vasculature, Ischemia, Behavior" and the State of California Department of Health Services.

E-mail address: chui@hsc.usc.edu

doi:10.1016/j.ncl.2007.04.003 *neurologic.theclinics.com*

Lacunar state

The syndrome of lacunar state first was described by Marie [1] and Ferrand [2] in 50 residents of a chronic care facility. Clinical features included sudden hemiparesis, dementia, dysarthria, pseudobulbar palsy and affect, crying, small-stepped gait, and urinary incontinence. Aphasia and heminopsia rarely were seen. The distribution of lacunes in subcortical gray matter and diffuse softening of the white matter, particularly of the frontal lobe, were noted [3–5]. Behavioral features including lack of volition and akinetic mutism, typically were attributed to prefrontal lobe lesions.

Strategic infarction dementia (eg, thalamic dementia)

Bilateral infarction in the distribution of the paramedian thalamic artery is associated with a dementia syndrome. At times, a single paramedian branch arising from basilar artery often supplies both anteromedial thalamic regions. This region includes the dorsomedial nuclei (closely connected with the prefrontal lobes) and the mammillothalamic tracts (integral components of the limbic-diencephalic memory system) [6]. The dementia syndrome associated with such strategic infarctions is characterized by marked apathy, impaired attention and mental control, and anterograde and retrograde amnesia [7,8], a picture characteristic of executive dysfunction.

Binswanger's syndrome

Otto Binswanger [9] described eight cases of slowly progressive mental deterioration and pronounced white matter changes and secondary dilatation of the ventricles. Alzheimer [10] subsequently reported the microscopic features, including severe gliosis of the white matter and hyalination, intimal fibrosis, and onion skinning of the long medullary arteries. Chronic hypoperfusion of the periventricular and deep white matter border zones is postulated as the mechanism of injury [11].

The clinical features of Binswanger's syndrome include insidiously progressive dementia, persistent hypertension or systemic vascular disease, lengthy clinical course with long plateaus, and accumulation of focal neurologic signs, including asymmetric weakness, pyramidal signs, pseudobulbar palsy, and gait disturbance. The neurobehavioral features of Binswanger's syndrome include apathy, lack of drive, mild depression, and alterations of mood. Readers are referred elsewhere for reviews [12,13]. The periods of slowly progressive dementia may be mistaken for Alzheimer's disease (AD). The presence of gait disturbance, urinary incontinence, and ventriculomegaly may be mistaken for normal pressure hydrocephalus, although cerebral atrophy and widening of the cortical sulci distinguish Binswanger's syndrome.

Evidence

Limited data are available regarding the prevalence of these three syndromes. In a longitudinal community survey of Japanese American men (Honolulu Asia Aging Study), 23% of vascular dementia was attributed to large-vessel, 50% to small-vessel, and 16% to mixed-vessel disease [14]. In the subsample with small-vessel distribution infarctions (n = 34), lacunar state was diagnosed in 85% and Binswanger's syndrome in 15%. In a hospital-based study, among the subset of patients who had lacunar-type MID (n = 39), 51% showed single and 49% showed multiple infarctions on CT scan [15]. Among the patients who had MID (n = 58), 12% had extensive white matter changes. According to these limited data, lacunar state (or multiple lacunes) is the phenotype of dementia associated with SVD recognized most commonly.

Unifying hypotheses: (A) disruption of frontal-subcortical loops and (B) disruption of long association fibers

All three classical SIVD syndromes (described previously) are associated with predominantly frontal type behavioral features. A unifying hypothesis based on disruption of frontal-subcortical circuits has been proposed [16]. Five parallel frontal-basal ganglia-thalamic circuits were delineated in anatomic studies of nonhuman primates [17]. Three of these circuits are relevant to nonmotor behavior: (1) a dorsomedial prefrontal circuit related to executive function, (2) a medial prefrontal circuit related to initiation and drive, and (3) an orbital prefrontal circuit related to social behavior. These three circuits share a common anatomic motif: prefrontal areas project somatotopically to the subcortical gray matter (ie, head of the caudate, globus pallidus, and dorsomedial or anterior thalamic nucleus) and then back to prefrontal cortex (Fig. 1). A unifying hypothesis is that SIVD results from disruption of these frontal-subcortical circuits by lacunar infarctions or deep white matter changes.

An alternate, nonmutually exclusive hypothesis is that deep white matter lesions disrupt white matter tracts important for cognition and emotion. These include association, commissural, striatal, and subcortical fibers that interconnect distributed neural circuits. Widespread lesions of the white matter have major effects on initiation and frontal executive function, because of preferential disruption of long association fibers (eg, cingulum, superior longitudinal fasciculus, and fronto-occipital fasciculus) [18,19].

There are two major scenarios by which small-artery disease leads to ischemic brain injury. The end-stages of the two pathways correspond with the classical syndromes of lacunar state and Binswanger's syndrome.

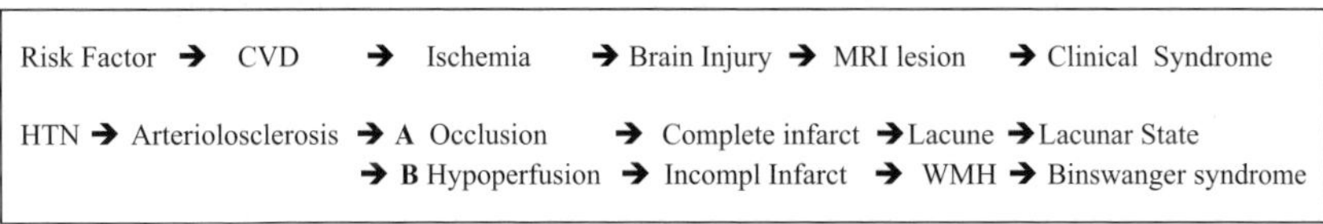

In scenario A, the lumen of a single artery becomes occluded, leading to a discrete lacunar infarction. The subcortical gray matter and white matter

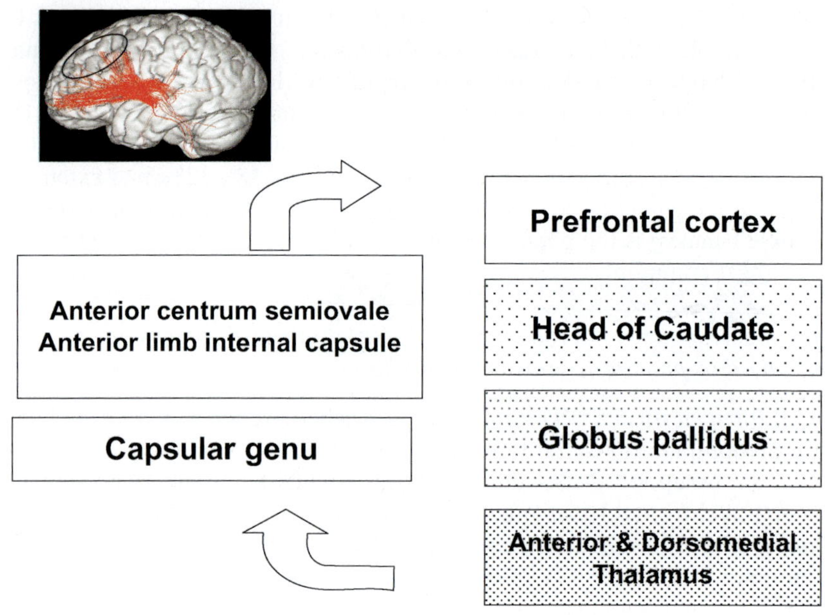

Fig. 1. SVD prefrontal-subcortical circuits.

are most vulnerable. In a meticulous study, Dozono and colleagues [5] tabulated the distribution of 2567 lacunar infarctions: frontal white matter (35%), putamen (16%), thalamus (8%), caudate (8%), and pons (9%) (Fig. 2) [17]. Note that 75% of these infarctions fall in locations that could disrupt frontal-subcortical loops.

In scenario B, the border zone between two or more arteries becomes ischemic, because of stenosis and hypoperfusion affecting multiple arteries simultaneously. The periventricular and deep white matter are most vulnerable [20,21], as these zones are perfused by long, narrow medullary arteries (Fig. 3). The added presence of high-grade carotid artery stenosis or systemic hypotension could exacerbate ischemia. Note that deep white matter changes can disrupt frontal-subcortical loops and long association fibers (eg, cingulum, superior longitudinal fasciculus, fronto-occipital fasciculus).

There is ample evidence from case studies that supports the plausibility of the frontal-subcortical loop hypothesis but few systematic studies that put this hypothesis to test. Case studies demonstrate that single, strategically placed lesions may result in dementia. Key locations include the head of the caudate [22], genu of the internal capsule [23], and thalamus [6,24]. Recently, Carrera and Bogousslavsky [25] described the behavioral patterns associated with infarction in each of the four main thalamic arterial territories: tuberothalamic, paramedian, inferolateral, and posterior choroidal. Infarction of the anterior thalamic nucleus results from occlusion of the

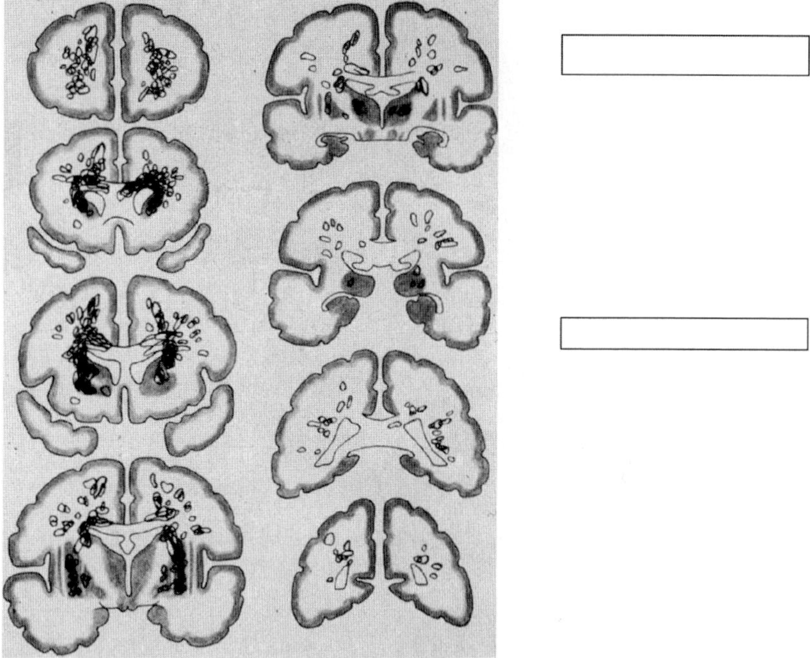

Fig. 2. Distribution of lacunes. Frontal WM = 35%, putamen = 16%, caudate = 8%, thalamus = 8%. (*Figure from* Ishii N, Nishihara Y, Imamura T. Why do frontal lobe symptoms predominante in vascular dementia with lacunes? Neurology 1986;36:340–5; with permission.)

tuberothalamic artery and is associated with apathy, amnesia, perseverations, and "palipsychism" (superimposition of unrelated information). Infarction of the dorsomedial nucleus of the thalamus follows occlusion of the paramedian artery and is associated with personality changes fluctuating between apathy, disinhibition, and at times manic psychosis.

Tullberg and colleagues [26] observed that the severity of white matter hyperintensities (WMH) (regardless of lobar distribution) correlates inversely with glucose metabolism in the dorsolateral frontal lobe. This finding is consistent with the notion that the long association fibers reaching the prefrontal cortex are vulnerable to the centrifugal spread of WMH, which begins in the periventricular end-arteriole zone and advances toward the cortical ribbon. Direct test of this hypothesis now is possible using diffusion tensor imaging and tractography.

Gold and colleagues [27] related lacunar and microvascular pathology to cognitive status in 72 elderly individuals who did not have significant neurofibrillary tangles or macrovascular lesions. In a multivariate model, cortical microinfarctions, and thalamic-basal ganglia lacunes explained 22% of variance and amyloid deposits and microvascular pathology 12%, whereas deep white matter lacunes were not significant contributors. These data

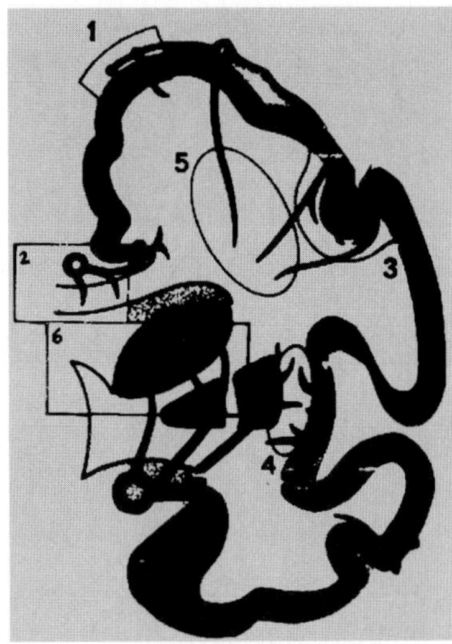

Fig. 3. Regional vulnerability to global ischemia. Less vulnerable are the (*1*) cerebral cortex, (*2*) the corpus callosum, (*3*) the subcortical cortical u-fibers, and (*4*) the external capsule. More vulnerable are (*5*) the deep white matter and (*6*) basal ganglia and thalamus. (*From* Moody DM, Bell MA, Challa VR. Features of the cerebral vascular pattern that predict vulnerability to perfusion or oxygenation deficiency: an anatomic study. Am J Neurorad 1990;11:431–9; with permission. Copyright © 1990, American Society of Neuroradiology.)

confirm the importance of lacunes in subcortical gray matter but indicate that other lesions, such as cortical microinfarctions and amyloid, may contribute to cognitive impairment in SIVD.

Diagnostic criteria

Sensitivity for detecting vascular brain injury widened significantly with the advent of modern imaging: CT in 1970s and MRI in the 1980s. Previously, the threshold occurred at the level of symptomatic stroke; nowadays, neuroimaging often reveals evidence of "silent" vascular brain injury without a history of corresponding clinical event. Recently, criteria have been proposed for SVD (Box 1), which include criteria for brain imaging with CT or MRI (Box 2) [28].

Evidence-based studies that address sensitivity and specificity of clinical criteria against a reference standard are limited. In contrast to AD, there is no gold standard agreed on for the diagnosis of vascular dementia. In reference to idiosyncratic pathologic definitions of VCI, positive likelihood values in the range of 2 to 5 have been reported for Hachinski, *Diagnostic and Statistical Manual of Mental Disorders, Fourth Edition* (*DSM-IV*), *International Statistical Classification of Diseases, 10th Revision* (*ICD-10*), National Institute of Neurological Disorders and Stroke and the Association Internationale pour la Recherche et l'Enseignement en Neurosciences

Box 1. Criteria for subcortical vascular dementia

The criteria for the clinical diagnosis of subcortical vascular dementia include all of the following:

1. Cognitive syndrome, including both dysexecutive syndrome (impairment in goal formulation, initiation, planning, organizing, sequencing, executing, set-shifting and maintenance, abstracting) *and* memory deficit (may be mild) (impaired recall, relative intact recognition, less severe forgetting, and benefit from cues); *and* deterioration from a previous higher level of functioning, interfering with complex (executive) occupational and social activities not due to physical effects of CVD alone.
2. CVD, including both
   a. Evidence of relevant CVD by brain imaging *and*
   b. Presence or history of neurologic signs consistent with subcortical CVD (such as hemiparesis, lower facial weakness, Babinski's sign, sensory deficit, dysarthria, gait disorder, or extrapyramidal signs).

Clinical features supporting the diagnosis of subcortical vascular dementia include the following:

1. Episodes of mild upper motor neuron involvement such as drift, reflex asymmetry, incoordination
2. Early presence of a gait disturbance (small-step gait or marche à petits-pas magnetic, apraxic-ataxic or Parkinsonian gait)
3. History of unsteadiness and frequent, unprovoked falls
4. Early urinary frequency, urgency, and other urinary symptoms not explained by urologic disease
5. Dysarthria, dysphagia, extrapyramidal signs (hypokinesia or rigidity)
6. Behavioral and psychologic symptoms, such as depression, personality change, emotional incontinence, or psychomotor retardation

Features that make the diagnosis of subcortical vascular dementia uncertain or unlikely include

1. Early onset of memory deficit and progressive worsening of memory and other cognitive functions, such as language (transcortical sensory aphasia), motor skills (apraxia), *and* perception (agnosia), in the absence of corresponding focal lesions on brain imaging
2. Absence of relevant CVD lesions on brain CT or MRI

From Erkinjuntti T, Inzitari D, Pantoni L, et al. Research criteria for subcortical vascular dementia in clinical trials. J Neural Transm 2000;59(Suppl 1):23–30; with kind permission of Springer Science and Business Media.

Box 2. Brain imaging criteria for subcortical vascular disease

CT

1. Extensive periventricular and deep white matter lesions: patchy or diffuse symmetric areas of low attenuation (intermediate density between normal white matter and cerebrospinal fluid, with ill-defined margins extending to the centrum semiovale, *and* at least one lacunar infarction; *and*
2. Absence of hemorrhages, cortical, or corticosubcortical nonlacunar territorial infarctions and watershed infarctions (large-vessel disease stroke). No signs of normal pressure hydrocephalus and specific causes of white matter lesions (eg, multiple sclerosis, sarcoidosis, or brain irradiation).

MRI

1. Binswanger-type white matter lesions: hyperintensities extending into periventricular and deep white matter; extending caps (>10 mm as measured parallel to ventricle) or irregular halo (>10 mm with broad, irregular margins and extending into deep white matter) *and* diffusely confluent hyperintensities (>25 mm, irregular shape) or extensive white matter change (diffuse hyperintensity without focal lesions), *and* lacunes in the deep gray matter; *or*
   Lacunar cases: multiple lacunes (eg, >5) in the deep gray matter *and* at least moderate white matter lesions: extending caps or irregular halo or diffusely confluent hyperintensities or extensive white matter changes; *and*
2. Absence of hemorrhages, cortical, or corticosubcortical nonlacunar territorial infarctions and watershed infarctions, signs of normal pressure hydrocephalus, and specific causes of white matter lesions (eg, multiple sclerosis, sarcoidosis, or brain irradiation).

From Erkinjuntti T, Inzitari D, Pantoni L, et al. Research criteria for subcortical vascular dementia in clinical trials. J Neural Transm 2000;59(Suppl 1):23–30; with kind permission of Springer Science and Business Media.

(NINDS-AIREN), and Alzheimer's Disease Diagnostic and Treatment Centers (ADDTC) criteria (reviewed by Chui [29]). This range of positive likelihood ratios may produce small, but sometimes important, changes in pre- to post-test probability [30].

In an autopsy sample of AD, SIVD, and normal controls [31], Chui and colleagues reported that the clinical diagnosis of SIVD by modified ADDTC criteria showed a sensitivity of 57%, a specificity of 85%, and positive likelihood ratio of 3.8. In this same autopsy sample, Reed and colleagues [32] noted that the presence of a "low executive function profile" showed a sensitivity of 67%, a specificity of 86%, and a positive likelihood ratio of 4.8) for the diagnosis of pure SIVD. There are no published studies attempting to validate the criteria for SIVD.

An impasse seemingly has been reached in the traditional approach to clinical diagnosis. One hopes that clinical and pathologic correlations with rapidly accumulating neuroimaging data will suggest new approaches to characterizing the contribution of vascular brain injury to cognitive impairment.

Brain-behavior correlations: imaging-clinical-pathologic data

The versatility and power of MRI offer exciting clinical and research opportunities. High-field MRI at 3 or more tesla offers unprecedented anatomic resolution, functional MRI and perfusion MRI give excellent temporal resolution, and diffusion tensor imaging provides information about architectural integrity. This review focuses on new findings using structural MRI (ie, T1-weighted, T2-weighted, and proton density sequences).

When studies are designed to address specific hypotheses, a combination of imaging, clinical, and pathologic data promises to revolutionize the understanding of brain-behavior relationships. Cross-sectional studies provide correlative data but are noninformative about causality. Longitudinal study designs allow more inferences relevant to determining cause and effect. Autopsy studies still are necessary to assess microscopic changes, including microinfarctions, hippocampal sclerosis (HS), and the presence and severity of AD.

The brain-behavior question relevant to SIVD focuses on the relationship between vascular brain injury (ie, lacunar infarctions and deep white matter changes) and cognitive impairment. In clinical practice, however, answers to the question of how MRI signal hyperintensities relate to cognitive impairment are not straightforward. The likelihood that multiple pathologies contribute to cognitive impairment increases exponentially with age. The risk for AD doubles every 5 years; the risk for stroke every 10. For older persons who have a history of slowly progressive cognitive impairment and evidence of vascular brain injury on neuroimaging, the possibility of concomitant vascular and AD pathology is real.

Pure SVD occurs in young stroke patients and in the rare genetic disorder, known as cerebral autosomal dominant arteriopathy subcortical infarctions and leukoencephalopathy (CADASIL). In older persons who are at greatest risk for cognitive impairment, AD often obscures or confounds the relationship with vascular brain injury. Because the ability to characterize the presence and severity of AD in vivo still is limited, knowledge about the interaction between vascular brain injury and AD pathology (eg, either additive or synergistic) also is unclear.

MRI—neuropsychologic correlations

Loss of brain volume and accumulation of brain hyperintensities can be assessed by qualitative rating scales or volumetric analyses of structure MRI. In 2006, a workshop to harmonize data acquisition related to VCI recommended several rating scales for measuring white matter changes and classifying lacunes [33], including those developed by the Cardiovascular Health Study (CHS) (Fig. 4) [34]. Volumetric measures of cortical gray matter, white matter, and abnormal white matter can be obtained by computerized k-means cluster analyses and voxel-based morphometry (Fig. 5) [35]. Various semiautomated techniques are available to determine hippocampal volumes and number of lacunes.

Several large-scale epidemiologic studies include prospective longitudinal MRI, neuropsychologic measures, and sometimes neuropathology but rarely all three sources of information together. Semiquantitative rating scales are used in several longitudinal epidemiologic studies (eg, Rotterdam Scan Study, CHS, and Atherosclerosis Risk in Communities), whereas volumetric analyses are employed in the Framingham Heart Study and

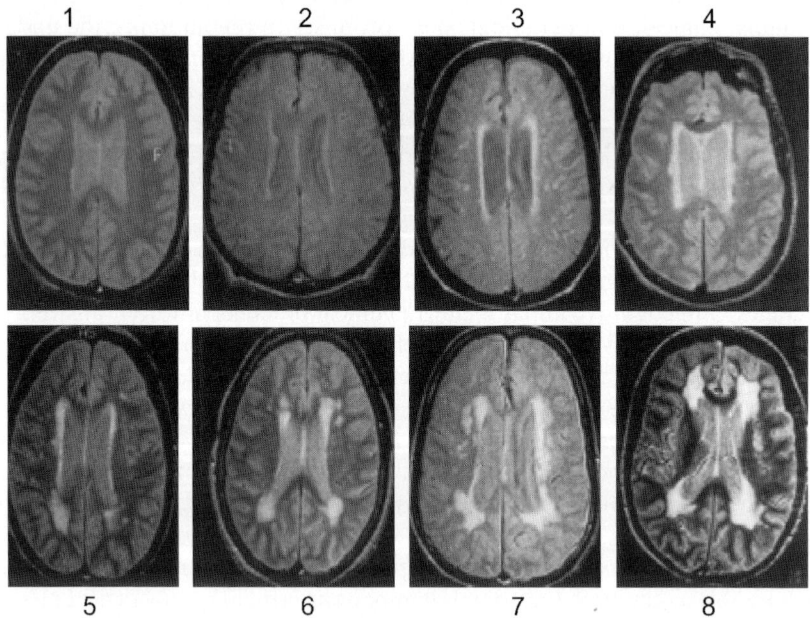

Fig. 4. CHS white matter grading scale. (*From* Longstreth WT, Manolio TA, Arnold A, et al, for the Cardiovascular Health Study Collaborative Research Group. Clinical correlates of white matter findings on cranial magnetic resonance imaging of 3301 elderly people. The Cardiovascular Health Study. Stroke 1996;27:1274–82; with permission.)

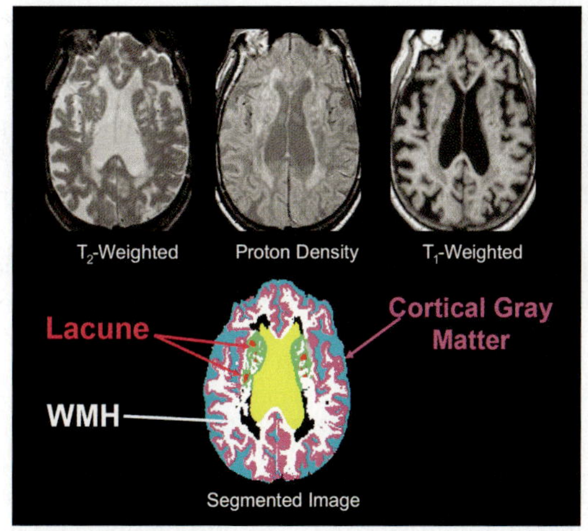

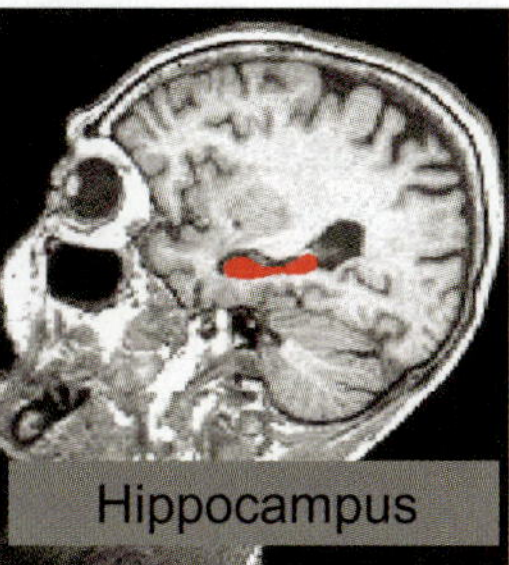

Fig. 5. Quantitative MRI measures (% intracranial volume): SIVD program project. (*From* Fein G, DiSclafani V, Tanabe J, et al. Hippocampal and cortical atrophy predict dementia in subcortical ischemic vascular disease. Neurology 2000;55:1626–35; with permission.)

Austrian Stroke Prevention Study. The Subcortical Ischemic Vascular Dementia (SIVD) program project is a longitudinal prospective study of SIVD, AD, and normal controls that acquires quantitative MRI, psychometric measures with linear response properties, and neuropathology.

Rotterdam Scan Study

From 1995 to 1996, 1077 subjects were selected randomly from two large epidemiologic studies (Rotterdam Study and Zoetermeer Study) to undergo longitudinal cranial MRI (Rotterdam Scan Study). Periventricular WMH, generalized brain atrophy, and brain infarctions on MRI were associated with steeper decline in information processing speed and executive function during 5.2 years' mean follow-up [36].

Atherosclerosis Risk in Communities

At visit 3 (1993–1995) of this prospective, biracial, population-based study, a subset of participants underwent brain MRI. WMH, ventricular size, and sulcal size were rated on a 10-point scale. Cognitive status was assessed using a delayed word recall test, digit symbol substitution test (DSS), and word fluency test. High-grade ratings on each of the MRI variables, including high-grade WMH, were associated independently with diminished cognitive functioning [37].

Cardiovascular Health Study (1989) and Cardiovascular Health Cognitive Study (1998)

From 1998 to 1999, the Cardiovascular Health Cognitive Study (CHCS) was implemented for 3608 participants who had undergone MRI in from

1991 to 1994. The CHS uses the Modified Mini–Mental State Examination (3MS) to assess cognitive status, a 0 to 9 point white matter grade (WMG) rating scale [34], and a stroke risk score [39]. Increasing severity of WMH was correlated with lower scores on 3MS and DSS at baseline [40]. Among a subset of 1919 subjects who had twp MRI scans separated by 5 years, 28% showed worsening of WMG and associated greater decline on 3MS and DSS (both, $P<.001$) (Fig. 6).

In summary, converging evidence from longitudinal epidemiologic studies indicate that progressive increase in WMH is associated with cognitive slowing and decline.

Subcortical Ischemic Vascular Dementia program project: MRI-cognitive-pathology

The SIVD program project is a prospective, longitudinal study to assess the inter-relationships between quantitative MRI, neuropsychologic testing, and, ultimately, neuropathology in subjects who have SIVD, AD, and normal aging. The independent MRI variables were the volumes (expressed as a percentage of intracranial volume) of WMH, lacunes (LAC), cortical gray matter (CGM), and hippocampii (HV) [35]. The dependent measures were neuropsychologic test results and composite measures of global cognition (GLOB), memory (MEM), and executive (EXEC) function, which had linear measurement properties. At the outset of the study, the author and colleagues hypothesized that lacunar infarctions and WMH would be markers of vascular brain injury and would predict decline in executive function, whereas hippocampal atrophy and gray matter atrophy would serve as a marker for AD and predict decline in memory and global cognitive function (Fig. 7).

MRI—cognition

The relationship between MRI measures and neuropsychologic test performance was examined using multistage, cross-sectional, regression models of the first 163 subjects enrolled in the study [41]. The best predictors of global cognition proved to CGM, which explained 14% of the variance in the Mattis Dementia Rating Scale, followed by HV, which explained an additional 11% of the variance. WMH independently, but weakly, explained 3% of the variance in verbal fluency. Lacune volume (most "silent lacunes" in this sample) was not a significant predictor of the cognitive measures.

Baseline MRI and cognitive decline

The relationship between baseline MRI measures and change in global cognition was assessed next among 120 subjects followed for 3 years [42]. CGM predicted decline in GLOB irrespective of the presence or absence of lacunes. HV predicted decline only in subjects who did not have lacunes (presumed AD) but not those who had lacunes (presumed SIVD). WMH, but not lacune volume, was a weak predictor of cognitive decline.

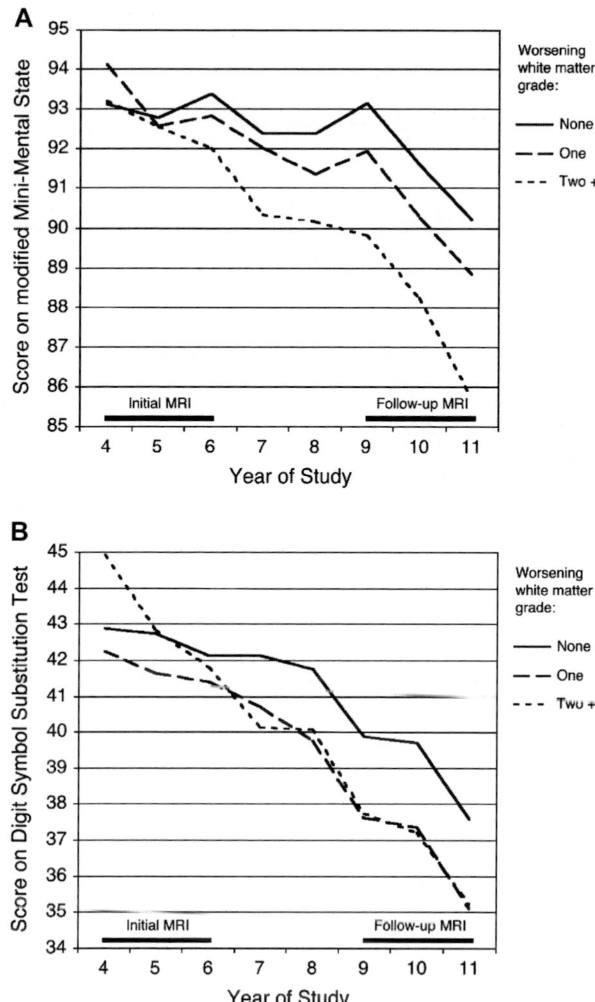

Fig. 6. Annualized changes in 3MS and DSS by groups of participants defined by worsening white matter. (*A*) Scores on the 3MS (maximum score 100). (*B*) DSS (number correct) for each year of study from initial to follow-up scans. (*From* Longstreth WT, Arnold Am, Beauchamp NJ, et al. Incidence, manifestations, and predictors of worsening white matter on serial cranial magnetic resonance imaging in the elderly: the Cardiovascular Health Study. Stroke 2005;36:56–61; with permission.)

Baseline and change in MRI versus cognitive decline

Finally, the relationships between baseline and change in MRI measures and change in MEM and EXEC function were examined among 103 subjects followed for 4.8 years [43]. HV at baseline and HV change predicted change in MEM. Decline in EXEC function was determined by multiple brain components, however, including CGM and change in CGM, HV,

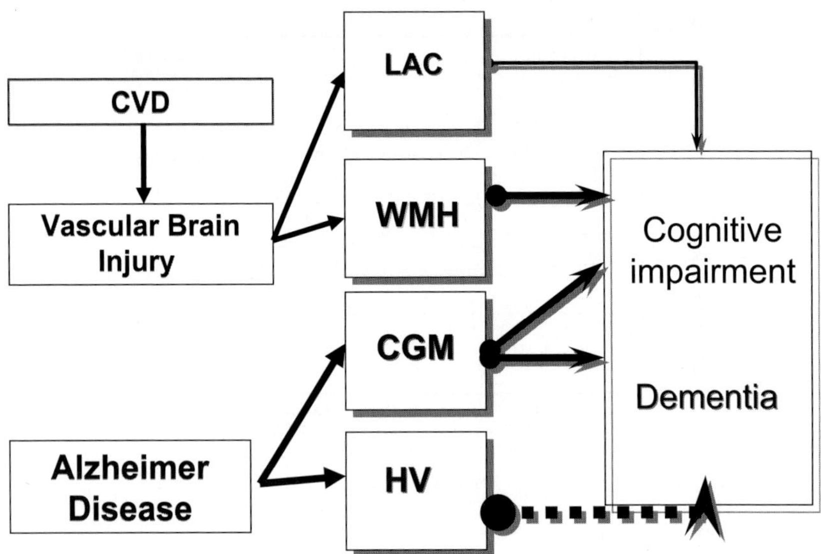

Fig. 7. A priori hypotheses: SIVD program project.

and LAC. The resulting model (shown graphically in Fig. 8) illustrates the expected change in MEM and EXEC in subjects who had AD (HV and CGM) versus AD plus SIVD (LAC). This shows not only the strong association between AD and decline and MEM and EXEC but also the added effect of LAC in years 2 and 4 on EXEC but not MEM function.

Pathology-cognitive correlations

The author and colleagues also examined the relative contribution of AD pathology, CVD pathology, and HS to cognitive status in 79 autopsy cases [31]. In an ordinal logistic regression analysis that included interaction terms to assess the effects of each pathologic variable when the other variables are interpolated to zero, each of the three pathology variables contributed independently to cognitive status: Braak & Braak stage (odds ratio [OR] 2.84; confidence intervals [CI] 1.81–4.45]), HS score (OR 2.43; CI 1.01–5.85), and cerebrovascular disease parenchymal score (CVDPS) (OR 1.02; CI 1.00–1.04). Advancing stages of AD pathology, however, overwhelmed the effects of CVDPS and HS to become the major determinant of dementia.

MRI-path correlations

MRI-path relationships were examined among 101 subjects who had been enrolled in the SIVD program project and came to autopsy [44]. WMH and number of lacunes were correlated with severity of CVD or vascular brain injury. Contrary to popular belief, however, CGM was determined not only by AD pathology but also by severity of vascular brain injury and arteriosclerosis. Hippocampal atrophy was determined not

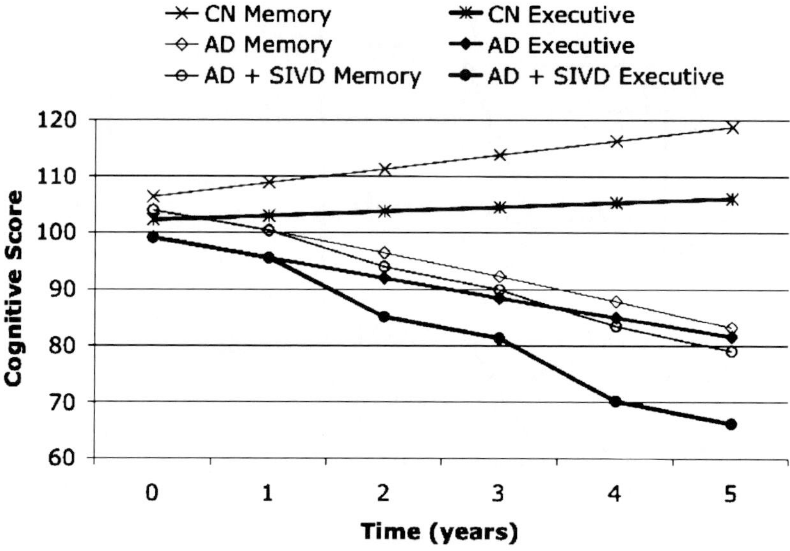

Fig. 8. Model-derived cognitive trajectories for hypothetical cases. (*From* Mungas D, Harvey D, Reed BR, et al. Longitudinal volumetric MRI change and rate of cognitive decline. Neurology 2005;65:565–71; with permission.)

only by AD pathology but also by HS, which is an alternate cause of amnesia but rarely is diagnosed premortem.

Summary

Some of the author and colleagues' a priori predictions were borne out. Baseline WMH, but not lacunes, which were silent for the most part, contribute to impairment verbal fluency and predict global cognitive decline. Baseline and change in HV are the primary determinants of baseline and change in MEM, particularly in subjects who do not have lacunes. Other data, however, led to important modifications of the author and colleagues' a priori hypotheses (Fig. 9). EXEC function is related complexly to baseline CGM and changes in CGM, HV, and LAC. The two major predictors of cognitive status, namely CGM and HV, are affected by multiple rather than single pathologies. Relatively speaking, AD pathology exerts a much greater impact than SIVD pathology on cognitive health.

Cerebral autosomal dominant arteriopathy with subcortical infarctions and leukoencephalopathy

CADASIL provides examples of pure SIVD without significant AD pathology. Resulting from mutations in the Notch3 gene on chromosome 19q12, CADASIL is associated with progressive degeneration of smooth muscle cells and the accumulation of granular osmiophilic deposits in the

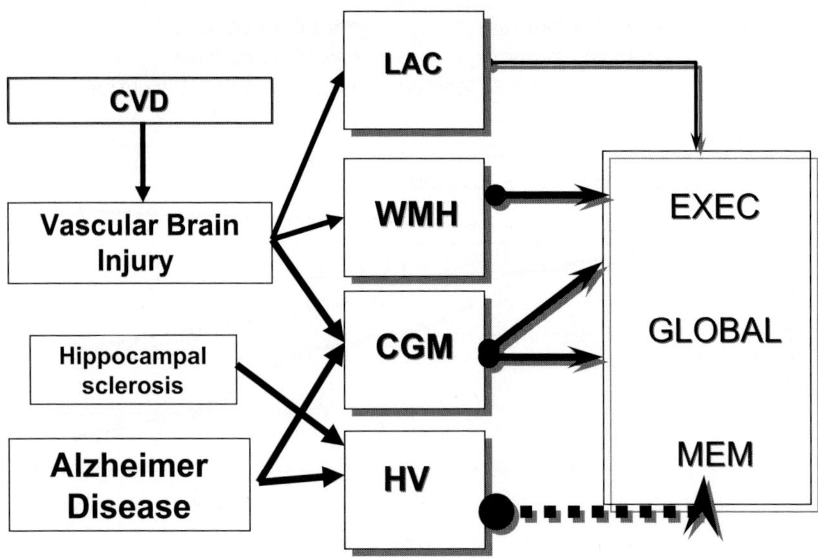

Fig. 9. Summary of SIVD project.

vascular basal lamina of small arteries [45]. This disorder may be diagnosed by skin biopsy or by genetic testing [46]. Patients experience migraine headaches, seizures, and progressive SIVD. MRI shows successive lacunar infarctions, microbleeds, and extensive WMH, which involve not only the periventricular white matter but also the temporal pole, external capsule, and corpus callosum (Fig. 10) [47,48]. Peters and colleagues [49] reported the results of neuropsychologic testing among 65 subjects who had CADASIL compared with 30 age-, sex-, and education-matched normal controls (Fig. 11). The greatest impairments were noted on Stroop III and Trails B and a compound executive score derived from symbol digit, digit span backward, and digit cancellation. O'Sullivan and colleagues [50] used diffusion tensor imaging to support the hypothesis that damage to the cingulum bundle may underlie these impairments in executive processing.

Prevention and treatment

Epidemiologic evidence

Many factors, such as age, hypertension, diabetes mellitus, smoking, high cholesterol, and heart disease, are risk factors for stroke, regardless of subtype (Fig. 12) [51]. In a recent meta-analysis of 16 studies, hypertension and diabetes seemed somewhat more common with lacunar versus nonlacunar or cardioembolic stroke, but this may be confounded by the circular inclusion of risk factor profiles in the definition of stroke subtype [52]. In the Atherosclerosis Risk in Communities study, the population-attributable risk for

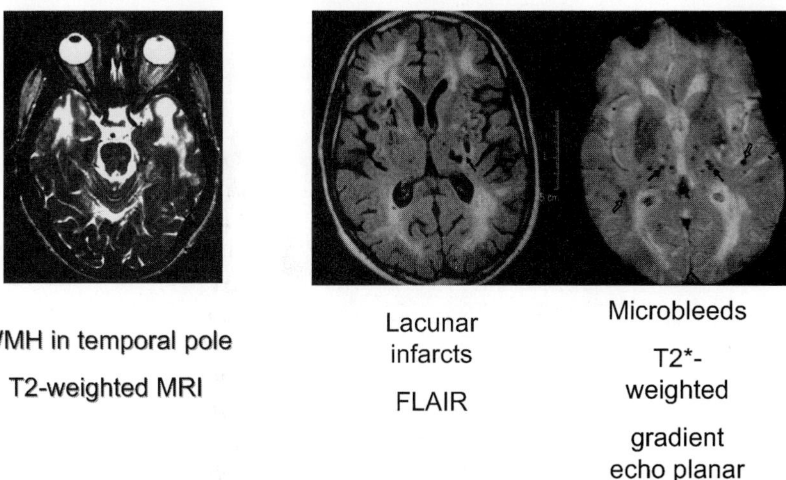

Fig. 10. CADASIL. (*From* O'Sullivan M, Jarosz JM, Martin RJ, et al. MRI hyperintensities of the temporal lobe and external capsule in patients with CADASIL. Neurology 2001;56:628–34; with permission; and Lesnik Oberstein SAJ, van den Boom R, van Buchem MA, et al, for the Dutch CADASIL research group. Cerebral microbleeds in CADASIL. Neurology 2001;57:1066–70; with permission.)

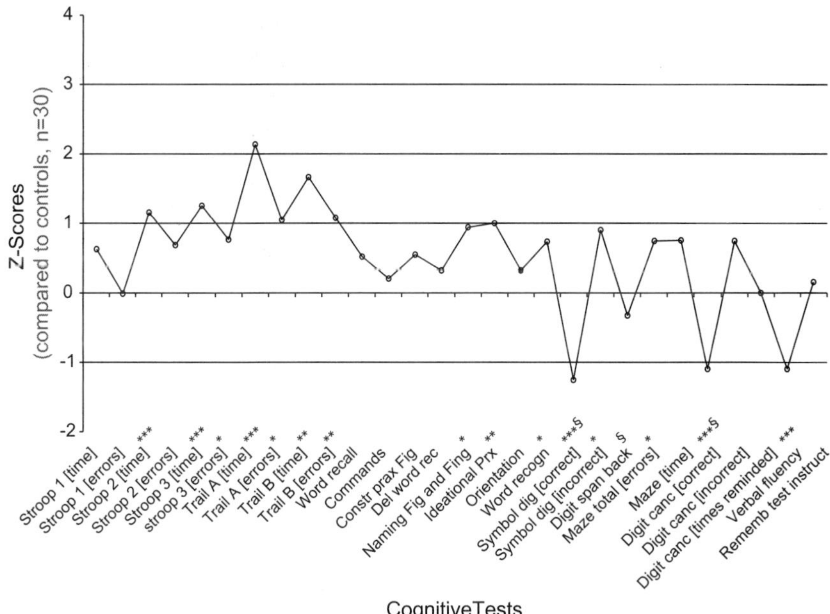

Fig. 11. Cognitive profile in CADASIL. Pronounced deficits in attention and processing speed. (*Data from* Peters N, Opherk C, Danek A, et al. The pattern of cognitive performance in CADASIL: a monogenic condition leading to subcortical ischemic vascular dementia. Am J Psychiatry 2005;162:2078–85.)

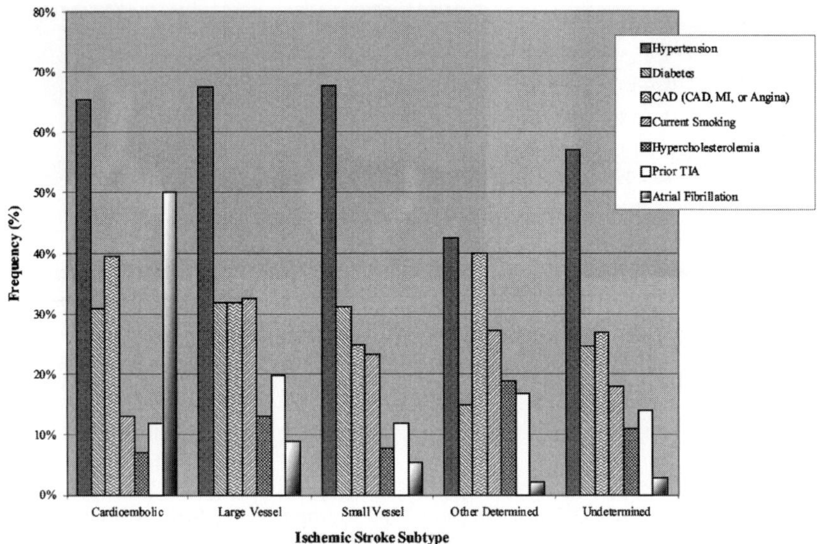

Fig. 12. Frequency of risk factors by ischemic stroke subtype. (*From* Schneider AT, Kissela B, Woo D, et al. Ischemic stroke subtypes: a population-based study of incidence rates among blacks and whites. Stroke 2004;35:1552–6; with permission.)

hypertension was 35% regardless of ischemic stroke subtype [53]. The population-attributable risks associated with diabetes mellitus and smoking, however, were higher for lacunar stroke (26% and 22%) compared with nonlacunar stroke (11.3 and 11.4%) and the definition of stroke subtype was risk-factor free.

Several longitudinal community-based studies provide evidence that identification and control of risk factors in midlife may reduce the risk for cognitive impairment in late life. Hypertension is the single most important modifiable risk factor.

In the Framingham Heart Study, 1695 stroke-free older participants, ages 55 to 85 years, were followed every 2 years from 1950. A significant age-related declined was observed in all neuropsychologic tests. In addition, lesser but independent declines in several tests (ie, immediate and delayed logical memory and visual reproduction) correlated with the magnitude and duration of hypertension in midlife [54].

In the Rotterdam Scan Study, current hypertension or established hypertension of 5- to 20-year duration were associated with significantly increased white matter lesions [38]. For participants who had more than 20 years of hypertension and were between ages 60 and 70 years at the time of follow-up, the relative risk (RR) for subcortical and periventricular white matter lesions was 24.3 (95% CI, 5.1–114.8) and 15.8 (95% CI, 3.4–73.5), respectively, compared with nonhypertensives. For subjects who had hypertension that was treated successfully, the RR for subcortical and periventricular white matter lesions was increased only moderately (RR 3.3, CI 1.3–8.4 and 2.6, CI 1.0–6.8, respectively).

In the Honolulu Asia Aging Study, 3734 Japanese-American men (average age 78 years) were followed every 5 years from 1965. For every 10–mm Hg increase in systolic blood pressure (from less than 110 to 160), there was a 7% increased risk for intermediate cognitive function and a 5% increase for poor cognitive function [55]. In prospective follow-up, for each additional year of antihypertensive treatment, there was a reduction in the risk for incident dementia (Hazard ratio 0.94; 95% CI, 0.89–0.99) [56].

Epidemiology of Vascular Ageing is a longitudinal study of vascular aging and cognitive decline. From 1991 to 1993, 1389 subjects, ages 59 to 72, were recruited from electoral rolls in Nantes, France, and followed every 2 years. Risk for severe WMH was reduced significantly in subjects who had normal blood pressure and were taking antihypertensive medications compared with those who had high blood pressure and were taking antihypertensive agents [57]. This study suggests that good control of blood pressure among hypertensives reduces the risk for severe WMH.

Austrian Stroke Prevention Study

From 1991 to 1994, 2007 individuals in Graz, Austria, were enrolled in a study of genes and vascular risk factors in normal aging. Every fourth study participant was invited to enter phase II of the study, which included MRI, Doppler sonography, SPECT, and neuropsychologic testing (n = 509). Glycated hemoglobin A was identified as a risk factor for greater rate of MRI-measured brain atrophy over 6 years in normal subjects (n = 201), explaining 13% of the variance [58].

Cardiovascular Health Study

In the CHS, independent predictors of worsening WMG include cigarette smoking and infarction on initial scan [40]. Among 622 elderly participants in the CHS, a linear trend was found between the top and bottom quintiles of total homocysteine level with a combined MRI rating of infarctions and high WMG (OR 3.3; 0.96–11.22) [59]. In the CHS among persons for whom lipid-lowering therapy was recommended, statin use was associated with 0.48 fewer points (95% CI, 0.06–0.89) decline per year in 3MS score compared with those who were untreated [60], a difference remaining after controlling for cholesterol level.

Primary prevention: clinical trials that include a cognition outcome measure

In a follow-up to the original Systolic Hypertension in Europe trial [61,62], long-term antihypertensive therapy over 3.9 years reduced the risk for dementia by 55%, from 7.4 to 3.3 cases per 1000 patient years (43 versus

21 cases, $P < .001$). Treatment of 1000 patients for 5 years can prevent 20 cases of dementia (95% CI, 7–33).

Secondary prevention: clinical trials to prevent recurrent stroke or transient ischemic attack

In the Perindopril Protection Against Recurrent Stroke Study (PROGRESS), 6105 subjects who had previous stroke or transient ischemic attack were randomized to perindopril plus or minus indapamide versus placebo and followed for 3.9 years [63]. The treatment group showed a 19% RR reduction versus placebo in cognitive decline as measured by the MMSE and a 43% reduction in new WMH [64].

Tertiary amelioration

Randomized, double-blind, placebo-controlled trials have been conducted for a wide variety of compounds in patients who have VCI, rarely distinguishing between the pathogenetic subtypes of VCI. The efficacy and safety of the calcium antagonist nimodipine versus placebo was studied in 230 patients who had subcortical vascular dementia [65]. At 52 weeks, no significant differences were noted in the Sandoz Clinical Assessment–Geriatric scale, but fewer dropouts and adverse events occurred in the nimodipine group, suggesting a possible beneficial effect on cardiovascular comorbidity.

Cholinesterase inhibitors have been studied in VCI (without distinction regarding subtype). Among patients who had probable vascular dementia or AD plus CVD, Erkinjuntti and colleagues [66] reported a 2.7-point difference in the Alzheimer's Disease Assessment Scale, cognitive subscale for the galantamine (n = 396) versus placebo (n = 196) group. Similarly, among subjects who had probable VCI (n = 616), Wilkinson and colleagues [67] reported a 2-point benefit in a randomized, double-blind, placebo-controlled, 24-week study of donepezil. By way of caveat, a meta-analysis undertaken by Schneider and colleagues [68] showed increased mortality associated with donepezil (OR 1.44; 95% CI, 0.68–3.02; $P = .04$) in two of three vascular dementia trials. Cholinergic deficits are demonstrated in Binswanger's syndrome [69] and CADASIL [70], which provide a biochemical rationale for cholinergic enhancement in at least these subgroups of SIVD. Cholinesterase inhibitors have been approved for the treatment of vascular dementia in some Asian countries but not in the United States.

Summary

Epidemiologic data suggest that prevention of SIVD is akin to prevention of stroke. Identification and treatment of vascular risk factors, such as hypertension, diabetes mellitus, and hyperlipidemia, is a high priority [71]. Overall, antihypertensive therapy is associated with a 35% to 44%

reduction in the incidence of stroke. Only 70% of Americans who have hypertension are aware of their condition, 60% are under treatment, and 34% are controlled successfully [72]. Lack of diagnosis and undertreatment are more common in elderly and minority populations. High priority must be given to reducing the vascular risk profiles.

References

[1] Marie P. Des foyers lacunaires de desintegration et de differents autres etats cavitaires du cerveau. Rev Med 1901;21:281–98 [in French].

[2] Ferrand J. Essai sur l'hemiplegie des vieillards: les lacunes de desintegration cerebrale. Paris These 1902 [in French].

[3] Fisher CM. Lacune: small deep cerebral infarcts. Neurology (Minneap) 1965;15:774–84.

[4] Ishii N, Nishihara Y, Imamura T. Why do frontal lobe symptoms predominante in vascular dementia with lacunes? Neurology 1986;36:340–5.

[5] Dozono K, Ishii N, Nishihara Y, et al. An autopsy study of the incidence of lacunes in relation to age, hypertension, and arteriosclerosis. Stroke 1991;22:993–6.

[6] Bogouslavsky J, Regli F, Uske A. Thalamic infarcts: clinical syndrome, etiology and prognosis. Neurology 1988;38:837–48.

[7] Katz DI, Alexander MP, Mandell AM. Dementia following strokes in the mesencephalon and diencephalon. Arch Neurol 1987;44:1127–33.

[8] Stuss DT, Guberman A, Nelson R, et al. The neuropsychology of paramedian thalamic infarction. Brain Cogn 1988;8:348–78.

[9] Binswanger O. Die Abgrenzung der allgemeinen progressiven Paralyse. Berl Klin Wochenschr 1894;31:1102–5, 1137–9 [in German].

[10] Alzheimer A. Die Seelenstorungen auf arterisclerotiсsher Grundlage. Allgem Z Psychiatr Psych Gerichtl Med 1902;59:695–711 [in German].

[11] DeReuck J, Crevits L, DeCoster W, et al. Binswanger chronic progressive subcortical encephalopathy. Neurology 1980;30:920–8.

[12] Román GC. Senile dementia of the Binswanger type. A vascular form of dementia in the elderly. JAMA 1987;258:1782–8.

[13] Pantoni L, Garcia JH. The significance of cerebral white matter abnormalities 100 years after Binswanger's report: a review. Stroke 1995;26:1293–301.

[14] Ross GW, Petrovitch H, White LR, et al. Characterization of risk factors for vascular dementia. The Honolulu Asia Aging Study. Neurology 1999;53:337–43.

[15] Gorelick PB, Chatterjee A, Patel D, et al. Cranial computed tomographic observations in multi-infarct dementia: a controlled study. Stroke 1992;23:804–11.

[16] Cummings JL. Frontal-subcortical circuits and human behavior. Arch Neurol 1993;50: 873–80.

[17] Alexander GE, DeLong MR, Strick PL. Parallel organization of functionally segregated circuits linking basal ganglia and cortex. Annu Rev Neurosci 1990;13:266–71.

[18] Schmahmann JD, Pandya DN. Fiber pathways of the brain. New York: Oxford University Press; 2006.

[19] Aralasmak A, Ulmer JL, Kocak M, et al. Association, commissural, and projection pathways and their functional deficit reported in the literature. J Comput Assist Tomogr 2006; 30:695–715.

[20] De Reuck J. The human periventricular arterial blood supply and the anatomy of cerebral infarctions. Eur Neurol 1971;5:321–34.

[21] Moody DM, Bell MA, Challa VR. Features of the cerebral vascular pattern that predict vulnerability to perfusion or oxygenation deficiency: an anatomic study. Am J Neurorad 1990; 11:431–9.

[22] Mendez MF, Adams NL, Lewandowski KS. Neurobehavioral changes associated with caudate lesions. Neurology 1989;39:349–54.

[23] Tatemichi TK, Desmond DW, Prohovnik I, et al. Confusion and memory loss from capsular genu infarction: a thalamocortical disconnection syndrome? Neurology 1992;42:1966–79.

[24] Graff-Radford RN, Damasio H, Yamada T, et al. Nonhaemorrhagic thalamic infarction. Brain 1985;108:485–516.

[25] Carrera E, Bogousslavsky J. The thalamus and behavior: effects of anatomically distinct strokes. Neurology 2006;66:1817–23.

[26] Tullberg M, Fletcher E, DeCarli C, et al. White matter lesions impair frontal lobe function regardless of their location. Neurology 2004;63:246–53.

[27] Gold G, Kovari E, Herrmann FR, et al. Cognitive consequences of thalamic, basal ganglia, and deep white matter lacunes in brain aging and dementia. Stroke 2005;36:1184–8.

[28] Erkinjuntti T, Inzitari D, Pantoni L, et al. Research criteria for subcortical vascular dementia in clinical trials. J Neural Transm 2000;59(Suppl 1):23–30.

[29] Chui HC, Lee AY. Clinical criteria for dementia subtypes. In: Qizilbash N, Schneider LS, Chui H, et al. editors. Evidence-Based Dementia Practice. Oxford: Blackwell Science, Inc. p. 106–19.

[30] Jaeschke R, Guyatt GH, Sackett DL, for the Evidence-Based Medicine Working Group. User's guide to the medical literature. III. How to use an article about a diagnostic test. A. What are the results and will they help me in caring for my patients? JAMA 1994;271: 703–7.

[31] Chui HC, Zarow C, Mack WJ, et al. Cognitive impact of subcortical vascular and Alzheimer disease pathology. Ann Neurol 2006;60:677–87.

[32] Reed BR, Mungas DM, Kramer JH, et al. Profiles of neuropsychological impairment in autopsy-defined Alzheimer's disease and cerebrovascular disease. Neurology 2007;130:731–9.

[33] Hachinski V, Iadecola C, Petersen RC, et al. National Institute of Neurological Disorders and Stroke–Canadian stroke network vascular cognitive impairment harmonization standards. Stroke 2006;37:2220–41.

[34] Longstreth WT, Manolio TA, Arnold A, et al, for the Cardiovascular Health Study Collaborative Research Group. Clinical correlates of white matter findings on cranial magnetic resonance imaging of 3301 elderly people. The Cardiovascular Health Study. Stroke 1996;27: 1274–82.

[35] Fein G, DiSclafani V, Tanabe J, et al. Hippocampal and cortical atrophy predict dementia in subcortical ischemic vascular disease. Neurology 2000;55:1626–35.

[36] Prins ND, van Dijk EJ, den Heijer T, et al. Cerebral small-vessel disease and decline in information processing speed, executive function and memory. Brain 2005;128:2034–41.

[37] Mosley TH, Knopman DS, Catellier DJ, et al. Cerebral MRI findings and cognitive functioning. The Atherosclerosis Risk in Communities Study. Neurology 2005;64:2056–62.

[38] De Leeuw F-E, de Groot JC, Oudkerk M, et al. Hypertension and cerebral white matter lesions in a prospective cohort study. Brain 2002;125:765–72.

[39] Manolio TA, Kronmal RA, Burke GL, et al. Short-term predictors of incident stroke in older adults. The Cardiovascular Health Study. Stroke 1996;27:1479–86.

[40] Longstreth WT, Arnold Am, Beauchamp NJ, et al. Incidence, manifestations, and predictors of worsening white matter on serial cranial magnetic resonance imaging in the elderly: the Cardiovascular Health Study. Stroke 2005;36:56–61.

[41] Mungas D, Jagust WJ, Reed BR, et al. MRI predictors of cognition in subcortical ischemic vascular disease and Alzheimer disease. Neurology 2001;57:2229–35.

[42] Mungas D, Reed BR, Jagust WJ, et al. Volumetric MRI predictors of cognitive decline related to Alzheimer's disease and cerebrovascular disease. Neurology 2002;59:867–73.

[43] Mungas D, Harvey D, Reed BR, et al. Longitudinal volumetric MRI change and rate of cognitive decline. Neurology 2005;65:565–71.

[44] Jagust WJ, Zheng L, Harvey DJ, et al. Neuropathological basis of MR images in aging and dementia. Ann Neurol, submitted for publication.

[45] Ishiko A, Shimuzu A, Nagata E, et al. Cerebral autosomal dominant arteriopathy with subcortical infarcts and leukoencephalopathy (CADASIL): a hereditary cerebrovascular disease which can be diagnosed by skin biopsy electron microscopy. Am J Dermatopathol 2005;27:131–4.
[46] Peters N, Opherk C, Bergmann T, et al. Spectrum of mutations in biopsy-proven CADASIL. Arch Neurol 2005;62:1091–4.
[47] O'Sullivan M, Jarosz JM, Martin RJ, et al. MRI hyperintensities of the temporal lobe and external capsule in patients with CADASIL. Neurology 2001;56:628–34.
[48] Lesnik Oberstein SAJ, van den Boom R, van Buchem MA, et al, for the Dutch CADASIL research group. Cerebral microbleeds in CADASIL. Neurology 2001;57:1066–70.
[49] Peters N, Opherk C, Danek A, et al. The pattern of cognitive performance in CADASIL: a monogenic condition leading to subcortical ischemic vascular dementia. Am J Psychiatry 2005;162:2078–85.
[50] O'Sullivan M, Barrick TR, Morris RG, et al. Damage within a network of white matter regions underlies executive dysfunction in CADASIL. Neurology 2005;65:1584–90.
[51] Schneider AT, Kissela B, Woo D, et al. Ischemic stroke subtypes: a population-based study of incidence rates among blacks and whites. Stroke 2004;35:1552–6.
[52] Jackson C, Sudlow C. Are lacunar strokes really different? A systematic review of differences in risk factor profiles between lacunar and nonlacunar infarcts. Stroke 2005;36: 891–904.
[53] Ohira T, Shahar E, Chambless LE, et al. Risk factors for ischemic stroke subtypes: the Atherosclerosis Risk in Community Study. Stroke 2006;37:2493–8.
[54] Elias MF, Wolf PA, D'Agostino RB, et al. Untreated blood pressure level is inversely related to cognitive functioning: the Framingham Study. Am J Epidemiol 1993;138:353–64.
[55] Launer LJ, Masaki K, Petrovich H, et al. The association between midlife blood pressure levels and late-life cognitive function. The Honolulu-Asia Aging Study. JAMA 1995;274: 1846–51.
[56] Peila R, White LR, Masaki K, et al. Reducing the risk of dementia. Efficacy of long-term treatment of hypertension. Stroke 2006;37:1165–70.
[57] Dufouil C, de Kersaint-Gilly A, Besancon V, et al. Longitudinal study of blood pressure and white matter hyperintensities. The EVA MRI Cohort. Neurology 2001;56:921–6.
[58] Enzinger C, Fazekas F, Matthews PM, et al. Risk factors for progression of brain atrophy in aging. Neurology 2005;64:1704–11.
[59] Longstreth WT, Katz R, Olson J, et al. Plasma total homocysteine levels and cranial magnetic resonance imaging findings in elderly persons. The cardiovascular Health Study. Arch Neurol 2004;61:67–72.
[60] Bernick C, Katz R, Smith NL, et al, for the Cardiovascular Health Study Collaborative Research Group. Statins and cognitive function in the elderly. The Cardiovascular Health Study. Neurology 2005;65:1388–94.
[61] Forette F, Seux ML, Staessen JA, et al. Prevention of dementia in randomized double-blind placebo-controlled Systolic Hypertension in Europe (Syst-Eur) trial. Lancet 1998;352: 1347–51.
[62] Forette F, Seux ML, Staessen JA, et al. The prevention of dementia with antihypertensive treatment: New evidence from the Systolic Hypertension in Europe (Syst-Eur) study. Arch Intern Med 2002;162:2046–52.
[63] The PROGRESS Collaborative Group. Effects of blood pressure lowering with perindopril and indapamide therapy on dementia and cognitive decline in patients with cerebrovascular disease. Arch Intern Med 2003;163:1069–75.
[64] Dufouil C, Chalmers J, Coskun O, et al. Effects of blood pressure lowering on cerebral white matter hyperintensities in patients with stroke. The PROGRESS magnetic resonance imaging substudy. Circulation 2005;112:1644–50.
[65] Pantoni L, del Ser T, Soglian AG, et al. Efficacy and safety of nimodipine in subcortical vascular dementia: a randomized placebo-controlled trial. Stroke 2005;36:619–24.

[66] Erkinjuntti T, Kurz A, Gauthier S, et al. Efficacy of galantamine in probable vascular dementia and Alzheimer's disease combined with cerebrovascular disease: a randomized trial. The Lancet 2002;359:1283–90.
[67] Wilkinson D, Dood R, Helme R, et al, the Donepezil 308 Study Group. Donepezil in vascular dementia: a randomized, placebo-controlled study. Neurology 2003;61:479–86.
[68] Schneider LS, Loy C, Birks J, et al. Cholinesterase inhibitors are associated with differential risks for death in vascular dementia and in severe Alzheimer's disease. Alzheimer's Association 10th International Conference on Alzheimer's Disease and Related Disorders, Madrid, July 15–20, 2006.
[69] Tomimoto H, Ohtani R, Shibata M, et al. Loss of cholinergic pathways in vascular dementia of the Binswanger type. Dement Geriatr Cogn Disord 2005;19:282–8.
[70] Keverne JS, Low WCR, Ziabreva I, et al. Cholinergic neuronal deficits in CADASIL. Stroke 2007;38:188–91.
[71] Goldstein LB, Adams R, Alberts MJ, et al. Primary prevention of ischemic stroke: a guideline from the American Heart Association/American Stroke Association Stroke Council; Cosponsored by the Atherosclerotic Peripheral Vascular Disease Interdisciplinary Work Group; Cardiovascular Nursing Council; Clinical Cardiology Council; Nutrition, Physical Activity, and Metabolism Council; and the Quality of Care and Outcomes Research Interdisciplinary Working Group. Stroke 2006;37:1583–633.
[72] Chobanian AV, Bakris GL, Black HR, et al. The seventh report of the Joint National Committee on Prevention, detection, evaluation, and treatment of high blood pressure: the JNC 7 report. JAMA 2003;289:2560–72.

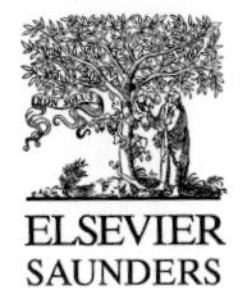

ELSEVIER
SAUNDERS

Neurol Clin 25 (2007) 741–760

NEUROLOGIC
CLINICS

Dementia with Lewy Bodies

Tanis J. Ferman, PhD[a,*], Bradley F. Boeve, MD[b]

[a]*Department of Psychiatry & Psychology, Mayo Clinic, Jacksonville, FL 32224, USA*

[b]*Mayo Clinic College of Medicine, Rochester MN 55905, USA*

Neocortical Lewy bodies are found in approximately 20% to 35% of elderly persons who have dementia [1–4] and do not occur commonly in normal brains [5]. Based on sensitive immunostaining techniques, dementia with Lewy bodies (DLB) is now considered the second most common cause of neurodegenerative dementia after Alzheimer's disease (AD) [5,6]. In 1996, consensus criteria for the clinical diagnosis of DLB were put forth that required dementia plus one or two of the following core features (two for probable DLB or one for possible DLB): recurrent fully formed visual hallucinations (VH), parkinsonism, and fluctuating cognition [7]. Using these criteria, diagnostic accuracy varies from poor to excellent [8–11]. Problems with reliable assessment of fluctuations, a lack of empiric data regarding when core features should occur relative to dementia onset, and limitations to study design (eg, circularity, absence of standardized assessment, and inclusion of cases with advanced dementia) contribute to this discrepancy [12–16]. The Third International Workshop meeting on DLB resulted in publication of revised consensus diagnostic criteria for DLB in December 2005 [17]. These criteria are presented in Box 1.

Neuropsychologic function

The dementias of DLB and AD are similar in insidious onset and progressive course, and before autopsy, many patients who have Lewy body disease are given the antemortem diagnosis of AD [3,13]. Despite some similarities, several studies show greater deficits in attention and visual perception in DLB, whereas AD is associated with worse memory and naming

Supported by NIH grants R01-AG15866, P50-AG16574, and P50-NS40256.

* Corresponding author.

E-mail address: ferman.tanis@mayo.edu (T.J. Ferman).

0733-8619/07/$ - see front matter

doi:10.1016/j.ncl.2007.03.001

Box 1. Revised criteria for the clinical diagnosis of dementia with Lewy bodies (DLB)

1. Central feature (essential for a diagnosis of possible or probable DLB)
   - Dementia defined as progressive cognitive decline of sufficient magnitude to interfere with normal social or occupational function
   - Prominent or persistent memory impairment may not necessarily occur in the early stages but usually is evident with progression
   - Deficits on tests of attention, executive function, and visuospatial ability may be especially prominent
2. Core features (two core features are sufficient for a diagnosis of probable DLB or one for possible DLB)
   - Fluctuating cognition with pronounced variation in attention and alertness
   - Recurrent VH that typically are well formed and detailed
   - Spontaneous features of parkinsonism
3. Suggestive features (If one or more of these is present in the presence of one or more core features, a diagnosis of probable DLB can be made. In the absence of any core features, one or more suggestive features is sufficient for possible DLB. Probable DLB should not be diagnosed on the basis of suggested features alone.)
   - REM sleep behavior disorder (RBD)
   - Severe neuroleptic sensitivity
   - Low dopamine transporter uptake in the basal ganglia demonstrated by single photon emission CT or positron emission tomographic imaging

From McKeith IG, Dickson DW, Lowe J, et al. Diagnosis and management of dementia with Lewy bodies: third report of the DLB consortium. Neurology 2005;65:1863–72; with permission.

[3,18–20]. Logistic regression modeling was done to determine the diagnostic usefulness of cognitive assessment in the differentiation of a prospective sample of persons who had DLB (n = 87) from those who did not have AD (n = 138) and those who had normal aging (n = 103) [21]. Patient groups did not differ in age, education, or dementia severity. The logistic models reveal that impairment in basic attention, visual perception, visual construction, and memory distinguished DLB from normal aging (sensitivity of 88.6% and specificity of 96.1%). In contrast, impaired visual construction and attention plus preserved memory and naming skills distinguished DLB from AD (sensitivity of 83.3% and a specificity of 91.4%). These results confirm the authors' prior findings of a double dissociation in neurocognitive function between early DLB and AD [21].

The higher-order visual processing deficits in DLB is a finding not attributable to motor slowness associated with parkinsonism [3,20,22–26]. The perceptual deficits evident in DLB may be responsible for some misperceptions (ie, illusions) and delusional misidentification (ie, reduplicative paramnesia, Capgras phenomena or not recognizing family). DLB patients with VH tend to do more poorly on visual tasks [19–25,27]. Nonetheless, some studies have not found differences between AD and DLB on visual tasks [28,29], although this may be because of methodologic issues, such as the inclusion of patients in the advanced stages of dementia, which can obfuscate group differences resulting from generalized impairment. Alternately, differential impairment of other task demands may be a factor. For example, visual problem solving may be affected negatively by executive difficulties in AD and by perceptual difficulties in DLB. Mori and colleagues examined this issue and revealed deficits in DLB but not AD on basic visual tasks that do not require executive function [30]. A distinction between spatial and perceptual processing also seems to be a distinguishing factor, with patients who have DLB showing greater deficits in the latter [31]. There may be group differences in how the information initially is encoded. Reflexive saccadic eye movements responsible for repositioning the fovea show greater impairment for DLB compared with AD [32], and regional blood flow is shown to be lower in occipital regions in DLB despite the relative absence of Lewy pathology there [33–36]. Overall, visual processing deficits in DLB may be the result of disruption of the cortical extrastriate association areas (especially the ventral visual pathway), but there also may be disruption to the afferent system (perhaps via mechanisms subserving saccadic foveation) before reaching the primary visual cortex.

Memory difficulties, when present in early DLB, seem to be fairly mild and stand in direct contrast to the pronounced amnestic disturbance of AD [18–20]. Neuropathologic and imaging studies also show significant atrophy in the hippocampus in AD, whereas patients who have DLB show little difference from normal controls [37–39]. Salmon and colleagues [18] demonstrated a pattern of poor initial learning and retrieval in four of five patients who had DLB without the rapid forgetting that typically is observed in AD. In a sample of nine cases of pure DLB, 57 of mixed DLB/AD, and 66 of pure AD, patients who had AD pathology performed worse on tasks of verbal memory, whereas patients who had LB pathology performed worse on tasks of visual spatial skills, and combined pathology affected visual spatial performance but not verbal memory [40].

Spontaneous motor features of parkinsonism

For diagnostic clarity, parkinsonian signs must be spontaneous and not attributable to neuroleptics [7]. Cognitive impairment in Parkinson's disease (PD) and DLB is associated more often with rigidity and bradykinesia than tremor [41–50]. Postural instability/gait difficulty is over-represented in DLB and Parkinson's disease dementia (PDD) compared with PD [51], and this has led some to speculate that extrapyramidal signs associated with dementia may have a dopaminergic and a nondopaminergic basis. In general, the parkinsonism associated with DLB tends to be less severe than that observed in PD or PDD, at least initially. Tremor, bradykinesia, and rigidity tend to be more symmetric than asymmetric, and tremor tends to be maximal with posture/action rather than at rest. One study of 14 patients who had DLB, 28 who had PD, and 30 who had PDD showed improvement in the Unified Parkinson's Disease Rating Scale score for all three groups in response to levodopa but less so for the patients who had DLB [52]. The possibility that this effect may be mediated by greater initial motor deficits in the PDD and PD groups should be considered.

Visual hallucinations

VH in DLB consist of fully formed, detailed, 3-dimensional objects, people, or animals that are not attributable to perceptual distortion or illusion [3,47,53]. Patients who have DLB with auditory hallucinations typically experience VH, but auditory hallucinations rarely occur in patients who do not have VH [54,55]. Hallucinations in DLB do not occur as a function of AD pathology [56] and are not associated with levodopa dose or the presence of "on" (able to move) and "off" (unable to move) states [57]. VH have been documented to occur in 59% to 85% of autopsy-confirmed DLB samples and in 11% to 28% of autopsy-confirmed AD samples [5,15,58,59]. Autopsy studies reveal that VH are most likely to occur early in DLB disease course, whereas they tend to occur in the advanced stages of AD [5,60–62]. In an autopsy study of DLB (n = 41) and AD (n = 70), a cutoff of 4 years for the onset of hallucinations relative to dementia onset improved the positive and negative predictive values of DLB to 81% and 79%, respectively [63]. Patients who have VH typically have greater cognitive and functional impairment [64–68], but whether or not the presence of VH in DLB is associated with faster rate of disease progression has yet to be determined. The underlying cause of hallucinations most likely is associated with the severe depletion of acetylcholine in DLB, but other neurotransmitter systems may have a contributory role, including dopamine and serotonin. Involvement of the basal forebrain and the ventral temporal lobe are implicated in the causation of VH, given their respective cholinergic and visual perceptual roles [5,58]. Also, the dysregulation of rapid eye movement (REM) sleep in many patients who have DLB raises the possibility of intrusion of dream imagery into wakefulness as a potential mechanism [69,70]. These etiologies are not necessarily mutually exclusive.

Fluctuations

The fluctuations of DLB resemble signs of delirium without identifiable precipitants of such mental status changes. This phenomenon involves a waxing and waning of cognition, abilities, and arousal. It has been described as variable attention, incoherent speech, hypersomnolence, impaired awareness of surroundings, staring into space, or appearing "glazed" or "switched off." The prevalence of fluctuations in DLB samples is widely discrepant and ranges from 10% to 80% with poor inter-rater reliability [8,10,12,71,72]. Studies often do not specify how the presence of fluctuations is determined and the usefulness of this core clinical feature has been highly criticized. Available techniques to assess fluctuations include a brief interview rating scale relying on clinical expertise, a semistructured interview that inquires about the day before the assessment [16,73–76], and a set of four questions derived from a lengthier questionnaire [77]. The latter questionnaire is designed to determine whether or not there are salient features of fluctuations that reliably differentiate DLB (n = 70) from AD (n = 70) and normal elderly (n = 200). Results show that four items significantly differentiated DLB from AD, including (1) daytime drowsiness and lethargy, (2) daytime sleep of 2 or more hours, (3) staring into space for long periods, and (4) times when a patient's flow of ideas seems disorganized, unclear, or not logical. The presence of three or four features of this composite occurred in 63% of patients who had DLB compared with 12% of those who had AD and 0.5% normal elderly ($P < .01$). A score of 3 or 4 yields a positive predictive value of 83% for the clinical diagnosis of DLB against an alternate diagnosis of AD, and a score of less than 3 yields a negative predictive value of 70% for the absence of DLB in favor of AD. Because not all patients who have DLB have fluctuations, these values suggest reasonable diagnostic usefulness. No particular combination of VH, parkinsonism (presence or severity), or RBD was associated with a fluctuations composite score of 3 or 4 [77]. These data indicate that an informant-based questionnaire is sensitive to fluctuations in alertness and speech but fails to differentiate fluctuations in ability or cognition between DLB and AD. It may be worthwhile to distinguish between fluctuations in arousal and cognition, whereby the latter may be evaluated best with neuropsychometric tests. This is supported by findings that attention, vigilance, and reaction time show greater impairment and variability in DLB than in AD [20,73,75].

Excessive daytime drowsiness

Patients who have DLB often have daytime drowsiness or somnolence. As such, ruling out known causes of daytime sleepiness, including medications and primary sleep disorders (ie, sleep apnea), is critical. In a clinical referral sample of 78 patients with early DLB who underwent overnight polysomnography, approximately three quarters of the sample had a significant number of arousals not accounted for by medication, periodic limb movements of sleep, or sleep apnea [78,79]. In half of the DLB sample, sleep efficiency fell well below the expected 80% for this age group [80–82]. This raises the possibility that dysfunction of brainstem or hypothalamic neuronal networks subserving sleep and wakefulness may be producing daytime drowsiness. Further studies are needed that represent a random selection of patients who have DLB and an AD group matched for age, gender, and dementia severity.

Rapid eye movement sleep behavior disorder

The loss of normal muscle atonia during rapid eye movement (REM) sleep refers to the parasomnia of REM sleep behavior disorder (RBD). In RBD, augmented muscle activity during REM sleep occurs along with dream content and can range from elevated muscle tone to complex behavioral sequences, such as pantomiming various activities that may be subdued or vigorous [22,83]. The presumed pathophysiologic mechanism of RBD involves damage to the descending pontine-medullary reticular formation (including the magnocellular reticular formation) or sublaterodorsal nucleus that leads to a loss of the normal REM sleep inhibition of the spinal alpha-motoneurons [84–87]. In humans, polysomnographic evidence of REM sleep without atonia is considered the electrophysiologic substrate of RBD and is found in patients with or without florid RBD [88,89]. RBD can precede the onset of neurodegenerative diseases with alpha-synuclein inclusions (ie, DLB, PD, or multiple system atrophy [MSA]) by years and even decades [22,89–94]. It rarely occurs in tau-predominant neurodegenerative conditions, such as AD [92]. Neuropathologic confirmation of Lewy body disease has been demonstrated in a patient who had a 20-year history of idiopathic RBD [93] and in a patient who had a 15-year history of idiopathic RBD [94], neither of whom had any other neurologic signs or symptoms or evidence of psychosis. Of 36 patients with clear clinical histories of RBD, 31 had Lewy body disease, four had MSA and one had progressive supranuclear palsy, providing further evidence that RBD usually reflects an underlying synucleinopathy [95].

The estimated onset of RBD typically precedes the onset of dementia, VH, and parkinsonism by many years and often decades (range, 6 months to 55 years) [19,20,22]. Despite this relationship, patients who present initially with dementia and RBD do not meet the 1996 DLB criteria until parkinsonism or hallucinations become apparent. The authors examined the neurocognitive performance of 25 patients who had RBD and dementia (without parkinsonism or hallucinations) and compared them to 37 patients with clinically probable DLB and 30 cases of autopsy-confirmed AD of matched dementia severity [19]. Results indicate that the DLB and RBD plus dementia groups were cognitively indistinguishable, but both groups differed significantly from autopsy-confirmed AD group of matched dementia severity. Follow-up data from a subset of patients who had RBD plus dementia revealed the subsequent development of parkinsonism or VH 1 to 6 years later. Thus, a clinical history of RBD in the context of dementia with disproportionate visual deficits and relatively preserved memory and naming is likely to represent the earliest stages of DLB.

Dysautonomia

Autonomic abnormalities, in particular orthostatic hypotension and carotid sinus sensitivity, are more common in DLB than AD or elderly controls [17]. A comparison of dysautonomia in DLB, PD, and MSA shows that orthostatic hypotension is affected most severely in MSA, least severely in PD, and of intermediate severity in DLB [96]. The DLB group tended to respond better to medications than the MSA group. The frequency of urinary symptoms and pattern of sweat loss in DLB was comparable to that of PD but much less than MSA.

Rate of decline in dementia with Lewy bodies

Several studies of DLB indicate a more rapid progression than that of pure AD, and earlier studies of AD suggest extrapyramidal features and psychosis are predictors of decline [13,48,97–100]. Some recent data, however, show no difference in the rate of cognitive decline between DLB and AD [101,102]. In an autopsy study of patients who were part of the Florida Alzheimer's Disease Initiative Brain Bank, there was a shorter duration of illness for DLB compared with AD [63]. In a longitudinal study of 63 patients who had DLB and 252 who had AD, psychometric performance and clinical staging methods did not distinguish groups in terms of rate of cognitive decline, but DLB was associated with increased risk of mortality. Extrapyramidal signs were a strong predictor of mortality [103].

Description and distribution of pathology in dementia with Lewy bodies

Lewy bodies are concentric, intracytoplasmic neuronal inclusions that have long been a recognized pathology of brainstem monoaminergic and cholinergic nuclei in idiopathic PD [104,105]. Subcortical Lewy bodies are distributed in the dorsal motor nucleus of the vagus, medullary magnocellular reticular nuclei, locus coeruleus, raphe nucleus and midbrain tegmentum, and are adequately detected by hematoxylin and eosin (H & E) histologic staining [106–109]. Neocortical Lewy bodies are less eosinophilic, less circumscribed, and are best detected by alpha-synuclein immunohistochemistry [106]. The hypothalamus, basal forebrain, amygdale and temporal cortex are particularly vulnerable to cortical Lewy bodies, with lesser involvement of frontal and posterior cortical regions [108–111]. Spongiosis also is observed in the amygdala and basal forebrain [106]. Similarly, using MRI, the rates of whole brain atrophy and ventricular expansion during a 1- to 2-year interval do not differ between a sample of DLB later confirmed by autopsy and normal controls [112]. When compared with AD, MRI voxel-based morphometry reveals that DLB has little cortical involvement but does show a discrete cluster of gray matter loss in the cholinergic-rich regions of the nucleus basalis of Meynert in the basal forebrain and dorsal midbrain [113].

Lewy neurites are widespread alpha-synuclein–positive inclusions that are located in neural processes and preferentially affect limbic and temporal lobe structures [37,38,107].

A portion of DLB cases has AD-type pathology that includes neurofibrillary tangles (NFTs) and neuritic plaques [3,4,13]. Plaques are composed of extracellular beta-amyloid (Aβ) protein deposits comprised of 40 and 42 amino acid peptides. The neuritic plaques that accompany AD include a dense core of Aβ40 with neuritic processes composed of the protein tau [114]. In contrast, plaques in Lewy body disease typically are diffuse (although some may contain a core) and are composed primarily of Aβ42 with a paucity or absence of tau-positive neuritis [115–119]. Diffuse plaques also are numerous in brains of cognitively normal elderly [37,120,121]. Most clinicopathologic studies of DLB and AD do not take this distinction into account, and as such, it is not known whether or not differences in plaque type influence clinical presentation. When NFTs are present in Lewy body disease, they are far less frequent than in AD, and regional distribution using Braak staging often is at Braak IV or less, indicating confinement to limbic regions [3,47,122–125]. Clinical diagnostic accuracy of DLB is significantly better in those who have low Braak stages and lower tangle density [126,127].

Clinicopathologic correlates in dementia with Lewy bodies and Alzheimer's disease

Dementia severity is not associated with neocortical plaque density but is related to NFT burden in AD [123,128,129]. In DLB, Lewy body density but not plaque or NFT density is correlated with dementia severity [123,130,131]. Lewy neurite density also is associated with the degree of cognitive impairment in DLB [132], suggesting that these inclusions may interfere with neuronal function, but further investigation is needed.

In AD, the CA1 region and subiculum of the hippocampus are affected severely, whereas the CA2/3 region is considered the "resistant zone" and typically is spared [133–135]. In DLB, it is the CA2/3 region that is affected, whereas the CA1 and subiculum regions typically are spared [37,136]. Similarly, AD is associated with a near total loss of perforant pathway neurons, whereas in DLB, the perforant pathway is more comparable to that of normal controls [137]. Although damage to the CA1 region is associated with memory impairment, is not known if CA2/3 pathology affects memory function.

The ventral temporal lobe is burdened heavily by prominent Lewy body pathology and spongiosis [48,106]. This neuroanatomic pattern seems to occur well before the onset of Lewy body pathology in other cortical regions, including the parietal lobe [110]. Thus, early specific visual perceptual deficits may be associated with disruption of the pattern/object recognition pathway. Patients who have VH have higher LB densities in amygdala, parahippocampus, and inferior temporal cortex [136], suggesting the involvement of these regions in the development of VH. Nonetheless, VH occur in patients with limbic-only Lewy body pathology [63] indicating that temporal lobe dysfunction is not required to elicit VH, though it certainly may have a modulating role.

The cholinergic hypothesis fits dementia with Lewy bodies better than Alzheimer's disease

The use of new cholinergic toxins to selectively target the nucleus basalis of Meynert (which is 90% cholinergic and widely projects to the cortex) [138] reveals no impairment of memory but does indicate deficits in sustained and divided attention [139–143]. In addition, profound cholinergic neuronal loss and severely depleted choline acetyltransferase levels occur early in DLB disease course, whereas AD and normal controls show little difference until the advanced stage of dementia [144–147]. In addition, anticholinergic agents can elicit hallucinations and disturbed consciousness that vary as a function of cholinergic deficiency [148–153]. Not surprisingly, one hypothesized mechanism for fluctuations and VH in DLB includes cholinergic depletion of the basal forebrain alone [5,145,149,154]. Increasing acetylcholine availability with cholinesterase inhibitors improves attention, hallucinations, and alertness in early DLB [154–159]. Thus, cholinergic depletion is a critical factor in the symptom manifestation of early DLB but may be less so in early AD. This highlights the importance of differentiating between early versus late stages of different dementias, because patients who have advanced AD may have similar clinical features as those who have early DLB.

Pharmacologic treatment of dementia with Lewy bodies

When faced with a challenging behavior, it is critical first to evaluate for potential medical contributors (eg, pain, medication side effects, injury, underlying sleep disorder, depression, dehydration, metabolic disturbance, and so on) and treat accordingly.

Neuroleptic medication is frequently administered to patients with dementia for episodic confusion, hallucinations, delusions, and agitation [160,161]. These clinical features are observed commonly in DLB, but there is convincing evidence that patients who have DLB can harbor neuroleptic sensitivity to traditional and to some atypical neuroleptics [59,162–166]. Specifically, antipsychotic agents with D2 antagonism and anticholinergic properties precipitate or exacerbate extrapyramidal signs and cognitive impairment, respectively [167,168]. Unfortunately, discontinuation of the neuroleptic does not necessarily lead to a reversal of the adverse reaction [59]. There is a mixed literature on the relationship between atypical antipsychotics and cognition, but quetiapine has a better response profile overall in DLB relative to AD [169–174]. Olanzepine does not seem to worsen parkinsonism [169], but its anticholinergic properties may exacerbate cognitive impairment [172].

Levodopa-carbidopa is generally well tolerated in DLB, does diminish extrapyramidal signs and does not seem to precipitate a profound worsening of psychosis as seen in the dopamine agonists or amantadine. There is some data to suggest that the levodopa-carbidopa response in DLB may not be at the same magnitude as in PD [51], but further study is needed to confirm and better characterize this [175,176].

Brain acetylcholine is severely depleted in the early stages of DLB compared with early AD [5,145–147]. This is concerning because drugs with anticholinergic properties are commonly prescribed to the elderly to treat mood, psychosis, movement disorders, incontinence, and pulmonary disease [150]. Several studies clearly demonstrate adverse reactions to anticholinergic agents that mimic delirium [151–153,177]. Alternately, improvement (sometimes dramatic) in delirium-like symptoms, fluctuations and VH can occur with the use of cholinesterase inhibitors [146,178–181]. Studies of cholinesterase inhibitors [157,182,183] reveal improved cognition in DLB and AD and detrimental effects when withdrawn suddenly [184]. A comparison of DLB (n = 30) and Parkinson's disease with dementia (n = 40) who were taking donepezil revealed improved Mini–Mental State Examination scores by a mean of 3.9 points in the DLB group and by 3.2 points in the PDD group by 20 weeks [185]. Extrapyramidal side effects of cholinesterase inhibitors are low, and it is recommended as a first-line treatment for DLB [186].

The goals of therapy for RBD are to minimize the injuries to patients and their bed partners and to reduce the likelihood of disrupted nighttime sleep. Clonazepam at a very low dose usually is effective [187]. Melatonin also may be effective, either as monotherapy or in conjunction with clonazepam [188].

Excessive daytime sleepiness is challenging, and the first approach is to try to identify if the cause may be a medication side effect, mood, or a primary sleep disorder. Although psychostimulants would be expected to exacerbate hallucinations and delusions in DLB, experience has shown that daytime somnolence in some patients can be managed with agents, such as modafinil and methylphenidate [69].

Nonpharmacologic treatment

Behaviors should be recognized as a form of communication and not as random, unpredictable, or meaningless events. It may be helpful to determine in the situations where challenging behaviors occur (who is present, when do they happen, what makes them better or worse, and what maintains them) and to focus on the emotions that accompany behaviors. For example, aggressive behavior often represents frustration, fear, pain, a reaction to not being taken seriously, or even mirroring a caregiver's behavior (ie, impatience or agitation). Addressing these feelings may help alleviate a patient's agitation.

In terms of nonmedical interventions, managing challenging behaviors should be shifted from trying to change patients to modifying other factors that may be causing or exacerbating a problem [189]. Put differently, patients cannot change, and therefore, it is up to those around them to change. This includes modifying the environment (eg, reduce clutter, increase illumination, reduce distracting noise), modifying responses to behavior (eg, validate patient concerns, apologize, reassure patients, model calm, avoid correcting, quizzing, and "reality orienting"), and modifying task demands (eg, provide structure and routine, break down tasks into manageable parts, focus on success and not failure, refrain from giving tasks that are too hard, provide guided exercise).

Before treating hallucinations or delusions (false beliefs), it must be determined if these symptoms are harmful or distressing to patients. Educating family members about ways to cope with these behaviors includes encouraging them to validate patients' feelings and devising strategies that go along with behaviors (eg, checking the house for intruders or appearing to call somebody to see what time is check-out time) that provide reassurance and that do not involve arguing or trying to reason with patients.

Providing information for caregivers is an important part of helping to manage challenging behaviors. Psychoeducation intervention groups for caregivers are associated with significant improvements in agitation and anxiety for patients who have dementia [190]. Using available support services, including adult day programs and companion services, also are shown to reduce caregiver-related stress and reported feelings of overload, strain, depression, and anger [191].

Summary

Clinical features that may be helpful in distinguishing early DLB from AD include neurocognitive presentation, VH, extrapyramidal signs, fluctuations, neuroleptic sensitivity, RBD, and dysautonomia. Early and accurate detection of DLB has implications for symptom management and for providing education and support to patients who have DLB and their caregivers.

References

[1] Galasko D, Hansen LA, Katzman R, et al. Clinical-neuropathological correlations in Alzheimer's disease and related dementias. Arch Neurol 1994;51:888–95.

[2] Joachim CL, Morris JH, Selkoe DJ. Clinically diagnosed Alzheimer's disease: autopsy results in 150 cases. Ann Neurol 1988;24:50–6.

[3] Hansen L, Salmon D, Galasko D, et al. The Lewy body variant of Alzheimer's disease: a clinical and pathologic entity. Neurology 1990;40:1–8.

[4] Hulette C, Mirra S, Wilkinson W, et al. The consortium to establish a registry for Alzheimer's Disease (CERAD). Part IX. A prospective cliniconeuropathologic study of Parkinson's features in Alzheimer's disease. Neurology 1995;45:1991–5.

[5] Perry EK, Marshall E, Perry RH, et al. Cholinergic and dopaminergic activities in senile dementia of Lewy body type. Alzheimer Dis Assoc Disord 1990;4:87–95.

[6] Lennox G, Lowe J, Landon M, et al. Diffuse Lewy body disease: correlative neuropathology using anti-ubiquitin immunocytochemistry. J Neurol Neurosurg Psychiatry 1989;52: 1236–47.

[7] McKeith IG, Galasko D, Kosaka K, et al. Consensus guidelines for the clinical and pathologic diagnosis of dementia with Lewy bodies (DLB): report of the consortium on DLB international workshop. Neurology 1996;47:1113–24.

[8] McKeith IG, Ballard CG, Perry RH, et al. Prospective validation of consensus criteria for the diagnosis of dementia with Lewy bodies. Neurology 2000;54:1050–8.

[9] Lopez OL, Becker JT, Kaufer DI, et al. Research evaluation and prospective diagnosis of dementia with Lewy bodies. Arch Neurol 2002;59:43–6.

[10] Verghese J, Crystal HA, Dickson DW, et al. Validity of clinical criteria for the diagnosis of dementia with Lewy bodies. Neurology 1999;53:1974–82.

[11] Litvan I, MacIntyre A, Goetz CG, et al. Accuracy of the clinical diagnoses of Lewy body disease, Parkinson disease, and dementia with Lewy bodies: a clinicopathologic study. Arch Neurol 1998;55:969–78.

[12] Mega MS, Masterman DL, Benson DF, et al. Dementia with Lewy bodies: reliability and validity of clinical and pathologic criteria. Neurology 1996;47:1403–9.

[13] Lippa CF, Smith TW, Swearer JM. Alzheimer's disease and Lewy body disease: a comparative clinicopathological study. Ann Neurol 1994;35:81–8.

[14] Kuzuhara S, Yoshimura M. Clinical and neuropathological aspects of diffuse Lewy body disease in the elderly. Adv Neurol 1993;60:464–9.

[15] Klatka LA, Louis ED, Schiffer RB. Psychiatric features in diffuse Lewy body disease: a clinicopathologic study using Alzheimer's disease and Parkinson's disease comparison groups. Neurology 1996;47:1148–52.

[16] Walker MP, Ayre GA, Cummings JL, et al. The clinician assessment of fluctuation and the one day fluctuation assessment scale. Two methods to assess fluctuating confusion in dementia. Br J Psychiatry 2000;177:252–6.

[17] McKeith IG, Dickson DW, Lowe J, et al, for the consortium on DLB. Diagnosis and management of dementia with Lewy bodies: third report of the DLB consortium. Neurology 2005;65:1863–72.

[18] Salmon DP, Galasko D, Hansen LA, et al. Neuropsychological deficits associated with diffuse Lewy body disease. Brain Cogn 1996;31:148–65.

[19] Ferman TJ, Boeve BF, Smith GE, et al. Dementia with Lewy bodies may present as dementia and REM sleep behavior disorder without parkinsonism or hallucinations. J Int Neuropsychol Soc 2002;8:907–14.

[20] Ferman TJ, Boeve BF, Smith GE, et al. REM sleep behavior disorder and dementia: cognitive differences when compared with AD. Neurology 1999;52:951–7.

[21] Ferman TJ, Smith GE, Boeve BF, et al. Neuropsychological differentiation of dementia with Lewy bodies from normal aging and Alzheimer's disease. Clin Neuropsychol 2006; 20:623–36.

[22] Boeve BF, Silber MH, Ferman TJ, et al. REM sleep behavior disorder and degenerative dementia: an association likely reflecting Lewy body disease. Neurology 1998;51: 363–70.

[23] Calderon J, Perry RJ, Erzinclioglu SW, et al. Perception, attention, and working memory are disproportionately impaired in dementia with Lewy bodies compared with Alzheimer's disease. J Neurol Neurosurg Psychiatry 2001;70:157–64.

[24] Ballard C, Holmes C, McKeith I, et al. Psychiatric morbidity in dementia with Lewy bodies: a prospective clinical and neuropathological comparative study with Alzheimer's disease. Am J Psychiatry 1999;156:1039–45.

[25] Shimomura T, Mori E, Yamashita H, et al. Cognitive loss in dementia with Lewy bodies and Alzheimer disease. Arch Neurol 1998;55:1547–52.

[26] Connor DJ, Salmon DP, Sandy TJ, et al. Cognitive profiles of autopsy-confirmed Lewy body variant vs pure Alzheimer disease. Arch Neurol 1998;55:994–1000.

[27] Simard M, van Reekum R, Myran D. Visuospatial impairment in dementia with Lewy bodies and Alzheimer's disease: a process analysis approach. Int J Geriatr Psychiatry 2003;18:387–91.

[28] Forstl H, Burns A, Luthert P, et al. The Lewy-body variant of Alzheimer's disease. Clinical and pathological findings. Br J Psychiatry 1993;162:385–92.

[29] Gnanalingham KK, Byrne EJ, Thornton A, et al. Motor and cognitive function in Lewy body dementia: comparison with Alzheimer's and Parkinson's diseases. J Neurol Neurosurg Psychiatry 1997;62:243–52.

[30] Mori E, Shimomura T, Fujimori M, et al. Visuoperceptual impairment in dementia with L'wy bodies. Arch Neurol 2000;57:489–93.

[31] Mosimann UP, Mather G, Wesnes KA, et al. Visual perception in Parkinson disease dementia and dementia with Lewy bodies. Neurology 2004;63:2091–6.

[32] Mosimann UP, Muri RM, Burn DJ, et al. Saccadic eye movement changes in Parkinson's disease dementia and dementia with Lewy bodies. Brain 2005;128:1267–76.

[33] Mito Y, Yoshida K, Yabe I, et al. Brain 3-D-SSP SPECT analysis in dementia with Lewy bodies, Parkinson's disease with and without dementia and Alzheimer's disease. Clinical Neurology and Neurosurgery 2005;107:396–403.

[34] Shimuzu S, Hanyu H, Kanetaka H, et al. Differentiation of dementia with Lewy bodies from Alzheimer's disease using brain SPECT. Dementia and Geriatric Cognitive Disorders 2005;20:25–30.

[35] Lobotesis K, Fenwick JD, Phipps A, et al. Occipital hypoperfusion on SPECT in dementia with Lewy bodies but not AD. Neurology 2001;56:643–9.

[36] Imamura T, Ishii K, Hirono N, et al. Occipital glucose metabolism in dementia with lewy bodies with and without Parkinsonism: a study using positron emission tomography. Dement Geriatr Cogn Disord 2001;12:194–7.

[37] Dickson DW, Ruan D, Crystal H, et al. Hippocampal degeneration differentiates diffuse Lewy body disease (DLBD) from Alzheimer's disease: light and electron microscopic immunocytochemistry of CA2-3 neurites specific to DLBD. Neurology 1991;41: 1402–9.

[38] Dickson DW, Schmidt ML, Lee VM, et al. Immunoreactivity profile of hippocampal CA2/3 neurites in diffuse Lewy body disease. Acta Neuropathol (Berl) 1994;87:269–76.

[39] Barber R, Gholkar A, Scheltens P, et al. Medial temporal lobe atrophy on MRI in dementia with Lewy bodies. Neurology 1999;52:1153–8.

[40] Johnson DK, Morris JC, Galvin JE. Verbal and visuospatial deficits in dementia with Lewy bodies. Neurology 2005;65:1232–8.

[41] Huber SJ, Paulson GW, Shuttleworth EC. Relationship of motor symptoms, intellectual impairment, and depression in Parkinson's disease. J Neurol Neurosurg Psychiatry 1988; 51:855–8.
[42] Richards M, Stern Y, Marder K, et al. Relationships between extrapyramidal signs and cognitive function in a community-dwelling cohort of patients with Parkinson's disease and normal elderly individuals. Ann Neurol 1993;33:267–74.
[43] Pearce J. The extrapyramidal disorder of Alzheimer's disease. Eur Neurol 1974;12:94–103.
[44] Molsa PK, Marttila RJ, Rinne UK. Extrapyramidal signs in Alzheimer's disease. Neurology 1984;34:1114–6.
[45] Rinne UK, Laakso K, Molsa PK. Relationship between Parkinson's and Alzheimer's diseases. Involvement of extrapyramidal, dopaminergic, cholinergic, and somatostatin mechanisms in relation to dementia. Acta Neurol Scand 1984;69:59–60.
[46] Mayeux R, Stern Y, Spanton S. Heterogeneity in dementia of the Alzheimer type: evidence of subgroups. Neurology 1985;35:453–61.
[47] Crystal HA, Dickson DW, Lizardi JE, et al. Antemortem diagnosis of diffuse Lewy body disease. Neurology 1990;40:1523–8.
[48] Byrne EJ, Lennox G, Lowe J, et al. Diffuse Lewy body disease: clinical features in 15 cases. J Neurol Neurosurg Psychiatry 1989;52:709–17.
[49] Galasko D, Katzman R, Salmon DP, et al. Clinical and neuropathological findings in Lewy body dementias. Brain Cogn 1996;31:166–75.
[50] Gibb WR, Esiri MM, Lees AJ. Clinical and pathological features of diffuse cortical Lewy body disease (Lewy body dementia). Brain 1987;110(Pt 5):1131–53.
[51] McKeith I, Mintzer J, Aarsland D, et al, on behalf of the International Psychogeriatric Association Expert Meeting on DLB. Dementia with Lewy bodies. Lancet Neurol 2004; 3:19–28.
[52] Molloy S, McKeith IG, O'Brien JT, et al. The role of levodopa in the management of dementia with Lewy bodies. J of Neurol, Neurosurg and Psychiatry 2005;76:1200–3.
[53] McKeith IG, Fairbairn AF, Perry RH, et al. The clinical diagnosis and misdiagnosis of senile dementia of Lewy body type (SDLT). Br J Psychiatry 1994;165:324–32.
[54] Ferman TJ, Boeve BF, Silber MH, et al. Hallucinations and delusions associated with the REM sleep behavior disorder/dementia syndrome. J Neuropsychiatry Clin Neurosci 1997; 9:692.
[55] Ferman TJ, Boeve BF, Smith GE, et al. The phenomenology of psychotic features in Dementia with Lewy bodies (DLB) and Alzheimer's disease (AD). Neurology 2005; 64:A257.
[56] Cercy SP, Bylsma FW. Lewy bodies and progressive dementia: a critical review and meta-analysis. J Int Neuropsychol Soc 1997;3:179–94.
[57] Sanchez-Ramos JR, Ortoll R, Paulson GW. Visual hallucinations associated with Parkinson disease. Arch Neurol 1996;53:1265–8.
[58] Harding AJ, Broe GA, Halliday GM. Visual hallucinations in Lewy body disease relate to Lewy bodies in the temporal lobe. Brain 2002;125:391–403.
[59] McKeith I, Fairbairn A, Perry R, et al. Neuroleptic sensitivity in patients with senile dementia of Lewy body type. BMJ 1992;305:673–8.
[60] Rockwell E, Choure J, Galasko D, et al. Psychopathology at initial diagnosis in dementia with Lewy bodies versus Alzheimer disease: comparison of matched groups with autopsy-confirmed diagnoses. Int J Geriatr Psychiatry 2000;15:819–23.
[61] Ala TA, Yang KH, Sung JH, et al. Hallucinations and signs of parkinsonism help distinguish patients with dementia and cortical Lewy bodies from patients with Alzheimer's disease at presentation: a clinicopathological study. J Neurol Neurosurg Psychiatry 1997; 62:16–21.
[62] Hope T, Keene J, Fairburn CG, et al. Natural history of behavioural changes and psychiatric symptoms in Alzheimer's disease. A longitudinal study. Br J Psychiatry 1999;174: 39–44.

[63] Ferman TJ, Dickson DW, Graff-Radford N, et al. Early onset of visual hallucinations in dementia distinguishes pathologically-confirmed Lewy body disease from AD. Neurology 2003;60(5):A264.

[64] Salmon DP, Kwo-on-Yuen PF, Heindel WC, et al. Differentiation of Alzheimer's disease and Huntington's disease with the Dementia Rating Scale. Arch Neurol 1989;46: 1204–8.

[65] Ballard C, Bannister C, Graham C, et al. Associations of psychotic symptoms in dementia sufferers. Br J Psychiatry 1995;167:537–40.

[66] Klein C, Kompf D, Pulkowski U, et al. A study of visual hallucinations in patients with Parkinson's disease. J Neurol 1997;244:371–7.

[67] Lopez OL, Becker JT, Brenner RP, et al. Alzheimer's disease with delusions and hallucinations: neuropsychological and electroencephalographic correlates. Neurology 1991;41: 906–12.

[68] Lopez OL, Brenner RP, Becker JT, et al. EEG spectral abnormalities and psychosis as predictors of cognitive and functional decline in probable Alzheimer's disease. Neurology 1997;48:1521–5.

[69] Boeve B, Silber M, Ferman T. REM sleep behavior disorder in Parkinson's disease and dementia with Lewy bodies. J Geriatr Psychiatry Neurol 2004;17:146–57.

[70] Boeve BF, Silber MH, Parisi JE, et al. Synucleinopathy pathology and REM sleep behavior disorder plus dementia or parkinsonism. Neurology 2003;61:40–5.

[71] Lopez OL, Hamilton RL, Becker JT, et al. Severity of cognitive impairment and the clinical diagnosis of AD with Lewy bodies. Neurology 2000;54:1780–7.

[72] Hohl U, Tiraboschi P, Hansen LA, et al. Diagnostic accuracy of dementia with Lewy bodies. Arch Neurol 2000;57:347–51.

[73] Walker MP, Ayre GA, Perry EK, et al. Quantification and characterization of fluctuating cognition in dementia with Lewy bodies and Alzheimer's disease. Dement Geriatr Cogn Disord 2000;11:327–35.

[74] Ballard CG, Aarsland D, McKeith I, et al. Fluctuations in attention: PD dementia vs DLB with parkinsonism. Neurology 2002;59:1714–20.

[75] Ballard C, Walker M, O'Brien J, et al. The characterisation and impact of 'fluctuating' cognition in dementia with Lewy bodies and Alzheimer's disease. Int J Geriatr Psychiatry 2001; 16:494–8.

[76] Ballard C, O'Brien J, Gray A, et al. Attention and fluctuating attention in patients with dementia with Lewy bodies and Alzheimer disease. Arch Neurol 2001;58: 977–82.

[77] Ferman TJ, Smith GE, Boeve BF, et al. DLB fluctuations: specific features that reliably differentiate DLB from AD and normal aging. Neurology 2004;62:181–7.

[78] Ferman TJ, Boeve BF, Silber MH, et al. Is fluctuating cognition in dementia with sleep. Sleep 2001;24:374.

[79] Boeve BF, Ferman TJ, Silber MH, et al. Sleep disturbances in dementia with Lewy bodies involve more than REM sleep behavior disorder. Neurology 2003;60(5):A79.

[80] Kales A, Ansel RD, Markham CH, et al. Sleep in patients with Parkinson's disease and normal subjects prior to and following levodopa administration. Clin Pharmacol Ther 1971;12: 397–406.

[81] Wetter TC, Collado-Seidel V, Pollmacher T, et al. Sleep and periodic leg movement patterns in drug-free patients with Parkinson's disease and multiple system atrophy. Sleep 2000;23:361–7.

[82] Bliwise DL. Sleep in normal aging and dementia. Sleep 1993;16:40–81.

[83] American Sleep Disorders Association. The international classification of sleep disorders diagnostic and coding manual. Rochester (MN): American Sleep Disorders Association; 1997.

[84] Jouvet M, Delorme F. [Locus coeruleus et sommeil paradoxal]. C R Seances Soc Biol Fil 1965;159:895–9.

[85] Lai YY, Siegel JM. Physiological and anatomical link between Parkinson-like disease and REM sleep behavior disorder. Mol Neurobiol 2003;27:137–52.
[86] Hendricks JC, Morrison AR, Mann GL. Different behaviors during paradoxical sleep without atonia depend on pontine lesion site. Brain Res 1982;239:81–105.
[87] Lu J, Sherman D, Devor M, et al. A putative flip-flop switch for control of REM sleep. Nature 2006;441:589–94.
[88] Plazzi G, Corsini R, Provini F, et al. REM sleep behavior disorders in multiple system atrophy. Neurology 1997;48:1094–7.
[89] Gagnon JF, Bedard MA, Fantini ML, et al. REM sleep behavior disorder and REM sleep without atonia in Parkinson's disease. Neurology 2002;59:585–9.
[90] Schenck CH, Bundlie SR, Mahowald MW. Delayed emergence of a parkinsonian disorder in 38% of 29 older men initially diagnosed with idiopathic rapid eye movement sleep behaviour disorder. Neurology 1996;46:388–93.
[91] Turner RS, Chervin RD, Frey KA, et al. Probable diffuse Lewy body disease presenting as REM sleep behavior disorder. Neurology 1997;49:523–7.
[92] Boeve BF, Silber MH, Ferman TJ, et al. Association of REM sleep behavior disorder and neurodegenerative disease may reflect an underlying synucleinopathy. Mov Disord 2001; 16:622–30.
[93] Uchiyama M, Isse K, Tanaka K, et al. Incidental Lewy body disease in a patient with REM sleep behavior disorder. Neurology 1995;45:709–12.
[94] Boeve BF, Dickson DW, Olson EJ, et al. Insights into REM sleep behavior disorder pathophysiology in brainstem-predominant Lewy body disease. Sleep Med 2007;8: 60–4.
[95] Boeve BF, Silber MH, Saper CB, et al. Pathophysiology of REM sleep behavior disorder and relevance to neurodegenerative disease. Brain, in press.
[96] Thaisetthawatkul P, Boeve BF, Benarroch EE, et al. Autonomic dysfunction in dementia with Lewy bodies. Neurology 2004;62:1804–9.
[97] Stern Y, Albert M, Brandt J, et al. Utility of extrapyramidal signs and psychosis as predictors of cognitive and functional decline, nursing home admission, and death in Alzheimer's disease: prospective analyses from the Predictors Study. Neurology 1994;44: 2300–7.
[98] Armstrong TP, Hansen LA, Salmon DP, et al. Rapidly progressive dementia in a patient with the Lewy body variant of Alzheimer's disease. Neurology 1991;41:1178–80.
[99] Olichney JM, Galasko D, Salmon DP, et al. Cognitive decline is faster in Lewy body variant than in Alzheimer's disease. Neurology 1998;51:351–7.
[100] Ballard C, Patel A, Oyebode F, et al. Cognitive decline in patients with Alzheimer's disease, vascular dementia and senile dementia of Lewy body type. Age Ageing 1996;25:209–13.
[101] Ballard C, O'Brien J, Morris CM, et al. The progression of cognitive impairment in dementia with Lewy bodies, vascular dementia and Alzheimer's disease. Int J Geriatr Psychiatry 2001;16:499–503.
[102] Helmes E, Bowler JV, Merskey H, et al. Rates of cognitive decline in Alzheimer's disease and dementia with Lewy bodies. Dement Geriatr Cogn Disord 2003;15:67–71.
[103] Williams MM, Xiong C, Morris JC, et al. Survival and mortality differences between dementia with Lewy bodies vs. Alzheimer's disease. Neurology 2006;67:1935–41.
[104] Dickson DW. Dementia with Lewy bodies: neuropathology. J Geriatr Psychiatry Neurol 2002;15:210–6.
[105] Pollanen MS, Dickson DW, Bergeron C. Pathology and biology of the Lewy body. J Neuropathol Exp Neurol 1993;52:183–91.
[106] Dickson DW, Davies P, Mayeux R, et al. Diffuse Lewy body disease. Neuropathological and biochemical studies of six patients. Acta Neuropathol (Berl) 1987;75:8–15.
[107] Dickson DW, Feany MB, Yen SH, et al. Cytoskeletal pathology in non-Alzheimer degenerative dementia: new lesions in diffuse Lewy body disease, Pick's disease, and corticobasal degeneration. J Neural Transm Suppl 1996;47:31–46.

[108] Kosaka K, Yoshimura M, Ikeda K, et al. Diffuse type of Lewy body disease: progressive dementia with abundant cortical Lewy bodies and senile changes of varying degree– a new disease? Clin Neuropathol 1984;3:185–92.

[109] Braak H, Braak E. Pathoanatomy of Parkinson's disease. J Neurol 2000;247(Suppl 2): II3–10.

[110] Braak H, Del Tredici K, Rub U, et al. Staging of brain pathology related to sporadic Parkinson's disease. Neurobiol Aging 2003;24:197–211.

[111] Kosaka K. Diffuse Lewy body disease in Japan. J Neurol 1990;237:197–204.

[112] Whitwell JL, Jack CR, Parisi JE, et al. Rates of cerebral atrophy differ in different degenerative pathologies. Brain 2007;130:1148–58.

[113] Whitwell JL, Weigand SD, Josephs KA, et al. Focal atrophy in dementia with Lewy bodies on MRI: a distinct pattern from Alzheimer's disease. Brain 2007;130:708–19.

[114] Dickson DW. Neuropathological diagnosis of Alzheimer's disease: a perspective from longitudinal clinicopathological studies. Neurobiol Aging 1997;18:S21–6.

[115] Lippa CF, Smith TW, Perry E. Dementia with Lewy bodies: choline acetyltransferase parallels nucleus basalis pathology. J Neural Transm 1999;106:525–35.

[116] Dickson DW, Crystal H, Mattiace LA, et al. Diffuse Lewy body disease: light and electron microscopic immunocytochemistry of senile plaques. Acta Neuropathol (Berl) 1989;78: 572–84.

[117] Dickson DW. The pathogenesis of senile plaques. J Neuropathol Exp Neurol 1997;56: 321–39.

[118] Armstrong RA, Cairns NJ, Lantos PL. Beta-amyloid deposition in the temporal lobe of patients with dementia with Lewy bodies: comparison with non-demented cases and Alzheimer's disease. Dement Geriatr Cogn Disord 2000;11:187–92.

[119] Jellinger KA. Morphological substrates of mental dysfunction in Lewy body disease: an update. J Neural Transm Suppl 2000;59:185–212.

[120] Katzman R, Brown T, Thal LJ, et al. Comparison of rate of annual change of mental status score in four independent studies of patients with Alzheimer's disease. Ann Neurol 1988;24; 384–9.

[121] Dickson DW, Crystal HA, Mattiace LA, et al. Identification of normal and pathological aging in prospectively studied nondemented elderly humans. Neurobiol Aging 1992;13: 179–89.

[122] Hansen LA, Masliah E, Galasko D, et al. Plaque-only Alzheimer disease is usually the lewy body variant, and vice versa. J Neuropathol Exp Neurol 1993;52:648–54.

[123] Samuel W, Galasko D, Masliah E, et al. Neocortical lewy body counts correlate with dementia in the Lewy body variant of Alzheimer's disease. J Neuropathol Exp Neurol 1996;55:44–52.

[124] Braak H, Braak E. Neuropathological stageing of Alzheimer-related changes. Acta Neuropathol (Berl) 1991;82:239–59.

[125] Samuel W, Alford M, Hofstetter CR, et al. Dementia with Lewy bodies versus pure Alzheimer disease: differences in cognition, neuropathology, cholinergic dysfunction, and synapse density. J Neuropathol Exp Neurol 1997;56:499–508.

[126] Merdes AR, Hansen LA, Jeste DV, et al. Influence of Alzheimer pathology on clinical diagnostic accuracy in dementia with Lewy bodies. Neurology 2003;60:1586–90.

[127] Del Ser T, Hachinski V, Merskey H, et al. Clinical and pathologic features of two groups of patients with Dementia with Lewy bodies: Effect of coexisting Alzheimer-type lesion load. Alzheimer Dis and Assoc Dis 2001;15:31–44.

[128] Samuel WA, Henderson VW, Miller CA. Severity of dementia in Alzheimer disease and neurofibrillary tangles in multiple brain regions. Alzheimer Dis Assoc Disord 1991;5:1–11.

[129] Arriagada PV, Growdon JH, Hedley-Whyte ET, et al. Neurofibrillary tangles but not senile plaques parallel duration and severity of Alzheimer's disease. Neurology 1992; 42:631–9.

[130] Haroutunian V, Serby M, Purohit DP, et al. Contribution of Lewy body inclusions to dementia in patients with and without Alzheimer disease neuropathological conditions. Arch Neurol 2000;57:1145–50.

[131] Hurtig HI, Trojanowski JQ, Galvin J, et al. Alpha-synuclein cortical Lewy bodies correlate with dementia in Parkinson's disease. Neurology 2000;54:1916–21.

[132] Churchyard A, Lees AJ. The relationship between dementia and direct involvement of the hippocampus and amygdala in Parkinson's disease. Neurology 1997;49:1570–6.

[133] Ransmayr G, Cervera P, Hirsch EC, et al. Alzheimer's disease: is the decrease of the cholinergic innervation of the hippocampus related to intrinsic hippocampal pathology? Neuroscience 1992;47:843–51.

[134] West MJ, Coleman PD, Flood DG, et al. Differences in the pattern of hippocampal neuronal loss in normal aging and Alzheimer's disease. Lancet 1994;344:769–72.

[135] Nagy Z, Jobst KA, Esiri MM, et al. Hippocampal pathology reflects memory deficit and brain imaging measurements in Alzheimer's disease: clinicopathologic correlations using three sets of pathologic diagnostic criteria. Dementia 1996;7:76–81.

[136] Harding AJ, Lakay B, Halliday GM. Selective hippocampal neuron loss in dementia with Lewy bodies. Ann Neurol 2002;51:125–8.

[137] Lippa CF, Pulaski-Salo D, Dickson DW, et al. Alzheimer's disease, Lewy body disease and aging: a comparative study of the perforant pathway. J Neurol Sci 1997;147:161–6.

[138] Mesulam MM, Mufson EJ, Levey AI, et al. Cholinergic innervation of cortex by the basal forebrain: cytochemistry and cortical connections of the septal area, diagonal band nuclei, nucleus basalis (substantia innominata), and hypothalamus in the rhesus monkey. J Comp Neurol 1983;214:170–97.

[139] Himmelheber AM, Sarter M, Bruno JP. The effects of manipulations of attentional demand on cortical acetylcholine release. Brain Res Cogn Brain Res 2001;12:353–70.

[140] McGaughy J, Kaiser T, Sarter M. Behavioral vigilance following infusions of 192 IgG-saporin into the basal forebrain: selectivity of the behavioral impairment and relation to cortical AChE-positive fiber density. Behav Neurosci 1996;110:247–65.

[141] McGaughy J, Everitt BJ, Robbins TW, et al. The role of cortical cholinergic afferent projections in cognition: impact of new selective immunotoxins. Behav Brain Res 2000;115: 251–63.

[142] Torres EM, Perry TA, Blockland A, et al. Behavioural, histochemical and biochemical consequences of selective immunolesions in discrete regions of the basal forebrain cholinergic system. Neuroscience 1994;63:95–122.

[143] Voytko ML, Olton DS, Richardson RT, et al. Basal forebrain lesions in monkeys disrupt attention but not learning and memory. J Neurosci 1994;14:167–86.

[144] Davis KL, Mohs RC, Marin D, et al. Cholinergic markers in elderly patients with early signs of Alzheimer disease. JAMA 1999;281(15):1401–6.

[145] Perry EK, Irving D, Kerwin JM, et al. Cholinergic transmitter and neurotrophic activities in Lewy body dementia: similarity to Parkinson's and distinction from Alzheimer disease. Alzheimer Dis Assoc Disord 1993;7:69–79.

[146] Perry EK, Haroutunian V, Davis KL, et al. Neocortical cholinergic activities differentiate Lewy body dementia from classical Alzheimer's disease. Neuroreport 1994;5:747–9.

[147] Tiraboschi P, Hansen LA, Alford M, et al. Early and widespread cholinergic losses differentiate dementia with Lewy bodies from Alzheimer disease. Arch Gen Psychiatry 2002;59: 946–51.

[148] Perry EK, Perry RH. Acetylcholine and hallucinations: disease-related compared to drug-induced alterations in human consciousness. Brain Cogn 1995;28:240–58.

[149] Perry R, McKeith I, Perry E. Lewy body dementia—clinical, pathological and neurochemical interconnections. J Neural Transm Suppl 1997;51:95–109.

[150] Tune LE, Egeli S. Acetylcholine and delirium. Dement Geriatr Cogn Disord 1999;10:342–4.

[151] Flacker JM, Cummings V, Mach JR Jr, et al. The association of serum anticholinergic activity with delirium in elderly medical patients. Am J Geriatr Psychiatry 1998;6:31–41.

[152] Han L, McCusker J, Cole M, et al. Use of medications with anticholinergic effect predicts clinical severity of delirium symptoms in older medical inpatients. Arch Intern Med 2001; 161:1099–105.

[153] Tune LE, Damlouji NF, Holland A, et al. Association of postoperative delirium with raised serum levels of anticholinergic drugs. Lancet 1981;2:651–3.

[154] Perry E, Walker M, Grace J, et al. Acetylcholine in mind: a neurotransmitter correlate of consciousness? Trends Neurosci 1999;22:273–80.

[155] Lebert F, Pasquier F, Souliez L, et al. Tacrine efficacy in Lewy body dementia. Int J Geriatr Psychiatry 1998;13:516–9.

[156] Wengel SP, Roccaforte WH, Burke WJ. Donepezil improves symptoms of delirium in dementia: implications for future research. J Geriatr Psychiatry Neurol 1998;11:159–61.

[157] Samuel W, Caligiuri M, Galasko D, et al. Better cognitive and psychopathologic response to donepezil in patients prospectively diagnosed as dementia with Lewy bodies: a preliminary study. Int J Geriatr Psychiatry 2000;15:794–802.

[158] Maclean LE, Collins CC, Byrne EJ. Dementia with Lewy bodies treated with rivastigmine: effects on cognition, neuropsychiatric symptoms, and sleep. Int Psychogeriatr 2001;13: 277–88.

[159] Bergman J, Lerner V. Successful use of donepezil for the treatment of psychotic symptoms in patients with Parkinson's disease. Clin Neuropharmacol 2002;25:107–10.

[160] Francis J, Martin D, Kapoor WN. A prospective study of delirium in hospitalized elderly. Jama 1990;263:1097–101.

[161] Moore DP. Rapid treatment of delirium in critically ill patients. Am J Psychiatry 1977;134: 1431–2.

[162] Allen RL, Walker Z, D'Ath PJ, et al. Risperidone for psychotic and behavioural symptoms in Lewy body dementia. Lancet 1995;346:185.

[163] Miller CH, Mohr F, Umbricht D, et al. The prevalence of acute extrapyramidal signs and symptoms in patients treated with clozapine, risperidone, and conventional antipsychotics. J Clin Psychiatry 1998;59:69–75.

[164] Burke WJ, Pfeiffer RF, McComb RD. Neuroleptic sensitivity to clozapine in dementia with Lewy bodies. J Neuropsychiatry Clin Neurosci 1998;10:227–9.

[165] Sechi G, Agnetti V, Masuri R, et al. Risperidone, neuroleptic malignant syndrome and probable dementia with Lewy bodies. Prog Neuropsychopharmacol Biol Psychiatry 2000;24:1043–51.

[166] Rosebush PI, Mazurek MF. Neurologic side effects in neuroleptic-naive patients treated with haloperidol or risperidone. Neurology 1999;52:782–5.

[167] Piggott MA, Perry EK, Marshall EF, et al. Nigrostriatal dopaminergic activities in dementia with Lewy bodies in relation to neuroleptic sensitivity: comparisons with Parkinson's disease. Biol Psychiatry 1998;44:765–74.

[168] Court JA, Piggott MA, Lloyd S, et al. Nicotine binding in human striatum: elevation in schizophrenia and reductions in dementia with Lewy bodies, Parkinson's disease and Alzheimer's disease and in relation to neuroleptic medication. Neuroscience 2000;98:79–87.

[169] Cummings JL, Street J, Masterman D, et al. Efficacy of olanzapine in the treatment of psychosis in dementia with Lewy bodies. Dementia and Geriatric Cognitive Disorders 2002;13: 67–73.

[170] Aarsland D, Larsen JP, Lim NG, et al. Olanzapine for psychosis in patinets with Parkinson's disease with and without dementia. J of Neuropsy and Clin Neurosc 1999;11: 392–4.

[171] Ellingrod VL, Schultz SK, Ekstam-Smith K, et al. Comparison of risperdone with olanzepine in elderly patients with dementia and psychosis. Pharmacotherapy 2002;22:1–5.

[172] Mulsant BH, Gharabawi GM, Bossie CA, et al. Correlates of anticholinergic activity in patients with dementia and psychosis treated with risperidone or olanzepine. J of Clinical Psychiatry 2004;65:1708–14.

[173] Ballard C, Margallo-Lana M, Juszczak E, Swann DS, et al. Quetiapine and rivastigmine and cognitive decline in Alzheimer's disease: randomised double blind placebo controlled trial. BMJ 2005;333:857–8.

[174] Juncos JL, Roberts VJ, Evatt ML, et al. Quetiapine improves psychotic symptoms and cognition in Parkinson's disease. Movement Disorders 2004;19:29–35.

[175] Morrison CE, Borod JC, Brin MF, et al. Effects of levodopa on cognitive functioning in moderate-to-severe Parkinson's disease (MSPD). J Neural Transm 2004;111:1333–41.

[176] Kulisevsky J, Garcia-Sanchez C, Berthier ML, et al. Chronic effects of dopaminergic replacement on cognitive function in Parkinson's disease: a two-year follow-up study of previously untreated patients. Movement Disorders 2000;15:613–26.

[177] Bedard MA, Pillon B, Dubois B, et al. Acute and long-term administration of anticholinergics in Parkinson's disease: specific effects on the subcortico-frontal syndrome. Brain Cogn 1999;40:289–313.

[178] McKeith I, Del Ser T, Spano P, et al. Efficacy of rivastigmine in dementia with Lewy bodies: a randomised, double-blind, placebo-controlled international study. Lancet 2000;356: 2031–6.

[179] Kaufer DI, Catt KE, Lopez OL, et al. Dementia with Lewy bodies: response of delirium-like features to donepezil. Neurology 1998;51:1512.

[180] Wilcock GK, Scott MI. Tacrine for senile dementia of Alzheimer's or Lewy body type. Lancet 1994;344:544.

[181] Levy R, Eagger S, Griffiths M, et al. Lewy bodies and response to tacrine in Alzheimer's disease. Lancet 1994;343:176.

[182] Grace J, Daniel S, Stevens T, et al. Long term use of rivastigmine in patients with dementia with Lewy bodies: an open-label trials. Int Psychogeriatr 2001;13:199–205.

[183] Bosboom JL, Stoffers D, Wolters ECh. Cognitive dysfunction and dementia in Parkinson's disease. J of Neural Transm 2004;111:1303–15.

[184] Minett TS, Thomas A, Wilkinson LM, et al. What happens when donepezil is suddently withdrawn? An open label trial in dementia with Lewy bodies and Parkinson's disease with dementia. International J of Geriatric Psychiatry 2003;18:988–93.

[185] Thomas AJ, Burn DJ, Rowan EN, et al. A comparison of the efficacy of donepezil in Parkison's'disease with dementia and dementia with Lewy bodies. Int J Geriatr Psychiatry 2005;20:938–44.

[186] Cummings J. Reconsidering diagnostic criteria for dementia with Lewy bodies. Highlights from the Third International Workshop on Dementia with Lewy bodies and Parkinson's disease dementia, September 17–20, 2003, Newcastle upon Tyne, United Kingdom. Rev Neurol Dis 2004;1(1):31–4.

[187] Boeve B, Silber M, Ferman TJ, et al. Current management of sleep disturbances in dementia. Curr Neurol Neurosci Rep 2001;2:169–77.

[188] Boeve B, Silber M, Ferman T. Melatonin for treatment of REM sleep behavior disorder in neurologic disorders: results in 14 patients. Sleep med 2003;4:281–4.

[189] Carlson D, Fleming K, Smith GE, et al. Management of dementia-related behavioral disturbances: a non-pharmacological approach. Mayo Clin Proc 1995;70:1108–15.

[190] Haupt M, Karger A, Janner M. Improvement of agitation and anxiety in demented patients after psychoeducative group intervention with their caregivers. International J of Geriatric Psychiatry 2000;15:1125–9.

[191] Zarit SH, Stephens MA, Townsend A, et al. Stress reduction for family caregivers: effect of adult day care use. J Gerontol 1998;53:S267–77.

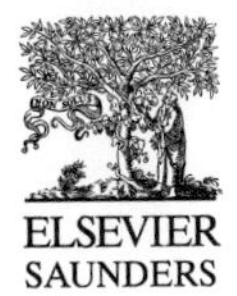

ELSEVIER
SAUNDERS

Neurol Clin 25 (2007) 761–781

NEUROLOGIC
CLINICS

Parkinson-Related Dementias

Bradley F. Boeve, MD[a,b,*]

[a]Divisions of Behavioral Neurology and Movement Disorders, Department of Neurology, Mayo Clinic, 200 First Street SW, Rochester, MN 55905, USA
[b]Department of Neurology, Mayo Clinic College of Medicine, Rochester, MN 55905

Overview

Recent advances in neurogenetics, molecular biology, and immunocytochemical staining methods have expanded the spectrum of neurodegenerative disorders now known to cause dementia associated with parkinsonism. A list of these disorders associated with the known dysfunctional proteins is presented in Box 1. This brief review concentrates on those rare disorders in which cognitive impairment/dementia and parkinsonism coexist: corticobasal syndrome (CBS)/corticobasal degeneration (CBD), progressive supranuclear palsy (PSP), multiple system atrophy (MSA), and frontotemporal dementia with parkinsonism linked to chromosome 17 (FTDP-17); dementia with Lewy bodies (DLB)—a common form of dementia often associated with parkinsonism—is reviewed in an article by Drs. Ferman and Boeve elsewhere in this issue. The clinical, neuropsychologic, neuroradiologic, and neuropathologic similarities and differences in these disorders are compared and contrasted along with Alzheimer's disease, Parkinson's disease, Parkinson's disease with dementia, and dementia with Lewy bodies, highlighting the features critical for identifying the correct diagnosis.

Corticobasal syndrome and corticobasal degeneration

Clinical features

The core clinical features considered characteristic of CBD include progressive asymmetric rigidity and apraxia, with other findings suggesting

Dr. Boeve is supported by National Institutes of Health grants P50 AG16574, UO1 AG06786, RO1 AG15866, RO1 AG23195, P50 NS40256, the Alzheimer's Association, and the Robert H. and Clarice Smith and Abigail Van Buren Alzheimer's Disease Research Program of the Mayo Foundation.

* Department of Neurology, Mayo Clinic, 200 First Street SW, Rochester, MN 55905.
E-mail address: bboeve@mayo.edu

doi:10.1016/j.ncl.2007.04.002 ***neurologic.theclinics.com***

Box 1. Neurodegenerative disorders and associated dysfunctional proteins that manifest as dementia with and without parkinsonism

Dysfunctional protein—amyloid (often termed, "amyloidopathies")
- Alzheimer's disease (AD) with extrapyramidal signs
- Down syndrome with parkinsonism

Dysfunctional protein—tau (often termed, "tauopathies")
- Pick's disease
- *CBD*
- *PSP*
- Argyrophilic grain disease
- Multisystem tauopathy
- *FTDP-17 with mutation in the microtubule-associated protein tau (FTDP-17*MAPT*)*
- AD

Dysfunctional protein—α-synuclein (often termed, "synucleinopathies")
- Lewy body disease (manifesting as the syndromes of Parkinson's disease [PD], DLB, or Parkinson's disease with dementia [PDD])
- *MSA*

Dysfunctional protein—huntingtin
- Huntington disease

Dysfunctional protein—α-internexin
- Neurofilament inclusion body dementia, also known as neuronal intermediate filament inclusion disease

Dysfunctional protein—TAR DNA-binding protein 43 (TDP-43)
- Frontotemporal lobar degeneration with ubiquitin-positive inclusions (FTLD-U), also known as FTD with inclusions, tau- and synuclein-negative, ubiquitinated; FTLD with motor neuron disease–type inclusions; and motor neuron disease–inclusion dementia
- *FTDP-17 with mutation in progranulin (FTDP-17*PGRN*)*

Note: the italicized disorders are the focus of this article.

Adapted from Boeve B. Diagnosis and management of the non-Alzheimer dementias. In: Noseworthy JW, editor. Neurological Therapeutics. London: Martin Dunitz; 2003. p. 2826–54.

additional cortical (eg, alien limb phenomena, cortical sensory loss, myoclonus, and mirror movements) and basal ganglionic (eg, bradykinesia, dystonia, and tremor) dysfunction [2–4]. The asymmetry of the findings is key, and some patients have elements of rigidity and spasticity in the affected limbs. Dystonia, tremor, myoclonus, choreiform movements, and alien limb features tend to be levodopa unresponsive.

Because of the considerable clinicopathologic heterogeneity between those who are diagnosed clinically and pathologically with CBD, some have suggested that the term, CBS, be used to describe the constellation of features believed most characteristic of CBD [3]. The proposed diagnostic criteria for the diagnosis of CBS are listed in Box 2.

Over time, some patients develop features of frontotemporal dementia (FTD), primary progressive aphasia (PPA), or posterior cortical atrophy (PCA). Also, some patients present with a focal cortical degeneration syndrome, such as FTD, PPA, or PCA, and subsequently develop CBS findings.

Neuropsychologic features

Neuropsychometric testing typically shows impairment in those domains subserved by frontal or frontostriatal and parietal cognitive networks, namely attention and concentration, executive functions, verbal fluency, praxis, and visuospatial functioning [4–6]. The profile of impairment depends in part on which cerebral hemisphere is affected maximally. Performance on tests of learning and memory tends to be mildly impaired or not impaired at all. Underlying AD should be considered if performance on delayed recall and recognition measures is markedly abnormal in the setting of CBS.

Neuroradiologic features

The typical MRI findings in CBS include asymmetric cortical atrophy, especially frontoparietal, with the more prominent atrophy existing contralateral to the side most severely affected clinically (Fig. 1A, B) [4]. The lateral ventricle in the maximally affected cerebral hemisphere also can be slightly larger than opposite one. Other reported MRI findings in CBS include atrophy of the middle or posterior segment of the corpus callosum and subtle hyperintense subcortical signal changes in motor with or without somatosensory cortex [4]. These often are subtle findings and their presence or absence should not alter the clinical diagnosis of CBS. In the only series of patients who had CBS associated with CBD pathology, CBS associated with non-CBD pathology, and CBD pathology associated with non-CBS clinical features, none of these MRI findings was found adequately sensitive or specific for CBD—the disease [4,7]. Over time, progressive parietal with or without frontal atrophy and thinning of the middle and posterior portion of the corpus callosum often occur on serial MRI scans in patients who have CBS [4].

Box 2. Criteria for the clinical diagnosis of corticobasal syndrome

Core features

- Insidious onset and progressive course
- No identifiable cause (eg, tumor or infarction)
- Cortical dysfunction as reflected by at least one of the following:
  - Focal or asymmetric ideomotor apraxia
  - Alien limb phenomenon
  - Cortical sensory loss
  - Visual or sensory hemineglect
  - Constructional apraxia
  - Focal or asymmetric myoclonus
  - Apraxia of speech or nonfluent aphasia
- Extrapyramidal dysfunction as reflected by at least one of the following:
  - Focal or asymmetric appendicular rigidity lacking prominent and sustained levodopa response
  - Focal or asymmetric appendicular dystonia

Supportive investigations

- Variable degrees of focal or lateralized cognitive dysfunction, with relative preservation of learning and memory, on neuropsychometric testing
- Focal or asymmetric atrophy on CT or MRI, typically maximal in parietofrontal cortex
- Focal or asymmetric hypoperfusion on single photon emission CT (SPECT) and hypometabolism on positron emission tomography (PET), typically maximal in parietofrontal cortex with or without basal ganglia with or without thalamus

---

From Boeve B, Lang A, Litvan I. Corticobasal degeneration and its relationship to progressive supranuclear palsy and frontotemporal dementia. Ann Neurol 2003;54:S15–9; with permission.

Asymmetric hypoperfusion on SPECT and asymmetric hypometabolism on PET involving the parietofrontal cortex with or without basal ganglia are reported (Fig. 1C, D) [4]. As on MRI, however, these findings are not specific for CBD—the disease.

Neuropathologic features

Consensus criteria for the pathologic diagnosis of CBD are published (Box 3) [8]. Asymmetric parietofrontal or frontotemporal cortical atrophy

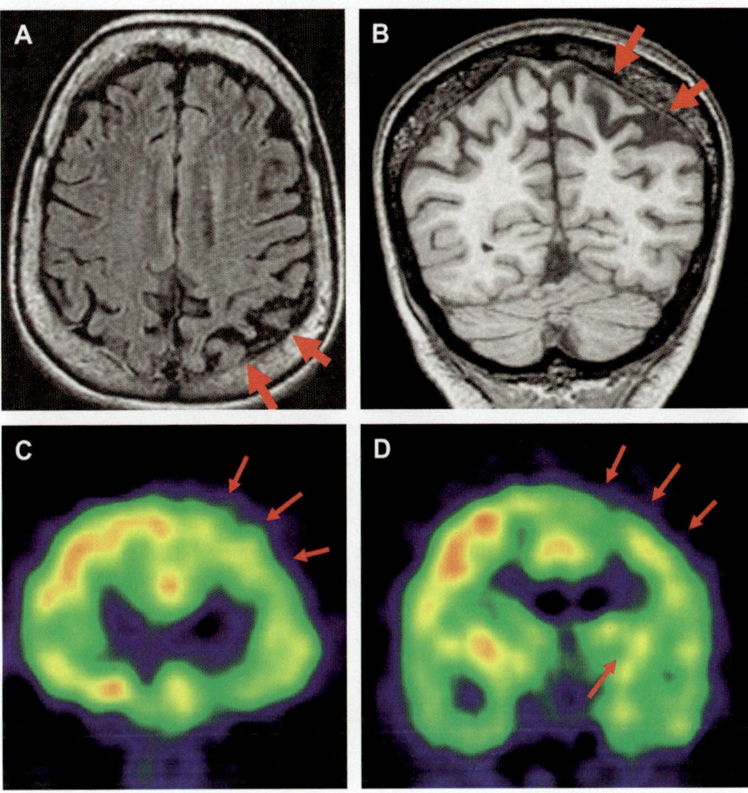

Fig. 1. Typical neuroimaging findings in CBS (FLAIR) (*A*) and coronal T1-weighted (*B*) MRI of a 67-year-old woman with right greater than left clinical findings, showing left parietal cortical atrophy (*thick arrows*). Coronal FDG-PET scans (*C, D*) in a 58-year-old woman who had similar clinical findings, showing left frontoparietal and left basal ganglia hypometabolism (*thin arrows*).

and pallor of the substantia nigra are the typical macroscopic pathologic findings. Neuronal loss, gliosis, and superficial spongiosus are prominent in the maximally affected cortical gyri. Immunocytochemistry with tau and phosphorylated neurofilament or αB-crystallin is critical when characterizing cases of possible CBD. The pathologic features of CBD—the disease—include tau-positive (tau^+) astrocytic plaques, oligodendroglial coiled bodies, and thread-like lesions in gray and white matter, most often in superior frontal gyrus, superior parietal gyrus, pre- and postcentral gyri, and striatum. Although achromatic, ballooned neurons that are immunoreactive to phosphorylated neurofilament or αB-crystallin typically are present in CBD, their absence does not preclude the diagnosis of CBD if the appropriate tau^+ lesions are present.

Box 3. Office of Rare Diseases neuropathologic criteria for the diagnosis of corticobasal degeneration

Core features

- Focal cortical neuronal loss, most often in frontal, parietal, or temporal regions
- Substantia nigra neuronal loss
- Gallyas/tau$^+$ neuronal and glial lesions, especially astrocytic plaques and threads, in white matter and gray matter, most often in superior frontal gyrus, superior parietal gyrus, pre- and postcentral gyri, and striatum

Supportive features

- Cortical atrophy, often with superficial spongiosis
- Ballooned neurons, usually numerous in atrophic cortices
- Tau$^+$ oligodendroglial coiled bodies

From Dickson D, Bergeron C, Chin S, et al. Office of Rare Diseases neuropathologic criteria for corticobasal degeneration. J Neuropathol Exp Neurol 2002;61:935–46; with permission.

Management

Because no therapy yet exists for CBD that affects the neurodegenerative process, management must be tailored toward symptoms [1,2,4,9]. Pharmacotherapy directed toward parkinsonism has been disappointing [10]. Levodopa, dopamine agonists, and baclofen tend to have little effect on rigidity, spasticity, bradykinesia, or tremor. Levodopa should be titrated upward, however, as tolerated (to at least 750 mg per day) in divided doses on an empty stomach (at least 45 minutes before or after meals) to provide an adequate trial. Some patients note significant improvement in parkinsonism but this rarely persists beyond several months. In those who do improve dramatically with levodopa therapy, it should be questioned if CBD is the underlying disorder, as levodopa-refractory parkinsonism is considered by many a characteristic feature of CBS and CBD. Botulinum toxin can alleviate pain from focal dystonia. Tremor may respond initially to propranolol or primidone, but their effects wane with progression of the disorder. Clonazepam or gabapentin may reduce myoclonus in some cases. Although intuitively, cholinesterase inhibitors would not be considered beneficial in this disorder, in rare cases, patients can experience improvement in psychomotor speed, concentration, and problem solving abilities with donepezil, rivastigmine, or galantamine. Vitamin E and other antioxidant agents have been tried in hopes of delaying progression of the disorder, but there is no evidence yet supporting a disease-altering effect.

Because of the poor response to pharmacotherapy, the mainstay of management, therefore, is physical, occupational, and speech therapies. A home assessment by an occupational therapist can aid in determining which changes can be made to facilitate functional independence (eg, replacing rotating doorknobs with handles, attaching specially formed pads around the handles of eating utensils and toothbrushes, purchasing clothing with Velcro instead of buttons or laces, and so forth). Passive range-of-motion exercises minimize development of contractures. In those who develop dystonic flexion of the hand musculature to form a "fisted hand," the fingernails can imbed in the palmar tissue, leading to cellulitis and even osteomyelitis of the hand. This can be avoided by clipping fingernails periodically and by placing a rolled-up washcloth or hand towel in the palm of the hand. All patients experience gait impairment at some point during their illness. A walker with handbrakes can improve ambulation for some patients. Wheelchair and handicap privileges are warranted in essentially every patient. Use of a bedside commode also is worthwhile. Apraxia often is the most debilitating feature of the disorder, and this feature can complicate the ability to operate a wheelchair or motorized scooter. Many patients are able to learn to operate these devices, however, and use them effectively for months or years. Some third-party payers have denied coverage for these devices and therapies, which is unfortunate, as any element of functional improvement and independence is important for these patients. Speech therapy and communication devices can optimize communication when dysarthria, apraxia of speech, or aphasia is present. Therapists also counsel patients and families on swallowing maneuvers and food additives to minimize aspiration when dysphagia occurs. Feeding gastrostomy should be discussed with all patients, although many decide not to undergo this procedure.

Constraint-induced movement therapy has been shown to be effective in the stroke population [11], and a few highly motivated patients who have CBS and who have used constraint-induced movement therapy have experienced a "useless hand made useful" by using this form of therapy [9].

Progressive supranuclear palsy

Clinical features

The classic presentation of PSP is the constellation of supranuclear gaze palsy, postural instability and falls, and parkinsonism. These same features form the core for the Neurological Disorders and Stroke–Society for Progressive Supranuclear Palsy (Box 4) clinical criteria [12].

Some of the qualitative features of parkinsonism are diagnostically relevant: wide-eyed stare, reduced eye blink frequency, axial greater than appendicular rigidity, and tendency to walk, turn, and sit en bloc.

Box 4. Clinical diagnosis of progressive supranuclear palsy: National Institute of Neurological Disorders and Stroke–Society for Progressive Supranuclear Palsy criteria

Core features (mandatory inclusion criteria)

Possible progressive supranuclear palsy

- Gradually progressive disorder
- Onset at age 40 or later
- Either vertical supranuclear palsy or both slowing of vertical saccades and prominent postural instability with falls in the first year of disease onset
- No evidence of other diseases that could explain the foregoing features, as indicated by mandatory exclusion criteria

Probable progressive supranuclear palsy

- Gradually progressive disorder
- Onset at age 40 or later
- Vertical supranuclear palsy and prominent postural instability with falls in the first year of disease onset
- No evidence of other diseases that could explain the foregoing features, as indicated by mandatory exclusion criteria

Definite progressive supranuclear palsy

- Clinically probable or possible PSP and histopathologic evidence of typical PSP

Supportive features

- Symmetric akinesia or rigidity, proximal more than distal
- Abnormal neck posture, especially retrocollis
- Poor or absence of response of parkinsonism to levodopa therapy
- Early dysphagia and dysarthria
- Early onset of cognitive impairment including at least two of the following: apathy, impairment in abstract thought, decreased verbal fluency, use or imitation behavior, or frontal release signs

Exclusion criteria

- Recent history of encephalitis
- Alien limb syndrome, cortical sensory deficits, focal frontal or temporoparietal atrophy
- Hallucinations or delusions unrelated to dopaminergic therapy
- Cortical dementia of Alzheimer type
- Prominent early cerebellar symptoms or prominent early unexplained dysautonomia
- Severe, asymmetric parkinsonian signs
- Neuroradiologic evidence of relevant structural abnormalities
- Whipple's disease, confirmed by polymerase chain reaction

From Litvan I, Agid Y, Calne D, et al. Clinical research criteria for the diagnosis of progressive supranuclear palsy (Steele-Richardson-Olszewski syndrome): report of the NINDS-SPSP international workshop. Neurology 1996;47:1–9; with permission.

Many cases have atypical features, including those mistaken for CBD; those with no gaze palsy, gait impairment, or parkinsonism; and those presenting with progressive aphasia, FTD, or obsessive-compulsive features [13–16].

Neuropsychologic features

The concept of "subcortical dementia" has been applied to those who have PSP, in which there is slowing of cognitive processing but "cortical" signs, such as significant amnesia and aphasia, tend to be mild at worst. Letter fluency (ie, word generation starting with a letter of the alphabet over a specific time period) and cognitive flexibility in particular tend to be impaired [5,17–19].

Those who have atypical presentations have the associated impairments in executive functioning, language, praxis, and visuospatial functioning typical of FTD, PPA, CBS, or some combination thereof.

Neuroradiologic features

Although no features on MRI or functional imaging studies are entirely specific for PSP, the following radiographic signs have been associated with PSP: the "morning glory sign," in which the lateral margin of the midbrain tegmentum has a concave rather than convex appearance resulting from atrophy in the midbrain tegmentum [20], and the "hummingbird sign," in which the shape of the rostral midbrain atrophy on midsagittal images looks like a hummingbird [21]. Longitudinal MRI studies show a rate of cerebral atrophy and ventricular expansion of 1.3% and 7.0% per year compared with 0.4% and 1.8% in control subjects [22]. Frontosubcortical hypoperfusion and hypometabolism on SPECT and PET imaging, respectively, are typical findings in PSP, and such changes tend to be symmetric in contrast to the asymmetric changes in those who have CBS (Fig. 2).

Neuropathologic features

The pathologic criteria for the diagnosis of PSP are shown in Box 5 [23].

Management

The management of the cognitive, motor, and gait aspects of PSP is challenging [24–26]. Parkinsonism responds poorly to carbidopa/levodopa, and gait assistance devices or confinement to a wheelchair often is necessary for management of gait impairment. The topography of cortical dysfunction tends to involve the frontal or frontosubcortical neural networks; thus, apathy and executive dysfunction often are present. Disinhibition, dysphoria, and anxiety also are common, but agitation and obsessive-compulsive

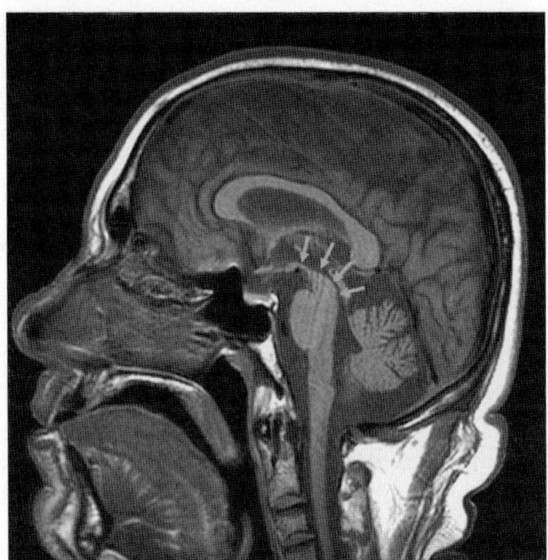

Fig. 2. Midsagittal MRI in a patient who had PSP. Note the thinning of the rostral midbrain (*arrows*) giving an appearance like the head and beak of a hummingbird ("hummingbird sign").

features are less frequent. Treatment is directed toward target symptoms [27]. Physical and occupational therapy, counseling on food preparation and swallowing to avoid aspiration, and gait assistance devices also are indicated in many.

Multiple system atrophy

Clinical features

Striatonigral degeneration, olivopontocerebellar atrophy, and Shy-Drager syndrome variants form the MSAs. The generally accepted criteria for the diagnosis of MSA are listed in Box 6 [28].

Functionally important cognitive impairment and cortical atrophy are not considered part of MSA, but rare cases of MSA have presented with some degree of cognitive impairment, progressive aphasia, frontal atrophy, or a combination of these [29–31]. Sleep disorders, in particular rapid eye movement sleep behavior disorder and nocturnal stridor, are becoming of increased interest in MSA because of the relevance of RBD associated with the synucleinopathies [32,33] and death associated with stridor [34] if not treated successfully.

Neuropsychologic features

As discussed previously, cognition generally is considered normal in MSA, but recent neuropsychologic studies have demonstrated impairment in this population. Executive functioning in particular is affected [35]. Impaired

Box 5. Pathologic diagnosis of progressive supranuclear palsy: National Institute of Neurological Disorders and Stroke criteria

Inclusion criteria

Typical progressive supranuclear palsy

- Many NFTs, NTs, or both in basal ganglia and brainstem
- At approximately ×250 magnification
  - Two or more neurons with NFTs or NTs must be found in the same field in three of the following brain areas: pallidum, subthalamic nucleus, substantia nigra, or pons
  - One or more neurons with NFTs or NTs must be found in the same field in at least three of the following brain areas: striatum, oculomotor complex, medulla, or dentate nucleus
  - The presence of tau^+ astrocytes or processes in these areas supports the diagnosis

Atypical progressive supranuclear palsy

- NFTs, NTs, or both in the basal ganglia and brainstem is mandatory
- At ×250 magnification
  - One or more neurons with NFTs or NTs must be found in the same field in at least five of the following brain areas: pallidum, subthalamic nucleus, substantia nigra, pons, medulla, or dentate nucleus
  - The presence of tau^+ astrocytes or processes in these areas support the diagnosis

Combined progressive supranuclear palsy

- The presence of typical neuropathologic changes of PSP together with findings that are diagnostic of another neurologicdisease

Exclusion criteria for progressive supranuclear palsy

- Lewy body–associated diseases
- AD
- MSA
- Pick's disease
- CBD

Abbreviations: NFT, neurofibrillary tangle; NT, neurophil thread.

From Hauw J-J, Daniel S, Dickson D, et al. Preliminary NINDS neuropathologic criteria for Steel-Richardson-Olszewski syndrome (progressive supranuclear palsy). Neurology 1994;44:2015–9; with permission.

Box 6. Criteria for the clinical diagnosis of multiple system atrophy

Core features

Sporadic, progressive, adult-onset disorder with following criteria:

- Autonomic dysfunction (orthostatic hypotension—>30 mm Hg systolic or 15 mm Hg diastolic—or urinary incontinence/ retention)
- Parkinsonism (bradykinesia plus one of the following: rigidity, postural instability, postural, or resting tremor)
- Cerebellar dysfunction (gait ataxia plus one of the following: ataxic dysarthria, limb ataxia, or sustained gaze-evoked nystagmus)
- Corticospinal tract signs (is a feature but not required for diagnosis of MSA)

Diagnostic categories

- Possible MSA: one criterion plus 2 features from other separate domains
- Probable MSA: criterion for autonomic failure/urinary incontinence plus poorly levodopa responsive parkinsonism or cerebellar dysfunction
- Definite MSA: pathology shows high density of glial cytoplasmic inclusions plus combination of nigrostriatal and olivopontocerebellar degeneration

Exclusion criteria

- Onset of symptoms before age 30
- Family history of similar disorder
- Other identifiable cause or systemic disease
- Hallucinations unrelated to medication
- *Diagnostic and Statistical Manual of Mental Disorders* criteria for dementia
- Prominent slowing of vertical saccades or vertical supranuclear gaze palsy
- Focal cortical dysfunction (aphasia, alien limb phenomenon, parietal lobe dysfunction)
- Metabolic, molecular genetic, and imaging evidence of an alternative cause

---

Adapted from Gilman S, Low P, Quinn N, et al. Consensus statement on the diagnosis of multiple system atrophy. J Neurol Sci 1999;163:94–8.

verbal memory and verbal fluency are found in MSA of the cerebellar type [31]. As in PSP, letter fluency and cognitive flexibility also are impaired [19].

Neuroradiologic features

Atrophy of the pons or cerebellum on MRI is typical, particularly in the olivopontocerebellar atrophy variant. The "hot cross bun sign" [36] and hyperintense signal lateral to the putamen [37] also are associated with MSA, although they are not entirely specific for the disorder. Many changes on PET are associated with MSA, depending on the radioligand used [38], but fluorodeoxyglucose (FDG)-PET tends to be more normal than not.

Neuropathologic features

The defining neuropathologic features of MSA are oligodendroglial inclusions, which are immunoreactive to α-synuclein. Various degrees of corticospinal tract, striatal, nigral, cerebellar, and autonomic nuclei degeneration also are typical of MSA [39,40].

Management

There is not even anecdotal or case study data regarding any agents that have been used in the management of cognitive impairment in MSA. Treatment, therefore, is directed at parkinsonism, orthostatism, and urinary incontinence. Nocturnal stridor is of concern whenever it develops in patients who have MSA [34]. Because this high-pitched musical sound that occurs during inspiration represents dystonic closure of the vocal cords, patients are at risk for sudden death [34]. Thus, they should be referred for urgent polysomnography and a trial of nasal continuous positive airway pressure (CPAP) therapy (CPAP may maintain laryngeal patency) or for possible tracheostomy [34]. For patients who have MSA with stridor and RBD, melatonin may be preferable to clonazepam.

Frontotemporal dementia with parkinsonism linked to chromosome 17

Clinical features

FTDP-17 is the term applied to those individuals within kindreds who have (1) FTD or parkinsonism and (2) linkage to a genetic alteration on chromosome 17 or an identified mutation on chromosome 17. The background on the genetics of FTDP-17 is discussed in the article by Dr. Josephs elsewhere in this issue.

Mutations in either of two genes that are in close proximity to each other on chromosome 17 are associated with FTDP-17—the genes are microtubule-associated protein tau (*MAPT*) [41] and progranulin (*PGRN*) [42].

For those who have FTDP-17*MAPT* (summarized from data and references in [43,44]), the typical age of onset is between 30 and 60, and penetrance seems to be close to 100%. The duration of symptoms from onset to death typically is 3 to 10 years. Symptomatology usually involves executive dysfunction and altered personality and behavior, with aphasia and parkinsonism evolving in many. Memory impairment occurs less frequently, and visuospatial impairment and limb apraxia are rare. Features of motor neuron disease also are infrequent. Over time, most patients develop other clinical features, such that two or more syndromic terms can be applied, reflecting the progressively expanding involvement of other brain regions [45].

For those who have FTDP-17*PGRN* (summarized from data in Refs. [46–55]), the typical age of onset is between 45 and 85, and the duration of disease varies from 1 to 13 years. The frequency of mutations in *PGRN* in FTD series is similar to that of *MAPT* [49]. The mode of inheritance follows an autosomal dominant pattern with a high but age-dependent penetrance (90% develop symptoms by age 70) [49]. There are known *PGRN* mutation carriers who are asymptomatic in their 70s and known affected individuals who developed symptoms after age 80, indicating some differences compared with what has been reported in *MAPT* mutation carriers. The clinical features have been more variable than in *MAPT* mutation carriers, with not only behavioral and cognitive features commonly present but also memory impairment, limb apraxia, parkinsonism, and visuospatial dysfunction. CBS also has been particularly frequent in the cases reported thus far. No *PGRN* mutation carrier is reported to date with an amyotrophic lateral sclerosis (ALS) phenotype.

Neuropsychologic features

Detailed neuropsychologic studies in patients who have FTDP-17*PGRN* are scant [47,52]; hence, additional studies are needed to determine the similarities and differences between FTDP-17 associated with *MAPT* versus *PGRN* mutations.

Neuroradiologic features

Structural neuroimaging studies in patients who have FTDP-17*MAPT* tend to show frontal or temporal atrophy, either symmetric or asymmetric, and parenchymal signal changes on MRI either are absent or mild (Fig. 3A) (reviewed in Ref. [56]). A similar topography of abnormalities typically is seen on SPECT and PET scans, often with basal ganglia or thalamic hypoperfusion or hypometabolism [57]. In those who have early and mild features in FTDP-17*MAPT*, PET scan findings tend to be more revealing than MRI (Fig. 4). Recent evidence suggests that subtle increased signal in the mesial temporal lobes on fluid attenuation inversion recovery (FLAIR) MRI scans can be seen in the symptomatic and asymptomatic patients

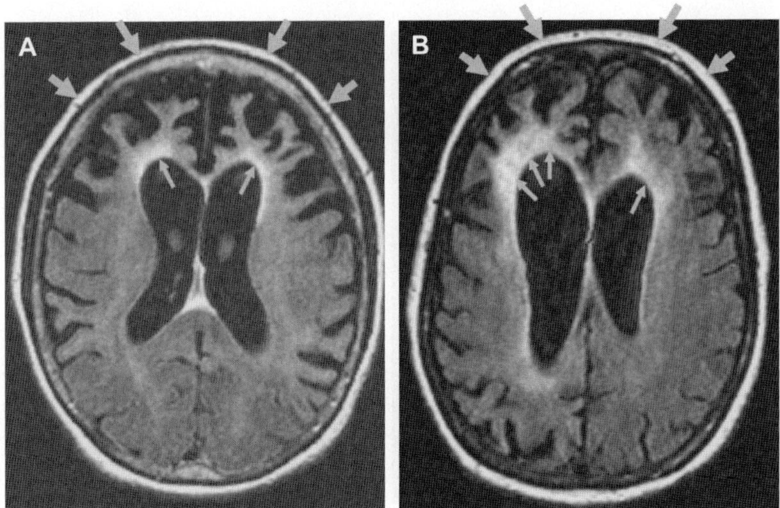

Fig. 3. Representative axial FLAIR MRI scans in a 68-year-old woman who had frontotemporal dementia associated with the P301L mutation in *MAPT* (*A*) and in a 60-year-old woman who had frontotemporal dementia and parkinsonism associated with the IVS1+1G>A mutation in *PGRN* (*B*). Note the bifrontal cortical atrophy in both cases (*thick arrows*), which happens to be symmetric in one and asymmetric in the other. Both also have increased signal changes in the subcortical white matter (*thin arrows*), which is more obvious in the patient who had the *PGRN* mutation (*B*).

who have the N279K mutation in *MAPT*, but it remains to be seen how sensitive and specific this finding is for this or any other mutation in *MAPT* [58].

MRI findings in FTDP-17*PGRN* are only starting to emerge. In one study, a variety of neuroimaging findings was seen in patients who had FTDP-17*PGRN*, with frontotemporal atrophy and parietal cortical atrophy; prominent subcortical white matter changes also were present in a minority of cases (see example in Fig. 3B) [47,59]. Voxel-based morphometry MRI comparing FTDP cases with and without mutations in *PGRN* showed significant gray matter loss in the posterior temporal lobes in the *PGRN*-positive and –negative subjects compared with controls [60]. Subjects who were *PGRN* positive showed significantly more gray matter loss in the lateral and medial frontal lobes, and less involvement of the temporal lobes, than subjects who were *PGRN* negative [60]. No direct comparison has been published to date that attempts to differentiate patients who have FTDP-17 and mutations in *MAPT* from such patients who have mutations in *PGRN* using any neuroimaging modality.

Neuropathologic features

In patients who have FTDP-17*MAPT*, cortical atrophy typically is maximal in the frontotemporal regions. Tau^{+} inclusions in neurons (eg, NFTs,

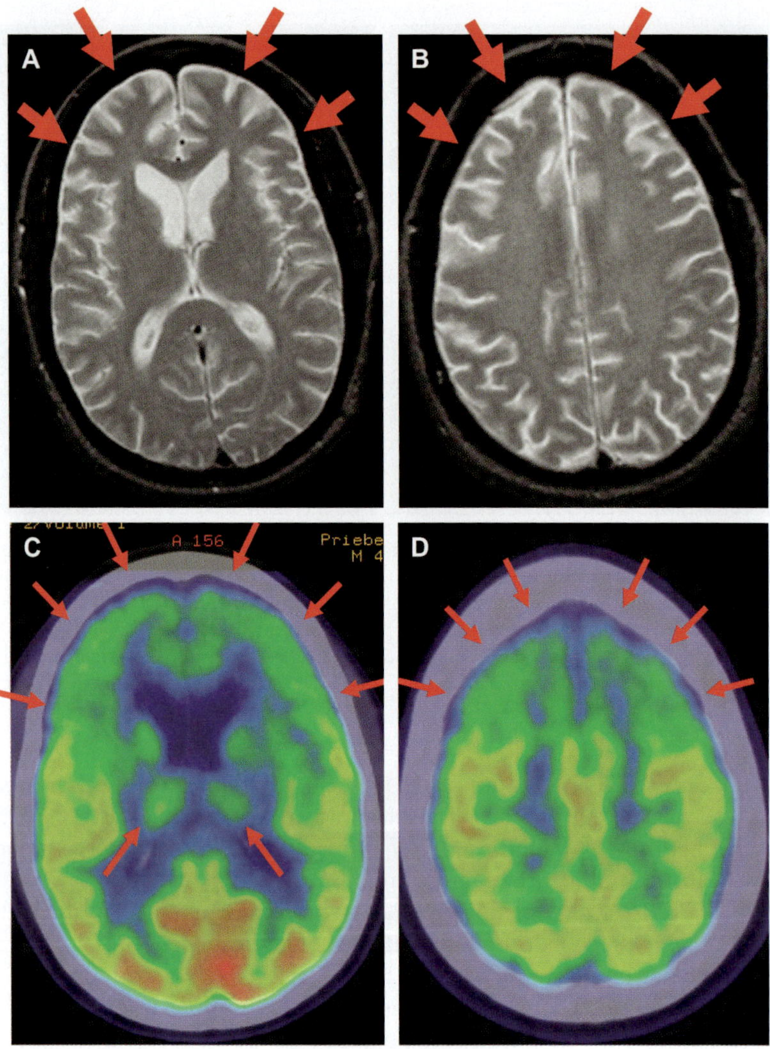

Fig. 4. Neuroimaging findings in early frontotemporal dementia with parkinsonism in a 26-year-old man. Axial T2-weighted images (*A, B*) showing mild bilateral and symmetric frontal cortical atrophy (*thick arrows*). Axial FDG-PET scans (*C, D*) in the same patient showing striking bilateral and symmetric frontal cortical and thalamic hypometabolism (*thin arrows*).

neuronal threads, or Pick's bodies) or glia (eg, astrocytic plaques or oligodendroglial coiled bodies) always are present on histologic examination, sometimes accompanied by argyrophilic grains. These tau^{+} inclusions often are in a distribution such that patients are diagnosed pathologically as having CBD, PSP, argyrophilic grain disease, or Pick's disease if the presence of a *MAPT* mutation is not known; the pathologic diagnosis of FTDP-17

Table 1
Comparison of specific parkinsonian findings in the various neurodegenerative disorders manifesting as dementia with or without parkinsonism

Disorder	Specific parkinsonian findings
AD	Parkinsonism tends to be later in course; rigidity, bradykinesia, tremor (resting aor postural) most obvious
PD	Masked facies, stooped posture, reduced arm swing. Unilateral or asymmetric rigidity, bradykinesia, resting tremor, and postural instablility; signs clearly are levodopa responsive
PDD	Same as in PD, but over time, bilateral involvement, marked postural instability, and loss of levodopa responsiveness
DLB	Masked facies, stooped posture, reduced arm swing similar to PD and PDD, but tremor is less asymmetric and more postural than at rest
CBS	Markedly asymmetric rigidity and apraxia, often with coexisting jerky tremor, myoclonus, dystonia, alien limb phenomenon, cortical sensory loss; parkinsonism is minimally levodopa responsive
PSP	Wide-eyed stare, reduced eye blink frequency, axial greater than appendicular rigidity, moves en bloc
MSA	Rigidity less asymmetric and minimally levodopa responsive in the striatonigral variant; ataxia and spasticity prominent in the olivopontocerebellar atrophy variant; orthostatic hypotension prominent in the Shy-Drager syndrome variant
FTDP-17	Parkinsonism variable, sometimes levodopa responsive, often similar findings to those in CBS

associated with a mutation in *MAPT* typically is used when a mutation is identified [61].

Cortical atrophy in patients with FTDP-17PGRN is similar to that in FTDP-17*MAPT*, although parietal lobe involvement is more prominent in FTDP-17*PGRN*. On histologic examination, the consistent finding is FTLD-U with neuronal intranuclear inclusions [42,47–49,51–55]. Immunostaining directed against progranulin stains normal structures and not the

Table 2
Patterns of impairment in cognitive domains based on neuropsychologic testing in the various neurodegenerative disorders manifesting as dementia with or without parkinsonism

Disorder	Learning and memory	Attention/ concentration	Executive functioning	Language functioning	Visuospatial functioning
AD	+++	+ to +++	+ to +++	+ to +++	+ to +++
PD	Nl to +	Nl to ++	Nl to ++	Nl	Nl
PDD	Nl to +++	++ to +++	++ to +++	Nl to ++	+ to +++
DLB	Nl to +++	++ to +++	++ to +++	Nl to ++	+ to +++
CBS	Nl to ++	Nl to +++	Nl to ++	Nl to ++	Nl to ++
PSP	Nl to ++	+ to +++	++ to +++	Nl to ++	Nl
MSA	Nl to +	+ to ++	+ to ++	Nl	Nl
FTDP-17	Nl to +++	+ to +++	+ to +++	Nl to +++	Nl to ++

Key: Nl = normal, + = mild impairment, ++ = moderate impairment, +++ = severe impairment.

Table 3
Comparison of findings on neuroimaging studies in the various neurodegenerative disorders manifesting as dementia with or without parkinsonism

Disorder	Pattern of atrophy on MRI	Pattern of hypoperfusion (SPECT) or hypometabolism (FDG-PET)
AD	Maximal in hippocampi, generalized cortical atrophy evolves over time	Maximal in temporoparietal cortex
PD	Minimal to no significant cortical or hippocampal atrophy	Normal or minimally abnormal
PDD	Minimal to no significant cortical or hippocampal atrophy	Maximal in frontoparieto-occipital cortex
DLB	Minimal to no significant cortical or hippocampal atrophy	Maximal in parieto-occipital cortex
CBS	Maximal in the parietal and posterior frontal cortex; asymmetric	Maximal in parietofrontal cortex ± BG ± thalamus; asymmetric
PSP	Maximal in the frontal cortex and midbrain	Maximal in frontosubcortical regions
MSA	Maximal in the pons or cerebellum	Normal or minimally abnormal
FTDP-17	Maximal in the frontotemporal cortex or amygdala	Maximal in the frontotemporal cortex ± amygdale ± basal ganglia

ubiquitinated protein that is presumed to be pathogenic; rather, TDP-43 recently was discovered to be the ubiquitinated protein in FTLD-U, FTLD with motor neuron disease, and clinical ALS [62]. How specific TDP-43 staining is for these inclusions remains to be seen.

Management

Management of patients who have FTDP-17 is discussed in the article by Dr. Graff-Radford elsewhere in this issue.

Summary

The specific clinical features relating to parkinsonism in the various neurodegenerative disorders are described in Table 1. The neuropsychologic profiles of impairment in CBS, PSP, MSA, and FTDP-17 compared and contrasted with those of AD and the Lewy body spectrum of phenotypes (PD, PDD, and DLB) are in Table 2. Patterns of atrophy on MRI, hypoperfusion on SPECT, and hypometabolism on FDG-PET in these same neurodegenerative disorders are listed in Table 3.

References

[1] Boeve B. Diagnosis and management of the non-Alzheimer dementias. In: Noseworthy JW, editor. Neurological Therapeutics: Principles and Practice, 2nd edition, volume 3. Abingdon: Informa Healthcare; 2006. p. 3156–206.

[2] Boeve B. Corticobasal degeneration. In: Adler C, Ahlskog J, editors. Parkinson's disease and movement disorders: diagnosis and treatment guidelines for the practicing physician. Totawa (NJ): Human Press Inc.; 2000. p. 253–61.
[3] Boeve B, Lang A, Litvan I. Corticobasal degeneration and its relationship to progressive supranuclear palsy and frontotemporal dementia. Ann Neurol 2003;54:S15–9.
[4] Boeve B. Corticobasal degeneration: the syndrome and the disease. In: Litvan I, editor. Atypical parkinsonian disorders. Totawa (NJ): Humana Press; 2005. p. 309–34.
[5] Pillon B, Blin J, Vidailhet M, et al. The neuropsychological pattern of corticobasal degeneration: comparison with progressive supranuclear palsy and Alzheimer's disease. Neurology 1995;45:1477–83.
[6] Massman P, Kreiter K, Jankovic J, et al. Neuropsychological functioning in cortical-basal ganglionic degeneration: differentiation from Alzheimer's disease. Neurology 1996;46: 720–6.
[7] Josephs KA, Tang-Wai DF, Edland SD, et al. Correlation between antemortem magnetic resonance imaging findings and pathologically confirmed corticobasal degeneration. Arch Neurol 2004;61(12):1881–4.
[8] Dickson D, Bergeron C, Chin S, et al. Office of Rare Diseases neuropathologic criteria for corticobasal degeneration. J Neuropathol Exp Neurol 2002;61:935–46.
[9] Boeve B, Josephs K, Drubach D. Current and future management of the corticobasal syndrome and corticobasal degeneration. In: Litvan I, Duyckaerts C, editors. Handbook of clinical neurology: dementias. Scotland: Danderhall: Elsevier Press, Inc.; in press.
[10] Kompoliti K, Goetz C, Boeve B, et al. Clinical presentation and pharmacological therapy in corticobasal degeneration. Arch Neurol 1998;55:957–61.
[11] Wolf S, Winstein C, Miller J, et al. Effect of constraint-induced movement therapy on upper extremity function 3 to 9 months after stroke: the EXCITE randomized clinical trial. JAMA 2006;296:2095–104.
[12] Litvan I, Agid Y, Calne D, et al. Clinical research criteria for the diagnosis of progressive supranuclear palsy (Steele-Richardson-Olszewski syndrome): report of the NINDS-SPSP international workshop. Neurology 1996;47:1–9.
[13] Litvan I, Mangone CA, McKee A, et al. Natural history of progressive supranuclear palsy (Steele-Richardson-Olszewski syndrome) and clinical predictors of survival: a clinicopathological study. J Neurol Neurosurg Psychiatry 1996;60(6):615–20.
[14] Boeve B, Duffy J, Bartleson J, et al. Progressive nonfluent aphasic and subsequent aphasic dementia associated with atypical progressive supranuclear palsy pathology. Eur Neurol 2003;49:72–8.
[15] Rippon G, Boeve B, Parisi J, et al. Late-onset frontotemporal dementia associated with progressive supranuclear palsy/argyrophilic grain disease/Alzheimer's disease pathology. Neurocase 2005;11:204–11.
[16] Josephs K, Boeve B, Duffy J, et al. Atypical progressive supranuclear palsy underlying progressive apraxia of speech and nonfluent aphasia. Neurocase 2005;11:283–96.
[17] Dubois B, Pillon B, Legault F, et al. Slowing of cognitive processing in progressive supranuclear palsy. A comparison with Parkinson's disease. Arch Neurol 1988;45:1194–9.
[18] Pillon B, Deweer B, Michon A, et al. Are explicit memory disorders of progressive supranuclear palsy related to damage to striatofrontal circuits? Comparison with Alzheimer's, Parkinson's, and Huntington's diseases. Neurology 1994;44:1264–70.
[19] Bak T, Crawford L, Hearn V, et al. Subcortical dementia revisited: similarities and differences in cognitive function between progressive supranuclear palsy (PSP), corticobasal degeneration (CBD) and multiple system atrophy (MSA). Neurocase 2005;11: 268–73.
[20] Adachi M, Kawanami T, Ohshima H, et al. Morning glory sign: a particular MR finding in progressive supranuclear palsy. Magn Reson Med Sci 2004;15:125–32.
[21] Kato N, Arai K, Hattori T. Study of the rostral midbrain atrophy in progressive supranuclear palsy. J Neurol Sci 2003;210:57–60.

[22] Josephs KA, Whitwell JL, Boeve BF, et al. Rates of cerebral atrophy in autopsy-confirmed progressive supranuclear palsy. Ann Neurol 2006;59:200–3.
[23] Hauw J-J, Daniel S, Dickson D, et al. Preliminary NINDS neuropathologic criteria for Steel-Richardson-Olszewski syndrome (progressive supranuclear palsy). Neurology 1994;44:2015–9.
[24] Nieforth KA, Golbe LI. Retrospective study of drug response in 87 patients with progressive supranuclear palsy. Clin Neuropharmacol 1993;16(4):338–46.
[25] Cole DG, Growdon JH. Therapy for progressive supranuclear palsy: past and future. J Neural Transm Suppl 1994;42:283–90.
[26] Kompoliti K, Goetz CG, Litvan I, et al. Pharmacological therapy in progressive supranuclear palsy. Arch Neurol 1998;55(8):1099–102.
[27] Boeve B. Diagnosis and management of the non-Alzheimer dementias. In: Noseworthy J, editor. Neurological therapeutics: principles and practice. 2nd edition. Abingdon (VA): Informa Healthcare; 2006. p. 3156–206.
[28] Gilman S, Low P, Quinn N, et al. Consensus statement on the diagnosis of multiple system atrophy. J Neurol Sci 1999;163:94–8.
[29] Konagaya M, Konagaya Y, Miwa S, et al. [Clinico-MRI study of hemispheric disorder in long-term follow-up cases of multiple system atrophy]. Rinsho Shinkeigaku 1998;38(12):1031–6 [in Japanese].
[30] Konagaya M, Sakai M, Matsuoka Y, et al. Multiple system atrophy with remarkable frontal lobe atrophy. Acta Neuropathologica 1999;97(4):423–8.
[31] Burk K, Daum I, Rub U. Cognitive function in multiple system atrophy of the cerebellar type. Mov Disord 2006;21:772–6.
[32] Boeve B, Silber M, Ferman T, et al. Association of REM sleep behavior disorder and neurodegenerative disease may reflect an underlying synucleinopathy. Mov Disord 2001;16:622–30.
[33] Boeve B, Silber M, Ferman T, et al. REM sleep behavior disorder in Parkinson's disease, dementia with Lewy bodies, and multiple system atrophy. In: Bedard M, Agid Y, Chouinard S, editors. Mental and behavioral dysfunction in movement disorders. Totowa (NJ): Humana Press; 2003. p. 383–97.
[34] Silber M, Levine S. Stridor and death in multiple system atrophy. Mov Disord 2000;15:699–704.
[35] Dujardin K, Defebvre L, Krystkowiak P, et al. Executive function differences in multiple system atrophy and Parkinson's disease. Parkinsonism Relat Disord 2003;9:205–11.
[36] Srivastava T, Singh S, Goyal V, et al. "Hot cross bun" sign in two patients with multiple system atrophy-cerebellar. Neurology 2005;64:128.
[37] Schrag A, Good CD, Miszkiel K, et al. Differentiation of atypical parkinsonian syndromes with routine MRI. Neurology 2000;54(3):697–702.
[38] Gilman S. Functional imaging with positron emission tomography in multiple system atrophy. J Neural Transm 2005;112:1647–55.
[39] Benarroch EE, Schmeichel AM. Depletion of cholinergic mesopontine neurons in multiple system atrophy: a substrate for REM behavior disorder? Neurology 2002;58:A345.
[40] Benarroch EE, Schmeichel AM, Sandroni P, et al. Brainstem respiratory control: substrates of respiratory failure of multiple system atrophy. Acta Neuropathol (Berl) 2007;113(1):75–80 [Epub 2006 Nov 2007].
[41] Hutton M, Lendon CL, Rizzu P, et al. Association of missense and 5'-splice-site mutations in tau with the inherited dementia FTDP-17. Nature 1998;393:702–5.
[42] Baker M, Mackenzie I, Pickering-Brown S, et al. Mutations in progranulin cause tau-negative frontotemporal dementia linked to chromosome 17. Nature 2006;442:916–9.
[43] Poorkaj P, Grossman M, Steinbart E, et al. Frequency of tau gene mutations in familial and sporadic cases of non-Alzheimer dementia. Arch Neurol 2001;58:383–7.
[44] MICROTUBULE-ASSOCIATED PROTEIN TAU; MAPT. Avialable at: http://www.ncbi.nlm.nih.gov/entrez/dispomim.cgi?id=157140; Accessed December 28, 2006.

[45] Kertesz A. Pick's complex and FTDP-17. Mov Disord 2003;18:S57–62.

[46] Benussi L, Binetti G, Sina E, et al. A novel deletion in progranulin gene is associated with FTDP-17 and CBS. Neurobiol Aging Dec 5, 2006 [Epub ahead of print].

[47] Boeve B, Baker M, Dickson D, et al. Frontotemporal dementia and parkinsonism associated with the IVS1+1G->A mutation in progranulin: a clinicopathologic study. Brain 2006;129: 3103–14.

[48] Cruts M, Gijselinck I, van der Zee J, et al. Null mutations in progranulin cause ubiquitin positive frontotemporal dementia linked to chromosome 17q21. Nature 2006;442:920–4.

[49] Gass J, Cannon A, Mackenzie I, et al. Mutations in progranulin are a major cause of ubiquitin-positive frontotemporal lobar degeneration. Hum Mol Genet 2006;15:2988–3001.

[50] Huey ED, Grafman J, Wassermann EM, et al. Characteristics of frontotemporal dementia patients with a Progranulin mutation. Ann Neurol 2006;60:374–80.

[51] Mackenzie I, Baker M, Pickering-Brown S, et al. The neuropathology of frontotemporal lobar degeneration caused by mutations in the progranulin gene. Brain 2006;129:3081–90.

[52] Masellis M, Momeni P, Meschino W, et al. Novel splicing mutation in the progranulin gene causing familial corticobasal syndrome. Brain 2006;129:3115–23.

[53] Mukherjee O, Pastor P, Cairns NJ, et al. HDDD2 is a familial frontotemporal lobar degeneration with ubiquitin-positive, tau-negative inclusions caused by a missense mutation in the signal peptide of progranulin. Ann Neurol 2006;60:314–22.

[54] Pickering-Brown S, Baker M, Gass J, et al. Mutations in progranulin explain atypical phenotypes with variants in MAPT. Brain 2006;129:3124–6.

[55] Snowden J, Pickering-Brown S, Mackenzie I, et al. Progranulin gene mutations associated with frontotemporal dementia and progressive non-fluent aphasia. Brain 2006;129: 3091–102.

[56] Boeve B, Tremont-Lukats I, Waclawik A, et al. Longitudinal characterization of two siblings with frontotemporal dementia and parkinsonism linked to chromosome 17 associated with the S305N tau mutation. Brain 2005;128:752–72.

[57] Pal P, Wszolek Z, Kishore A, et al. Positron emission tomography in pallido-ponto-nigral degeneration (PPND) family (frontotemporal dementia with parkinsonism linked to chromosome 17 and point mutation in tau gene). Parkinsonism Relat Disord 2001;7:81–8.

[58] Frank A, Wszolek Z, Jack CR, et al. Distinctive MRI findings in pallido-ponto-nigral degeneration (PPND). Neurology 2007;68:620–1.

[59] Boeve BF, Kelley BJ, Haidar W, et al. MRI findings in familial frontotemporal dementia and/or parkinsonism associated with mutations in progranulin. Neurology 2007;68(Suppl 1): A388.

[60] Whitwell JL, Jack CR Jr, Baker M, et al. Voxel-based morphometry in frontotemporal lobar degeneration with ubiquitin-positive inclusions with and without progranulin mutations. Arch Neurol 2007;64:371–6.

[61] McKhann GM, Albert MS, Grossman M, et al. Clinical and pathological diagnosis of frontotemporal dementia: report of the Work Group on Frontotemporal Dementia and Pick's Disease. Arch Neurol 2001;58(11):1803–9.

[62] Neumann M, Sampathu D, Kwong L, et al. Ubiquitinated TDP-43 in frontotemporal lobar degeneration and amyotrophic lateral sclerosis. Science 2006;314:130–3.

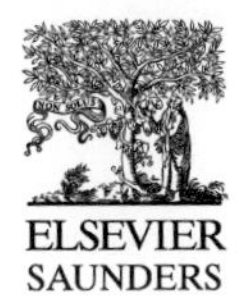
ELSEVIER
SAUNDERS

Neurol Clin 25 (2007) 783–807

NEUROLOGIC
CLINICS

Rapidly Progressive Dementia

Michael D. Geschwind, MD, PhD*,
Aissa Haman, MD, Bruce L. Miller, MD

Department of Neurology, Memory & Aging Center, Francisco, 350 Parnassus Avenue, Suite 706, San Francisco, CA 94117, USA

As a major prion disease referral center in the United States, the authors are referred several rapidly progressive dementia (RPD) cases every week, most of which are referred with a potential diagnosis of Creutzfeldt-Jakob disease (CJD). The number of referrals increased dramatically with the identification of quinacrine as a potential therapy for CJD and commencement of the first United States CJD treatment trail in May 2005 [1,2]. The authors recognized the need for a broader diagnostic approach to RPD after observing that 15% to 20% of these referrals were the result of other nonprion conditions, many of which were treatable. Physicians, and even neurologists, generally are not trained formally in the assessment of RPDs. This review hopes to provide a more thorough appreciation of the myriad etiologies for RPDS and to offer a possible diagnostic decision tree or algorithm, based largely on the experience of the authors' center.

Most dementias develop slowly, allowing an unhurried outpatient evaluation. Algorithms for the assessment of these patients have been developed and refined, and most neurologists are well acquainted with these approaches. A careful history usually detects dementia secondary to medications or depression, and routine laboratory assessments help to eliminate metabolic conditions that can cause dementia, including anemia, electrolyte imbalance, liver or kidney failure, thyroid disease, and vitamin B_{12} deficiency. The majority of slowly progressive dementias are secondary to Alzheimer's disease (AD), although there is an increasing recognition of non-AD dementias, including frontotemporal dementia (FTD) (see article by Josephs elsewhere in this issue), subcortical ischemia vascular disease (see article by Chui elsewhere in this issue), dementia with Lewy bodies

* Corresponding author. Department of Neurology, Memory & Aging Center, University of California, San Francisco Medical Center, 350 Parnassus Avenue, Suite 706, San Francisco, CA 94117

E-mail address: mgeschwind@memory.ucsf.edu (M.D. Geschwind).

doi:10.1016/j.ncl.2007.04.001 ***neurologic.theclinics.com***

(DLB) (see article by Boeve elsewhere in this issue), and other parkinsonian dementias, such as cortical basal degeneration (CBD) and progressive supranuclear palsy (see elsewhere in this issue) [3]. With the possible exceptions of DLB and CBD, however, the disorders that commonly lead to slowly progressive adult dementia, such as AD and FTD, rarely present as RPDs [4–6]. Patients who have a RPD often require consideration of a different set of disorders.

The primary aim of this article is to instruct clinicians in an approach to the differential diagnosis of RPD that will broaden their scope of inquiry and, particularly, identify RPDs that are treatable and potentially reversible. This article is organized around the following categories: neurodegenerative, autoimmune, toxic and metabolic, infectious, neoplastic, and vascular, emphasizing the RPDs most difficult to diagnose or least likely be recognized. As many types of conditions can cause RPD and they can progress quickly, it is important to have an organized, systematic approach to diagnosis. The mnemonic, VITAMINS, often is useful for summarizing some of the major categories of etiologies for RPDs (Box 1). Box 2 lists many etiologies of RPD (many of which are not discussed in this review). When considering patients who have a RPD, it may be helpful to use the information in Boxes 1 and 2 to ensure a complete differential is considered. RPDs that present with space-occupying brain lesions easily identified by CT or MRI scan are not discussed in this article. Figs. 1 and 2 provide an outline for the diagnostic approach that the authors use in evaluating patients who have RPD. Fig. 1 shows the overall approach, whereas Fig. 2 details an expanded evaluation when standard testing is inconclusive.

Over the past 5 years, the authors' dementia center has been referred approximately 825 RPD cases, many with a presumptive diagnosis of CJD. After reviewing records and in many cases evaluating the patients, determined the diagnostic breakdown of this group was determined as 54% prion disease (37% probable or definite sporadic, 15% genetic, and 2% acquired), 28% undetermined (because of insufficient records, although most met

Box 1. VITAMINS mnemonic for categories of conditions causing rapidly progressive dementias

*V*ascular
*I*nfectious
*T*oxic-metabolic
*A*utoimmune
*M*etastases/neoplasm
*I*atrogenic
*N*eurodegenerative
*S*ystemic

Box 2. Differential diagnosis of rapidly progressive dementias

Neurodegenerative
CJD (sporadic, iatrogenic, familial)
AD
DLB
FTD
CBD
Progressive supranuclear palsy (PSP)

Infectious
Viral encephalitis, including herpes simplex virus
HIV dementia
Progressive multifocal leukoencephalopathy
Subacute sclerosing panencephalitis (young adults)
Fungal infections (immunosuppression [eg, central nervous system (CNS) aspergillosis])
Syphilis
Parasites
Lyme disease (rarely encephalopathy)
Balamuthia
Whipple's disease

Toxic/metabolic
Vitamin B_{12} (cyanocobalamin) deficiency
Vitamin B_1 (thiamine) deficiency
Niacin deficiency
Folate deficiency (dementia rare)
Uremia
Wilson's disease
Portosystemic encephalopathy
Acquired hepatocerebral degeneration
Porphyria
Bismuth toxicity
Lithium toxicity
Mercury toxicity
Arsenic toxicity
Electrolyte abnormalities

Autoimmune
Hashimoto's encephalopathy (HE)
Paraneoplastic (autoimmune) limbic encephalopathy (PLE)
Nonparaneoplastic autoimmune (eg, anti–voltage-gated potassium channel [VGKC] antibodies mediated)
Lupus cerebritis

Other CNS vasculitides
Sarcoid

Endocrine abnormalities
Thyroid disturbances
Parathyroid abnormalities
Adrenal diseases

Neoplasm related
Nonautoimmune paraneoplastic conditions
Metastases to CNS
Primary CNS lymphoma (PCNSL)
Intravascular lymphoma
Lymphomatoid granulomatosis
Gliomatosis cerebri

criteria for possible CJD; see article by Eggenberger elsewhere in this issue), and, importantly, 18% who had other nonprion conditions, many of which were treatable. The diagnostic breakdown of these nonprion RPDs was 26% neurodegenerative, 15% autoimmune, 11% infectious, 11% psychiatric, and 9% miscellaneous other, whereas 28% still were undetermined, often

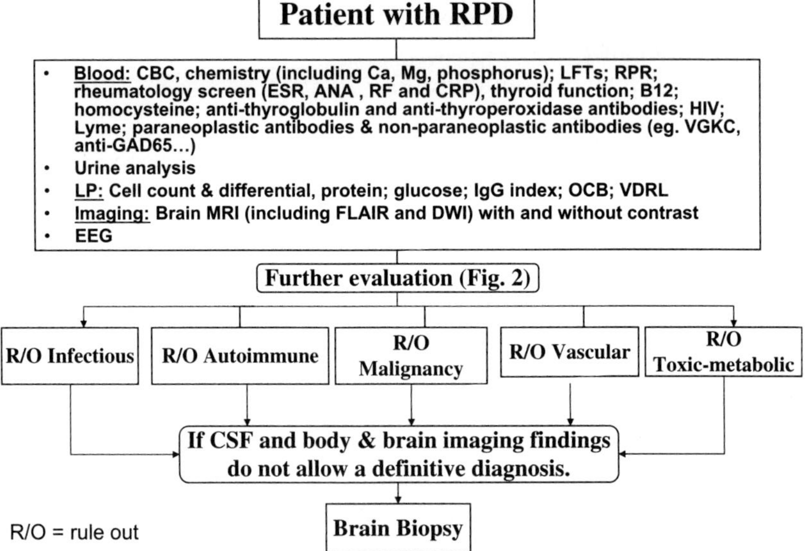

Fig. 1. RPD evaluation. AFB, acid-fast bacillus; Ca, calcium; CBC complete blood count; LDH, lactate dehydrogenase; LFT, liver function tests; LP, lumbar puncture; OCB, oligoclonal bands; Mg, magnesium.

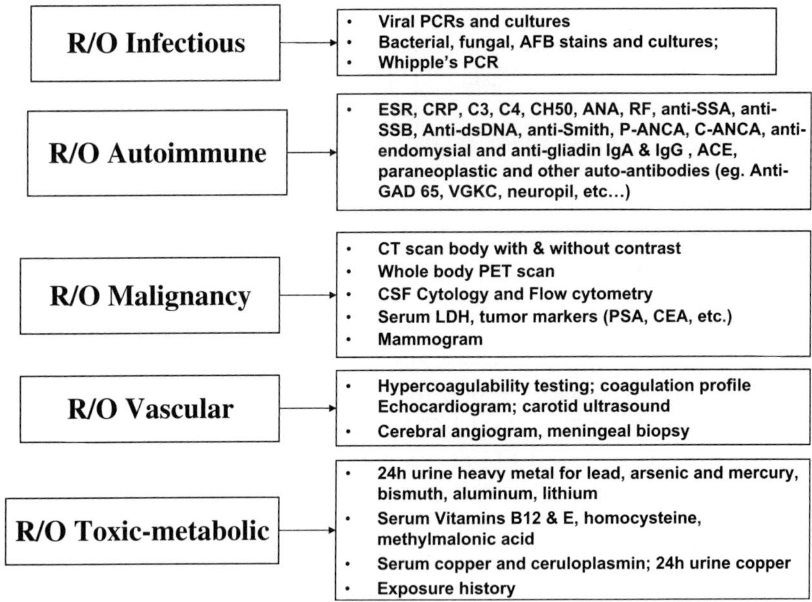

Fig. 2. Further RPD evaluation. AFB, acid-fast bacillus; CBC complete blood count; LDH, lactate dehydrogenase; LFT, liver function tests; LP, lumbar puncture; OCB, oligoclonal bands; Mg, magnesium.

leukoencephalopathies or encephalopathies of unknown etiology (M. Geschwind, MD, PhD, unpublished data, 2007). Because the authors' efforts in improving diagnosis of RPDs was prompted by the necessity to differentiate prion diseases from other causes of RPD, following is a brief discussion of some of the salient issues in diagnosis of the prototypical RPD, prion disease (discussed in detail in article by Eggenberger elsewhere in this issue).

Degenerative dementias as rapidly progressive dementias

Prion diseases

When considering a RPD in particular patients who have prominent motor or cerebellar dysfunction, CJD should be high on the differential. Some key features to consider with prion disease, based on the authors' experiences, are discussed in this article.

The most commonly used clinical criteria for probable sporadic CJD s(sCJD) [7,8] do not allow early diagnosis of CJD and use ancillary tests (electroencephalogram [EEG] and cerebrospinal fluid [CSF] protein 14-3-3) that many consider to have poor sensitivity or specificity and not useful in clinical practice [9–11]. A major problem with these criteria is that they include signs or symptoms, such as akinetic mutism and the characteristic

EEG, that often do not occur until late stages of the illness. These criteria also do not include features that often are early signs of the illness, such as behavioral changes or aphasia [12]. The authors identified the first symptom in 114 subjects who had sCJD referred to the center and found the most common were cognitive (39% of patients), followed by cerebellar (21%), behavioral (20%), constitutional (20%), sensory (11%), motor (9%), and visual (7%). Three of these categories—behavioral, constitutional, and sensory symptoms (headache, malaise, vertigo, and so forth)—are not included in current diagnostic criteria. Furthermore, the authors have found that ancillary tests in World Health Organization criteria that are required for a probable sCJD diagnosis, EEG or 14-3-3, are neither sensitive nor specific. In a recent evaluation of a RPD cohort (150 sCJD and 47 nonprion RPD subjects), the authors found the 14-3-3 to have a sensitivity of 48% and a specificity of 66%. The EEG had a sensitivity of less than 45% by the time patients had an EEG at the authors' institution, which generally was not their first EEG. This increased to approximately 50% when patients then were followed prospectively during their entire disease course (M. Geschwind, MD, PhD, unpublished data, 2007) [13]. In the authors' cohort, the preliminary data suggest that two other surrogate biomarkers for sCJD, total tau and neuron-specific enolase, have somewhat higher sensitivity and specificity for CJD than 14-3-3 or EEG. The authors believe these CSF biomarkers merely are signs of rapid neuronal injury, are not specific for prion disease, and, therefore, are of questionable diagnostic usefulness. A prion-specific test is needed [14–16].

Typically chronic degenerative dementias

AD rarely is rapid, but unusual presentations can be mistaken for CJD [4]. Several cases of AD are reported in conjunction with angiopathy (cerebral amyloid angiopathy) presenting as adult-onset RPD [17–19]. Other nonprion neurodegenerative diseases that also can present, albeit rarely, in a more fulminant fashion, include DLB, FTD (in particular the subtype with motor neuron disease), CBD, and PSP. Patients who have AD typically survive a median of 11.7 (SD ±0.6) years, patients who have FTD 11 years (SD ±0.9), patients who have PSP/CBD 11.8 years (SD ±0.6) [20], and patients who have PSP alone 5.6 years [21] from first symptom. More rapid onset or progression can occur [20,22–25]. In a large German study, of 413 autopsied suspected cases of CJD, 7% had AD and 3% had DLB. Myoclonus and extrapyramidal signs occurred in more than 70% of patients who had DLB and more than 50% of the patients who had AD [4]. Similarly, in a French pathologic study of 465 patients who had suspected CJD, the two most frequent non-CJD pathologic diagnoses were AD and DLB [26].

Parkinsonian dementias, such as DLB and FTD-spectrum disorders, including PSP, CBD, and FTD, are discussed in articles elsewhere in this issue and, thus, are mentioned only briefly in this article. DLB is a progressive dementia often associated with fluctuations in cognitive function, persistent well-formed visual hallucinations, or parkinsonism (see the article by Boeve elsewhere in this issue) [27]. Duration of DLB often is shorter than for many other neurodegenerative dementias; one study suggests 3-year survival [28], although rapid decline with death in 1 year can occur. Periodic sharp waves may be seen on EEG, leading to confusion with CJD [26,29]. In several large cohort studies, DLB was the second most common condition mistaken for CJD [4,26]. FTD rarely is rapidly progressive, although it typically has a faster course than AD. Patients typically present with a frontal syndrome, including behavioral, personality, and cognitive changes occurring over years, followed by dementia (see article by Josephs elsewhere in this issue). Fifteen percent or more of patients who have FTD develop amyotrophic lateral sclerosis and these patients typically die within 1.4 years from the time of diagnosis [30–33]. Corticobasal degeneration (CBD) is a clinically and pathologically heterogeneous atypical parkinsonian dementia often confused clinically with AD, PSP, or FTD (see article by Boeve elsewhere in this issue) [34–38]. Many features of CBD, including myoclonus; alien limb; and visual, sensory, and motor deficits, overlap with features of CJD. The converse also is true; CJD sometimes can present as a rapid cortical basal syndrome [39] or with a protracted course over 2 to 3 years with features indistinguishable from CBD; however, the fluid-attenuated inversion recovery (FLAIR) and diffusion-weighted imaging (DWI) MRI abnormalities seen in CJD are not found in CBD [40]. As in CJD, patients who have PSP develop dementia, akinetic-rigid parkinsonism (symmetric bradykinesia and axial rigidity), postural instability, and swallowing and speech problems and often progress to a hypokinetic, mute state [41–46]. Abnormalities of eye movements, particularly slowed velocity of saccades progressing to supranuclear gaze palsy, are part of the PSP syndrome (see article by Boeve elsewhere in this issue). CJD mimicking PSP has been reported [47].

Neurofilament inclusion body disease (NIBD) is a recently described pathologic condition that can present clinically as FTD or CBD. The four index cases were all more rapid than typical degenerative dementias, with duration of only 2 to 4 years. Brain MRI and pathology showed frontal, temporal, and caudate atrophy. A distinguishing feature of NIBD is the presence of intracytopasmic neuronal inclusions that stain strongly with antibodies to neurofilament proteins and ubiquitin, but not tau or α-synuclein [48]. One case of NIBD also presented as an early-onset rapidly progressive FTD with features of primary lateral sclerosis [49].

Fahr's disease is a neurodegenerative disease of unknown cause with basal ganglia calcification that typically presents with a movement and neuropsychiatric disorder. Although usually very slowly progressive, a 50-year-old patient was reported with a rapidly progressive frontal behavioral and cognitive presentation of Fahr's disease (idiopathic basal ganglia calcification) resulting in dementia within 6 months. Patients who have Fahr's disease have extensive basal ganglia calcification, a finding that is not present in CJD [50]. Rarely, genetic neurodegenerative diseases also may present as a RPD. A case recently was reported of a man who had the fragile X premutation who presented in his mid-60s with a rapid course of tremor, gait ataxia, parkinsonism, and cognitive deficits [51].

Autoimmune encephalopathies (paraneoplastic and nonparaneoplastic)

Over the past few years, there has been a growing awareness and identification of autoimmune causes of encephalopathy or RPDs. Initially, most of these autoimmune conditions were believed to be paraneoplastic—due to antibodies or other components of the immune system, against the cancer, cross-reacting with antigens of the nervous system. In many of these conditions, however, no cancers have been identified, despite repeated comprehensive searches for a tumor. This section dise cusses paraneoplastic and nonparaneoplastic autoimmune encephalopathies.

Paraneoplastic neurologic disorders (PNDs) often present as a rapidly progressive limbic encephalopathy. PNDs that involve the CNS often are divided into two forms: those with isolated involvement of one part of the nervous system (eg, limbic encephalitis/encephalopathy, cerebellar syndromes, or retinal degeneration) or those with more diffuse, multifocal symptoms, sometimes referred to as paraneoplastic encephalomyelitis (PEM). PLE can occur as an isolated syndrome or as PEM with involvement of other parts of the nervous system (ie, brainstem, cerebellum, or peripheral nerves). The most common symptoms are a subacute amnestic syndrome, presenting as problems with short-term anterograde memory or more variable retrograde amnesia. Depression, personality changes, anxiety, and emotional lability often precede the cognitive dysfunction. Seizures are common [52,53]. PNDs occur in patients who have a known diagnosis of a cancer or may precede the detection of the cancer by weeks, months, or, rarely, a few years. In patients who do not have a known cancer diagnosis, various signs or symptoms may suggest a PEM or PLE, including subacute development of multifocal neurologic symptoms, CSF evidence of inflammation, elevated tumor markers (carcinoembryonic antigen, cancer antigen 125, prostate-specific antigen, and so forth), a family history of cancer, unexplained anorexia or weight loss or other symptoms suggestive of cancer, and the presence of certain paraneoplastic antibodies in the serum or CSF [52,53].

The most common tumors associated with PLE are small cell lung cancer (SCLC) (75% of cases), germ-cell tumors (ovarian or testicular), thymoma, Hodgkin's lymphoma, and breast cancer [52,53], whereas the most common antibodies associated with PLE are anti-Hu (ANNA-1), anti-Ma2 (also called anti-Ta; antigen is Ma2), CV2 (anti–CMRP-5), Yo (PCA-1), and probably antineuropil [52,54–56]. Anti-Hu antibodies are found in 50% of cases of PLE with SCLC. Identification of antineural antibodies is highly suggestive of an underlying neoplasm. Furthermore, the type of autoantibody may suggest the tumor type rather than the neurologic syndrome [52,57]. Almost one third of patients who have a neurologic syndrome and autoantibodies have more than one autoantibody [57,58]. In PLE associated with anti-Ma2 (Ta) antibodies and testicular cancer, approximately half of patients have dramatic improvement of their neurologic syndrome after treatment of their cancer [56,59]. This may be in part because of the ability to remove all the cancer through orchiectomy [60]. Hypothalamic involvement is common in patients who have anti-Ma2 antibodies [56]. Antibodies to CRMP-5 (anti-CV2 or anti–CRMP-5), a protein in the collapsin response-mediator protein family, often are associated with PNDs, including PLE. Peripheral neuropathy (47%) and autonomic neuropathy (31%) are the most common neurologic signs. Subacute dementia and cerebellar ataxia each occur in approximately one quarter of patients, followed by neuromuscular junction disorders (12%), chorea (11%), and cranial neuropathy (17%, including optic neuropathy and loss of taste). Spinal fluid often is inflammatory. Anti-CV2 is seen most often with SCLCs, followed by thymomas [61,62]. FLAIR MRI in anti-CV2 antibody syndrome often shows caudate, anterior putamen with or without medial temporal lobe hyperintensity [58], although thalamic T2-weighted hyperintensity also can occur (M. Geschwind, MD, PhD, unpublished data, 2007). The striatal and thalamic involvement can appear similar to findings in CJD; however, unlike CJD, the T2-weighted hyperintensity may extend beyond the deep gray nuclei into adjacent white matter, and there are no diffusion-weighted abnormalities. Most patients who have limbic encephalopathy and thymoma (often anti-CV2 or anti-VGKC antibodies) have significant neurologic improvement after tumor removal and treatment [63]. Table 1 summarizes some of the major antibodies, with their clinical phenotypes, that are associated with limbic encephalopathy.

Recently, there has been increasing awareness of several immune-mediated encephalopathies that not always are associated with cancers [54,64]. In some of these syndromes, antibodies, and sometimes their antigens, have been identified. Two such syndromes of limbic encephalopathy are due to anti-VGKC antibodies and to antineuropil antibodies. Patients who have anti-VGKC antibodies present along a spectrum of nervous system involvement, from the peripheral to the CNS. Involvement of the peripheral nervous system alone may manifest as neuromyotonia (Isaacs syndrome). Isolated CNS involvement may present as a seizure disorder or limbic encephalopathy [54,65–69]. Combinations of peripheral and central involvement, however, such as in Morvan's syndrome, also occur. Some of these patients have limbic encephalopathy in isolation, whereas others also are shown to exhibit different degrees of Morvan's fibrillary chorea, a syndrome characterized by neuromyotonia, myalgias, hyperhydrosis, and disordered sleep [70]. Anti–glutamic acid decarboxylase (anti-GAD)

Table 1
Paraneoplastic and nonparaneoplastic antibodies often associated with limbic encephalopathy

Antibodies	Tumors	Usual age of onset	Gender	Associated symptoms
Anti-Hu	SCLC, neuroblastoma, prostate	55–65	F> = M	PEM, subacute sensory neuropathy
Anti- Ma2 (anti-Ta)	Germinoma, testicular, lung cancer	22–45	M> >F	PLE, brainstem, cerebellar, hypothalamic
Anti-CV2 (anti–CRMP-5)	Thymoma, lung cancer, renal cell	50–70	F = M	Neuropathy, cerebellar, PLE, chorea
Anti-VGKC	80% none, 20% tumor thymoma, lung	Variable	???	Isaac's and Morvan's syndromes, neuromyotonia, cramps, hyperhydrosis, sleep disorder, seizures PLE
Anti-amphiphysin	Breast, SCLC			PEM, stiff-person syndrome, opsoclonus-myoclonus
Anti-Yo	Gynecologic and breast, adenocarcinoma	26–85	F> >M	Paraneoplastic cerebellar degeneration, limbic encephalopathy
Anti-nCMAg (some antineuropil)	Teratomas, thymus	20–50s	F>M	Acute PLE, abnormal movements, decreased consciousness
Anti-Ma1	Lung, other (breast, parotid, colon)	60	F	Paraneoplastic cerebellar degeneration, brainstem
Anti-Ri (ANNA-2)	Breast, gynecologic, lung, bladder			Ataxia, opsoclonus/myoclonus

Abbreviations: >, greater than; > > much greater than.

antibodies, although commonly associated with stiff-person syndrome, also can cause subacute ataxia, sometimes with mild cognitive complaints [71]. Novel antibodies against components of the CNS continually are identified [54]. If autoimmune syndrome is strongly suspected, because of CSF or serologic findings or concurrent or family history of autoimmune disorders, one should have a low threshold for sending serum and CSF to a research laboratory that specializes in identifying such antibodies.

HE is a rare but probably underdiagnosed, treatable autoimmune disorder associated with chronic lymphocytic Hashimoto's thyroiditis [72,73].

Often, it begins with a prodrome of depression, personality change, or psychosis and progresses into a cognitive decline associated with myoclonus, ataxia, pyramidal and extrapyramidal signs, stroke-like episodes, altered levels of consciousness, confusion, or seizures. Hallucinations or other psychoses are common [72–74]. It often is confused with CJD because of their overlapping clinical profile [5,74]. Compared with CJD, HE is associated more frequently with seizures and tends to have a more fluctuating course [74]. For unclear reasons, more women (85%) than men have been diagnosed with HE [74]. Patients may be euthyroid, hypothyroid, and even hyperthyroid, although the diagnosis cannot be made until patients are euthyroid [74]. Elevated levels of either antithyroglobulin or antithyroperoxidase (anti-TPO) and neurologic and psychiatric symptoms when patients are euthyroid, in the absence of other possible causes, suggest the diagnosis. The EEG frequently shows nonspecific abnormalities with asynchronous background slowing and intermittent diffuse or focal slow activity; however, as in CJD, triphasic waves or periodic sharp waves may occur [72,75]. MRI is not specific but commonly shows increased T2-weighted subcortical, mesial-temporal, or white matter signal, which may disappear after treatment [72,76–78]. CSF often has increased protein, a nonspecific finding that occurs in many other RPDs, including CJD [13,72,73]. The cause of HE may be the result of the presence of a shared antigen in the brain and thyroid [72,73,79]. More than 90% of patients respond favorably to immunosuppression, typically high-dose steroids followed by a long, slow taper, although some patients may have persistent symptoms or a fluctuating course [72,75,80]. Plasmapharesis also may be helpful [81].

Many other autoimmune disorders present as RPDs and are important to consider because of potential for reversibility with immunosuppression. A new clinicopathologic entity, called "cerebral amyloid inflammatory vasculopathy," has been described recently. These patients show acute or rapid onset of dementia. MRI shows evidence of amyloid-related hemorrhages and sometime large confluent white matter hyperintensities. Brain biopsy revealed Aβ amyloid cerebral angiopathy associated with chronic nongranulomatous vasculitis. With two 4 mg doses of dexamethasone, a patient made a rapid and nearly complete recovery over a few months [82].

Collagen vascular and granulomatous diseases also affect the CNS through mechanisms other than vasculitis. Several of these disorders may cause an encephalopathy or RPD, including primary angiitis of the CNS, polyarteritis nodosa, sarcoidosis, systemic lupus erythematosus, Sjögren's syndrome, celiac disease (sprue), Behçet's disease, and hypereosinophilic syndrome [83–89]. Some investigators group these encephalopathies of nonvasculitic origin under the term, nonvasculitic autoimmune inflammatory meningoencephalopathies; this group includes HE and Sjogren's encephalopathy, which almost uniformly have abnormal EEGs and respond to high-dose steroids [90]. The heralding features of the disorder may be neurologic sarcoid, a systemic illness of unknown origin characterized by the formation of non-necrotizing granulomas, and can be treated successfully, like other autoimmune conditions, with immunosuppression. Only approximately 5% of patients who have sarcoidosis have involvement of the nervous system, but when it involves the CNS it sometimes presents as a RPD. When there is brainstem involvement, cranial neuropathies may occur. MRI is highly variable and may be normal and show enhancing granulomas (often at the base of the brain) or nonenhancing T2-weighted white matter hyperintensities consistent with a leukoencephalopathy. CT of the chest may reveal hilar lymphadenopathy. CSF may be normal but often shows elevated protein and a mild to severe pleiocytosis. CSF angiotensin-converting enzyme levels are elevated in only 33% to 58% of cases and this test also lacks specificity. Biopsy of affected tissue is needed for diagnosis. Steroid treatment or other immunosuppression may be helpful, as are plasmapheresis and intravenous immunoglobulin. It is important to rule out other granulomatosis diseases, in particular tuberculosis, before initiating immunosuppression (M. Geschwind, MD, PhD, unpublished data, 2007) [91].

Vascular etiologies of rapidly progressive dementia

Depending on the location, strokes can present as RPD. Large vessel occlusions and thalamic, anterior corpus callosal or multiple diffuse infarctions in particular all have presented as RPDs [92,93]. Thrombotic thrombocytopenic purpura can cause microangiopathic thromboses producing global cerebral ischemia, resulting in an encephalopathy. Hyperviscosity syndromes from blood dyscrasias, such as polycythemia, or gammopathies, such as Waldenström's macroglobulinemia, can present as RPDs by causing global cerebral microvessel ischemia.

Although it is an autoimmune condition, CNS vasculitis is discussed in this article because of its direct effect on the vasculature as the cause of RPD. Criteria for classification of certain vasculitides largely are based on a combination of clinical symptoms or signs and laboratory findings [94,95]. A vasculitis may be limited to the CNS without any systemic or peripheral nervous system signs or may present initially as a systemic disorder with accompanying fever, weight loss, rash, neuropathy, and other organ involvement. Urinalysis may contain red cells as a sign of renal involvement. Ophthalmologic examination may identify uveitis, scleritis, or signs of ophthalmic artery vasculitis. If a rash is present, a skin biopsy can be diagnostic. There may be signs of a hemolytic anemia. A basic rheumatologic screen may include erythrocyte sedimentation rate (ESR), C-reactive protein (CRP), complement (C3), complement (C4), total complement (CH50), antinuclear antibody (ANA), rheumatoid factor (RF), anti-SSA, anti-SSB, perinuclear antineutrophil cytoplasmic autoantibodies (p-ANCA), and cytoplasmic ANCA (c-ANCA) with other testing depending on results of this initial screen. Serologic testing likely is abnormal in systemic forms of vasculitis, but in primary CNS vasculitis, patients typically have normal nonspecific tests, such as ESR, ANA, and CRP [96]. Vasculitides often are distinguished from other RPDs by brain MRI abnormalities, such as strokes or hemorrhage involving the white or gray matter [96]. Similarly, body imaging for systemic involvement may be helpful [97]. When primary CNS vasculitis is suspected, cerebral angiogram or brain and meningeal brain biopsy of the affected area may be required for diagnosis. Intravascular lymphoma sometimes mimics CNS vasculitis on angiogram; if this condition is suspected (based on an elevated serum lactate dehydrogenase or MRI findings), then one should avoid the angiogram and go directly to biopsy [98,99].

Infectious Etiologies

AIDS-dementia complex, HIV encephalopathy, or HIV-associated dementia is a neurologic complication of acquired immunodeficiency syndrome, eventually occurring in one fourth of patients who have AIDS. It typically occurs in the later stages of HIV infection [100] and has diminished since the introduction of highly active antiretroviral therapy (HAART). Some individuals, however, develop RPD during seroconversion or immune reconstitution. In general, more rapid neurologic impairment is associated with symptomatic HIV seroconverting illness [101]. Concomitant use of methamphetamine or cocaine also may synergize with HIV infection to cause an accelerated course of HIV dementia [102]. As dementia can be a presenting feature of AIDS [103], HIV testing should be considered in the evaluation of every RPD.

Subacute and chronic opportunistic infections associated with HIV infection and other immunocompromised states always must be considered in the differential diagnosis of RPD. Cryptococcus and JC virus infections typically present with meningitis or progressive focal neurologic deficits, respectively; however, they also can present with rapid progression of dementia [104]. CNS infection with mycobacteria may present as an inflammatory meningitis. A recent case report identified an atypical acid-fast bacillus, *Mycobacterium neoaurum*, by polymerase chain reaction (PCR) in autopsy brain tissue from a patient who had RPD and was on low-dose steroids. CSF cell count, mycobacterial culture, and Ziehl-Neelsen staining all failed to demonstrate the presence of mycobacterium. It is possible that many undiagnosed RPDs could be caused by infectious organisms that escape detection using standard microbiologic techniques [9,105,106]. (For a review on diagnosis and etiology of encephalitis, see Glaser and colleagues [106]).

Spirochete infections are unusual causes of cognitive impairment but important to consider as they are treatable. No workup for dementia, including RPD, is complete without an evaluation for CNS infection with *Treponema pallidum*, or neurosyphilis. Cognitive dysfunction is the most common neurologic syndrome, although usually a late complication, of syphilis [107]. It occasionally presents with rapid progression, particularly in immunocompromised patients [108]. Serologic testing with rapid plasma regain and VDRL and CSF VDRL suggest the diagnosis. The CSF in neurosyphilis usually shows a pleiocytosis and an elevated protein [107]. Lyme disease is a systemic infection with the spirochette, *Borrelia burgdorferi*, which is transmitted to people from a tick bite. Neurologic manifestations are rare in Lyme disease but can include cranial nerve palsy, meningitis, polyradiculopathy, depression, psychosis, and dementia [109]. Although RPD caused by Lyme disease is reported, it is rare [110,111], but it is important to consider because it responds readily to treatment [112].

Subacute sclerosing panencephalitis is a chronic CNS infection from the virus that causes measles and still occurs in individuals from countries where measles infections are common. It typically occurs in children but can occur in adults [113]. Patients develop progressive dementia, seizures (focal or generalized), myoclonus, ataxia, rigidity, and visual disturbances. In the late stage of the illness, patients are unresponsive, with spastic quadriparesis, brisk deep tendon reflexes, and positive Babinski's signs. EEG often reveals periodic slow-wave complexes with associated sharp waves every 3 to 10 seconds that often are associated temporally with myoclonus. Definitive diagnosis is made with elevated antibody titers to the measles virus in the blood and CSF in the appropriate clinical setting [114].

Whipple's disease is a rare bacterial (*Tropheryma whippelii*) infection, involving many organ systems, that can present as a neuropsychiatric syndrome that, although typically insidious, can progress rapidly over months. More than 80% of the cases have been diagnosed in men. Although the age range varies from childhood to the elderly, onset typically is in the fifth through seventh decades, with an approximate mean age of onset of 50. Clinical presentation is varied. It most commonly presents as a malabsorption syndrome with diarrhea, abdominal pain, weight loss, arthralgias, wasting, fever, and lymphadenopathy; but as many as 15% of cases do not exhibit gastrointestinal symptoms. CNS involvement occurs in 5% to 45% of cases, with 5% of cases having neurologic presenting symptoms [115]. Dementia or mental status changes occur in more than 50% of the cases with neurologic involvement [115,116]. Cognitive impairment occurs in 71% and psychiatric signs in 44% of cases of CNS Whipple's [117]. Eye movement abnormalities, myoclonus or other abnormal involuntary movements, headache, and abnormal hypothalamic function frequently are seen. Seizures, aseptic meningitis, ataxia, and focal cerebral signs may occur [46,77,115–117]. Ataxia has been reported to occur in 45% of CNS Whipple's cases [118]. Approximately 10% of cases have a triad of dementia, ophthalmoplegia, and myoclonus, which is highly suggestive of this condition [115], Oculomasticatory myorrythymia is uncommon but pathognomic [46,118]. Clinically, Whipple's may be mistaken for CBD or PSP [35]. Brain imaging is nonspecific. CSF shows elevated protein or pleiocytosis in approximately half of cases with CNS involvement. Diagnosis is made by identification of PAS-positive inclusions or *T whipellii* in foamy macrophages on jejunal biopsy or by *T whipellii* PCR of CSF or jejunal biopsy. PCR in serum probably is less sensitive. Diagnosis can be challenging, as many of the symptoms are nonspecific, and is particularly difficult when Whipple's presents as an isolated neurologic syndrome without gastrointestinal symptoms [115]. Although rare, Whipple's is important to recognize, as it is readily treatable with antibiotics [115,117,119,120].

Malignancies causing rapidly progressive dementia

Several primary and secondary malignancies can cause an acute or subacute RPD. RPDs that can be identified readily by MRI are not discussed in detail in this article, as once identified, the work-up is somewhat routine. Three malignancies that often present as RPDs and present with varied abnormalities on MRI are PCNSL, intravascular lymphoma (ie, angiotropic lymphoma), and lymphomatoid granulomatosis (also known as angiocentric immunoproliferative lesions). Only the first two are discussed in this article.

PCNSL is an extranodal form of non-Hodgkin's lymphoma. It typically presents with symptoms of intracranial mass lesions, such as headaches, seizures, and focal neurologic deficits, but can present as a RPD [121]. A diffusely infiltrating PCNSL, sometimes called lymphomatosis cerebri, also occurs [122]. Symptoms of PCNSL include personality changes, irritability, memory loss, lethargy, confusion, disorientation, psychosis, dysphasia, ataxia, gait disorder, and myoclonus [121–124]. CNS lymphoma can mimic CJD [5,96,125]. PCNSL accounts for 2% to 3% of all CNS neoplasms. The vast majority of PCNSLs are non-Hodgkin's diffuse large B-cell type, but T-cell, Burkitt's lymphoma, and poorly characterized forms also occur [121,126]. The incidence increased from the mid-1970s to the mid-1980s because of an escalating number of immunocompromised patients from transplants, chemotherapy, and patients who had HIV before the era of HAART but seems to have stabilized during the past decade [126]. This article focuses on PCNSL in immunocompetent individuals. PCNSL occurs most commonly in the sixth to seventh decades but can occur at any age, with a slight male predominance [123]. Uveitis or vitreitisis present in approximately 10% of cases, sometimes preceding the tumor by months, in approximately 75% of cases; identifying the uveitis or vitreitis may allow earlier diagnosis of the cancer [127]. In immunocompetent individuals, brain MRI may show isointense to mildly hyperintense T2-weighted signal consistent with mass lesions with minimal to moderate edema, often involving the cerebral hemispheres, basal ganglia, periventricular white matter, or corpus callosum. Lesions may be isolated or multiple and generally show contrast enhancement [128]. When presenting as lymphomatosis cerebri, imaging reveals progressive, diffuse white matter signal abnormality without significant (or any) enhancement or mass effect—likely from a diffusely infiltrative process without interruption of the blood-brain barrier [122,123]. CSF can show a lymphocytosis, increased protein, and low glucose. Serial CSF cytologic evaluations typically are required to identify the lymphoma [126]. EEG may show symmetric or asymmetric nonspecific diffuse slowing [122,123]. Unfortunately, definitive diagnosis often requires brain biopsy. In cases of ocular involvement, diagnosis sometimes can be made by vitrectomy. When possible, avoid giving corticosteroids before biopsy, as steroids can cause tumor cell necrosis, resulting in temporary shrinkage of the tumor but preventing tissue diagnosis [96,126]. Prognosis is poor with patients surviving only a median of 4 months or fewer without treatment and 12 to 18 months with whole-brain radiation therapy (WBRT) alone; however, survival is upwards of 40 or more months with a combination of aggressive chemo- and radiotherapy. Chemotherapy includes high-dose systemic methotrexate. The use of chemotherapy alone versus chemotherapy plus WBRT is controversial. Because of the increased risk of neurotoxicity, WBRT in patients over 60 is not recommended. Neurotoxicity presents as a RPD with dementia, ataxia, and incontinence, with median onset just over 1 year post WBRT [126,129].

Intravascular lymphoma can occur in almost any organ but commonly has one of four presentations: CNS, skin, reticuloendothelial, or fever of unknown origin. It is caused by the proliferation of clonal lymphocytes within blood vessels, with relative sparing of parenchyma [130]. The more acute form of CNS intravascular lymphoma typically presents in middle age as an acute or subacute dementia, often with transient ischemic attacks or strokes. Systemic symptoms (eg, fever and weight loss) may be present. The tumor cells are believed to be activated or transformed lymphocytes and typically are an angiotropic large B-cell lymphoma, although cell-type forms also occur. These clonal lymphocytes preferentially bind endothelium. Imaging in CNS intravascular lymphoma is variable. MRI may show multiple areas of T2-weighted hyperintensity with patchy enhancement on T1 weighting, with or without edema [131]. Unfortunately, most cases reported in the literature were diagnosed post mortem; therefore, a high index of suspicion, and a low threshold for brain biopsy, is required for patients who have a RPD and focal T2-weighted abnormalities on MRI [99,127,132]. Laboratory findings can include elevated ESR, serum lactate dehydrogenase, CSF pleiocytosis, and increased protein [132,133]. Survival in intravascular lymphoma usually is poor, especially without treatment. Aggressive treatment is needed for PCNSL and intravascular lymphoma. The combination of chemo- and radiotherapy is better than radiotherapy alone [127,130,132].

At the authors' center, several patients referred with potential CJD were determined to have encephalopathy resulting from metastatic cancers, including lymphoma. A recently published case of a 79-year-old woman who had a RPD presenting with early visual hallucinations, followed by severe memory impairment, and extrapyramidal signs was believed to be CJD because of her course and a positive 14-3-3. Unfortunately, the diagnosis of miliary adenocarcinoma was only made at autopsy [134].

Toxic-metabolic conditions

Metabolic causes of RPD include vitamin deficiences, endocrinologic disturbances, and adult presentations of inborn errors of metabolism. Vitamin deficiencies can result in significant neurologic deficits, including cognitive impairment. Pellagra ("rough skin") results from niacin deficiency and classically is described by the three Ds: *d*ermatitis, *d*iarrhea, and *d*ementia (on a historical note, the original term, nicotinic acid, was changed to niacin because of its confusion with nicotine). Niacin deficiency causes abnormalities of the skin and gastrointestinal tract, peripheral neuropathy, myelopathy, and cognitive dysfunction. With a careful history, the dementia of pellagra typically is found to be insidious, not rapid. In industrialized nations, niacin deficiency should be considered in patients who have nutritional deficiency, such as alcoholics and patients who have anorexia nervosa, and in those taking isoniazid [135–138]. Although diagnosis can be made by finding nicotinic acid metabolites in the urine, given the ease of treatment with niacin (40 to 250 mg per day), diagnosis usually is based on clinical suspicion. Treatment often results in rapid resolution of symptoms [135,139]. Deficiency of thiamine (vitamin B_1), a necessary cofactor in oxidative metabolism, can cause Wernicke's encephalopathy, which presents classically as a triad of ophthalmoparesis (with vertical or horizontal nystagmus), ataxia, and memory loss. DWI MRI can show diffusion abnormalities in mammilary bodies and dorsomedial nucleus of the thalamus, areas in which hemorrhagic necrosis is found pathologically. The thalamic involvement on DWI MRI can appear similar to that seen in CJD [40,140–142]. All patients who have dementia should be screened for vitamin B_{12} deficiency, as potentially it is reversible.

Adult presentations of metabolic disorders that typically afflict children in rare instances also can present as dementia in adults. These dementias usually are associated with a constellation of symptoms, such as weakness, spasticity, and ataxia, and tend to be more slowly progressive. They can present with rapid cognitive decline. In the proper clinical context of gastrointestinal disturbance, fluctuating course, an unexplained pain syndrome, or worsening after use of new medicines, porphyria should be ruled out. Adult-onset metachromatic leukodystrophy presented as a RPD in a woman who developed psychiatric symptoms and severe cognitive decline over 18 months with no weakness or ataxia [143]. Other leukodystrophies also can present as RPD. Orthochromatic leukodystrophies are a heterogeneous group of metabolic disorders in which the specific enzymatic defects have not been found. Most are sporadic, but dominant inheritance is reported. One report describes two family members (57 and 38 at presentation) who had a dominantly inherited orthochromatic leukodystrophy and developed rapid dementia progressing to death over 2 to 3 years [144]. Finally, Kufs' disease, the rare adult form of neuronal ceroid lipofuscinoses, can present as RPD. Kufs' is an autosomal recessive lysosomal storage disease in which acid phosphatase-staining ceroid and lipofuscins accumulate in neurons, causing a progressive encephalopathy. Kufs' disease typically presents in early adulthood. Patients who have type A Kufs' disease present with a progressive myoclonic epilepsy, whereas those who have type B present with dementia, which often begins with psychosis. A case reported in 1997 involved a 49-year-old woman who presented initially with alternating catatonia and acute psychosis over 5 months before the development of dementia over the next 2 months. Diagnosis was made by acid phosphatase staining of brain and skin biopsies [145]. The authors recently diagnosed a 50-year-old woman who had a methylmalonic (and malonic) academia who had developed significant cognitive impairment after a several months prodrome of gastrointestinal disturbance and psychiatric disturbance. She had low normal vitamin B_{12} levels and normal homocysteine. Despite thorough evaluation of her vitamin B_{12} pathways, the cause of her metabolic disorder still is unknown (M. Geschwind, MD, PhD, unpublished data, 2007).

Several toxins can cause RPD. Exposure to heavy metals, such as arsenic, mercury, aluminum, lithium, or lead, can lead to cognitive decline, particularly after acute exposure. Most cases of acute exposures result in florid encephalopathies that progress over hours to days and thus would not be confused with RPDs, which progress over weeks to months. Manganese toxicity, found usually in miners, can present with significant parkinsonism [138].

Bismuth is a metal used to treat gastrointestinal disorders, principally peptic ulcer disease and diarrhea. Bismuth intoxication, typically caused by overdosing on bismuth-containing products, such as Pepto-Bismol, can cause a disorder mimicking CJD. Patients initially manifest with apathy, mild ataxia, and headaches, which progress to myoclonus, dysarthria, severe confusion, hallucinations (auditory and visual), seizures, and, in severe cases, even death [146–149]. Blood levels of bismuth, greater than 50 μg/L, are considered in the toxic range [147,149] . The condition usually is reversible; however, extremely prolonged use can result in permanent tremors [146,147]. A careful history may be needed to make the diagnosis.

Nonorganic (psychiatric) causes of rapidly progressive dementia

Psychologic processes sometimes can mimic RPD, although it is essential to rule out a neurologic cause in these cases. Pseudodementia, resulting from depression, occurs in patients who have a past history of major depression. There usually are signs that patients are severely depressed, and cognitive dysfunction, particularly on testing, is found to be the result of decreased effort. Many of the features of patients who have true dementia are seen in atypical psychiatric disorders, including personality disorders, conversion disorders, psychosis, and malingerers [150], and a full assessment is required to rule out potentially treatable or organic disorders. These cases can have many of the features of a true dementia. Furthermore, psychiatric features may be an early symptom of many neurodegenerative conditions, including CJD, DLB, CBD, and others [12].

Summary

Although the evaluation of patients who have RPD may seem daunting, it can be facilitated greatly through a structured approach. Common things being common, most cases of RPD in elderly persons probably are the result of urinary infection or pneumonia causing a delirium. When simple causes are ruled out, however, it is helpful to consider various categories of potential etiologies and rule out each category systematically. As many tests may be necessary, an inpatient evaluation can expedite the process. The authors often find that a body CT with and without contrast is of assistance in diagnosing many difficult cases, helping to identify such conditions as sarcoid, malignancies, and paraneoplastic conditions. Unfortunately, in many cases, a standard laboratory evaluation is not sufficient and brain biopsy may be necessary. If prion disease is in the differential, prion precautions must be used in the operating room and when handling brain tissue.

References

[1] Korth C, Peters PJ. Emerging pharmacotherapies for Creutzfeldt-Jakob disease. Arch Neurol 2006;63(4):497–501.

[2] Korth C, May BCH, Cohen FE, et al. Acridine and phenothiazine derivatives as pharmacoptherapeutics for prion disease. Proc Natl Acad Sci U S A 2001;98(17):9836–41.

[3] Greicius MD, Geschwind MD, Miller BL. Presenile dementia syndromes: an update on taxonomy and diagnosis. J Neurol Neurosurg Psychiatry 2002;72(6):691–700.

[4] Tschampa HJ, Neumann M, Zerr I, et al. Patients with Alzheimer's disease and dementia with Lewy bodies mistaken for Creutzfeldt-Jakob disease. J Neurol Neurosurg Psychiatry 2001;71(1):33–9.

[5] Poser S, Mollenhauer B, Kraubeta A, et al. How to improve the clinical diagnosis of Creutzfeldt-Jakob disease. Brain 1999;122(Pt 12):2345–51.

[6] Olichney JM, Galasko D, Salmon DP, et al. Cognitive decline is faster in Lewy body variant than in Alzheimer's disease. Neurology 1998;51(2):351–7.

[7] WHO. Global surveillance, diagnosis and therapy of human transmissible spongiform encephalopathies: report of a WHO consultation. Paper Presented at the World Health Organization: Emerging and other communicable diseases, surveillance and control. Geneva (Switzerland), February 9–11, 1998.

[8] Masters CL, Harris JO, Gajdusek DC, et al. Creutzfeldt-Jakob disease: patterns of worldwide occurrence and the significance of familial and sporadic clustering. Ann Neurol 1979; 5(2):177–88.

[9] Geschwind MD, Martindale J, Miller D, et al. Challenging the clinical utility of the 14-3-3 protein for the diagnosis of sporadic Creutzfeldt-Jakob disease. Arch Neurol 2003;60(6): 813–6.

[10] Chapman T, McKeel DW Jr, Morris JC. Misleading results with the 14-3-3 assay for the diagnosis of Creutzfeldt-Jakob disease. Neurology 2000;55(9):1396–7.

[11] Huang N, Marie SK, Livramento JA, et al. 14-3-3 protein in the CSF of patients with rapidly progressive dementia. Neurology 2003;61(3):354–7.

[12] Rabinovici GD, Wang PN, Levin J, et al. First symptom in sporadic Creutzfeldt-Jakob disease. Neurology 2006;66(2):286–7.

[13] Geschwind MD, Haman A, Torres-Chae C, et al. Astract P03.135. CSF findings in a large United States sporadic CJD cohort. Neurology 2007;68(Suppl 1):A142.

[14] Safar J, Wille H, Itri V, et al. Eight prion strains have PrP(Sc) molecules with different conformations. Nat Med 1998;4(10):1157–65.
[15] Safar JG, Geschwind MD, Deering C, et al. Diagnosis of human prion disease. Proc Natl Acad Sci U S A 2005;102(9):3501–6.
[16] Safar JG, Wille H, Geschwind MD, et al. Human prions and plasma lipoproteins. Proc Natl Acad Sci U S A 2006;103:11312–7.
[17] Lopez O, Claassen D, Boller F. Alzheimer's disease, cerebral amyloid angiopathy, and dementia of acute onset. Aging (Milano) 1991;3(2):171–5.
[18] Barcikowska M, Mirecka B, Papierz W, et al. A case of Alzheimer's disease simulating Creutzfeldt-Jakob disease [Polish]. Neurol Neurochir Pol 1992;26(5):703–10.
[19] Caselli RJ, Couce ME, Osborne D, et al. From slowly progressive amnesic syndrome to rapidly progressive Alzheimer disease. Alzheimer Dis Assoc Disord 1998;12(3):251–3.
[20] Roberson ED, Hesse JH, Rose KD, et al. Frontotemporal dementia progresses to death faster than Alzheimer disease. Neurology 2005;65(5):719–25.
[21] Litvan I, Mangone CA, McKee A, et al. Natural history of progressive supranuclear palsy (Steele-Richardson-Olszewski syndrome) and clinical predictors of survival: a clinicopathological study. J Neurol Neurosurg Psychiatry 1996;60(6):615–20.
[22] Caine D, Patterson K, Hodges JR, et al. Severe anterograde amnesia with extensive hippocampal degeneration in a case of rapidly progressive frontotemporal dementia. Neurocase 2001;7(1):57–64.
[23] Kleiner-Fisman G, Lang AE, Bergeron C, et al. Rapidly progressive behavioral changes and parkinsonism in a 68-year-old man. Mov Disord 2004;19(5):534–43.
[24] Hodges JR, Davies R, Xuereb J, et al. Survival in frontotemporal dementia. Neurology 2003;61(3):349–54.
[25] Catani M, Piccirilli M, Geloso MC, et al. Rapidly progressive aphasic dementia with motor neuron disease: a distinctive clinical entity. Dement Geriatr Cogn Disord 2004;17(1–2):21–8.
[26] Haik S, Brandel JP, Sazdovitch V, et al. Dementia with Lewy bodies in a neuropathologic series of suspected Creutzfeldt-Jakob disease. Neurology 2000;55(9):1401–4.
[27] McKeith IG, Galasko D, Kosaka K, et al. Consensus guidelines for the clinical and pathologic diagnosis of dementia with Lewy bodies (DLB): report of the consortium on DLB international workshop. Neurology 1996;47(5):1113–24.
[28] Walker Z, Allen R, Shergill S, et al. Three years survival in patients with a clinical diagnosis of dementia with Lewy bodies. Int J Geriatr Psychiatry 2000;15(3):267–73.
[29] Byrne EJ, Lennox G, Lowe J, et al. Diffuse Lewy body disease: clinical features in 15 cases. J Neurol Neurosurg Psychiatry 1989;52:709–17.
[30] Mitsuyama Y. Presenile dementia with motor neuron disease. Dementia 1993;4(3–4):137–42.
[31] Nasreddine ZS, Loginov M, Clark LN, et al. From genotype to phenotype: a clinical pathological, and biochemical investigation of frontotemporal dementia and parkinsonism (FTDP-17) caused by the P301L tau mutation. Ann Neurol 1999;45(6):704–15.
[32] Levy ML, Miller BL, Cummings JL, et al. Alzheimer disease and frontotemporal dementias. Behavioral distinctions. Arch Neurol 1996;53(7):687–90.
[33] Rosen HJ, Lengenfelder J, Miller B. Frontotemporal dementia. Neurol Clin 2000;18(4):979–92.
[34] Schneider JA, Watts RL, Gearing M, et al. Corticobasal degeneration: neuropathologic and clinical heterogeneity. Neurology 1997;48(4):959–69.
[35] Litvan I, Agid Y, Goetz C, et al. Accuracy of the clinical diagnosis of corticobasal degeneration: a clinicopathologic study. Neurology 1997;48(1):119–25.
[36] Gimenez-Roldan S, Mateo D, Benito C, et al. Progressive supranuclear palsy and corticobasal ganglionic degeneration: differentiation by clinical features and neuroimaging techniques. J Neural Transm Suppl 1994;42:79–90.

[37] Mathuranath PS, Xuereb JH, Bak T, et al. Corticobasal ganglionic degeneration and/or frontotemporal dementia? A report of two overlap cases and review of literature. J Neurol Neurosurg Psychiatry 2000;68(3):304–12.
[38] Kertesz A, Martinez-Lage P, Davidson W, et al. The corticobasal degeneration syndrome overlaps progressive aphasia and frontotemporal dementia. Neurology 2000;55(9): 1368–75.
[39] Avanzino L, Marinelli L, Buccolieri A, et al. Creutzfeldt-Jakob disease presenting as corticobasal degeneration: a neurophysiological study. Neurol Sci 2006;27(2):118–21.
[40] Young GS, Geschwind MD, Fischbein NJ, et al. Diffusion-weighted and fluid-attenuated inversion recovery imaging in Creutzfeldt-Jakob disease: high sensitivity and specificity for diagnosis. AJNR Am J Neuroradiol 2005;26(6):1551–62.
[41] Grafman J, Litvan I, Stark M. Neuropsychological features of progressive supranuclear palsy. Brain Cogn 1995;28(3):311–20.
[42] Litvan I, Agid Y, Calne D, et al. Clinical research criteria for the diagnosis of progressive supranuclear palsy (Steele-Richardson-Olszewski syndrome): report of the NINDS-SPSP international workshop. Neurology 1996;47(1):1–9.
[43] Litvan I, Agid Y, Jankovic J, et al. Accuracy of clinical criteria for the diagnosis of progressive supranuclear palsy (Steele-Richardson-Olszewski syndrome). Neurology 1996;46(4): 922–30.
[44] Litvan I, Mega MS, Cummings JL, et al. Neuropsychiatric aspects of progressive supranuclear palsy. Neurology 1996;47(5):1184–9.
[45] Yagishita A, Oda M. Progressive supranuclear palsy: MRI and pathological findings. Neuroradiology 1996;38(Suppl 1):S60–6.
[46] Leigh RJ, Zee DS. The neurology of eye movements. 3rd edition. New York: Oxford University Press; 1999.
[47] Josephs KA, Tsuboi Y, Dickson DW. Creutzfeldt-Jakob disease presenting as progressive supranuclear palsy. Eur J Neurol 2004;11(5):343–6.
[48] Josephs KA, Holton JL, Rossor MN, et al. Neurofilament inclusion body disease: a new proteinopathy? Brain 2003;126(Pt 10):2291–303.
[49] Mackenzie IR, Feldman H. Neurofilament inclusion body disease with early onset frontotemporal dementia and primary lateral sclerosis. Clin Neuropathol 2004;23(4): 183–93.
[50] Benke T, Karner E, Seppi K, et al. Subacute dementia and imaging correlates in a case of Fahr's disease. J Neurol Neurosurg Psychiatry 2004;75(8):1163–5.
[51] Mothersead P, Conrad K, Hagerman R, et al. An atypical progressive dementia in a male carrier of the fragile X premutation: an example of fragile X-associated Tremor/Ataxia syndrome. Appl Neuropsychol 2005;12(3):169–78.
[52] Dropcho EJ. Paraneoplastic diseases of the nervous system. Curr Treat Options Neurol 1999;1(5):417–27.
[53] Gultekin SH, Rosenfeld MR, Voltz R, et al. Paraneoplastic limbic encephalitis: neurological symptoms, immunological findings and tumour association in 50 patients. Brain 2000; 123(Pt 7):1481–94.
[54] Ances BM, Vitaliani R, Taylor RA, et al. Treatment-responsive limbic encephalitis identified by neuropil antibodies: MRI and PET correlates. Brain 2005;128(Pt 8):1764–77.
[55] Rosenfeld MR, Eichen JG, Wade DF, et al. Molecular and clinical diversity in paraneoplastic immunity to Ma proteins. Ann Neurol 2001;50(3):339–48.
[56] Dalmau J, Graus F, Villarejo A, et al. Clinical analysis of anti-Ma2-associated encephalitis. Brain 2004;127(Pt 8):1831–44.
[57] Pittock SJ, Kryzer TJ, Lennon VA. Paraneoplastic antibodies coexist and predict cancer, not neurological syndrome. Ann Neurol 2004;56(5):715–9.
[58] Vernino S, Tuite P, Adler CH, et al. Paraneoplastic chorea associated with CRMP-5 neuronal antibody and lung carcinoma. Ann Neurol 2002;51(5):625–30.

[59] Burton GV, Bullard DE, Walther PJ, et al. Paraneoplastic limbic encephalopathy with testicular carcinoma. A reversible neurologic syndrome. Cancer 1988;62(10):2248–51.
[60] Mathew RM, Vandenberghe R, Garcia-Merino A, et al. Orchiectomy for suspected microscopic tumor in patients with anti-Ma2-associated encephalitis. Neurology 2007;68(12): 900–5.
[61] Yu Z, Kryzer TJ, Griesmann GE, et al. CRMP-5 neuronal autoantibody: marker of lung cancer and thymoma-related autoimmunity. Ann Neurol 2001;49(2):146–54.
[62] Honnorat J, Antoine JC, Belin MF. Are the "newly discovered" paraneoplastic anticollapsin response-mediator protein 5 antibodies simply anti-CV2 antibodies? Ann Neurol 2001; 50(5):688–91.
[63] Antoine JC, Honnorat J, Anterion CT, et al. Limbic encephalitis and immunological perturbations in two patients with thymoma. J Neurol Neurosurg Psychiatry 1995;58(6): 706–10.
[64] Vernino S, Geschwind MD, Boeve B. Autoimmune encephalopathies. Neurologist 2007; 13(3):140–7.
[65] Buckley C, Oger J, Clover L, et al. Potassium channel antibodies in two patients with reversible limbic encephalitis. Ann Neurol 2001;50(1):73–8.
[66] Pozo-Rosich P, Clover L, Saiz A, et al. Voltage-gated potassium channel antibodies in limbic encephalitis. Ann Neurol 2003;54(4):530–3.
[67] Thieben MJ, Lennon VA, Boeve BF, et al. Potentially reversible autoimmune limbic encephalitis with neuronal potassium channel antibody. Neurology 2004;62(7):1177–82.
[68] Vincent A, Buckley C, Schott JM, et al. Potassium channel antibody-associated encephalopathy: a potentially immunotherapy-responsive form of limbic encephalitis. Brain 2004;127(Pt 3):701–12.
[69] Bataller L, Kleopa KA, Wu GF, et al. Autoimmune limbic encephalitis in 39 patients: immunophenotypes and outcomes. J Neurol Neurosurg Psychiatry 2007;78(4):381–5.
[70] Liguori R, Vincent A, Clover L, et al. Morvan's syndrome: peripheral and central nervous system and cardiac involvement with antibodies to voltage-gated potassium channels. Brain 2001;124(Pt 12):2417–26.
[71] Chang CC, Eggers SD, Johnson JK, et al. Anti-GAD antibody cerebellar ataxia mimicking Creutzfeldt-Jakob disease. Clin Neurol Neurosurg 2007;109:54–7.
[72] Kothbauer-Margreiter I, Sturzenegger M, Komor J, et al. Encephalopathy associated with Hashimoto thyroiditis: diagnosis and treatment. J Neurol 1996;243(8):585–93.
[73] Ghika-Schmid F, Ghika J, Regli F, et al. Hashimoto's myoclonic encephalopathy: an underdiagnosed treatable condition? Mov Disord 1996;11(5):555–62.
[74] Seipelt M, Zerr I, Nau R, et al. Hashimoto's encephalitis as a differential diagnosis of Creutzfeldt- Jakob disease. J Neurol Neurosurg Psychiatry 1999;66(2):172–6.
[75] Henchey R, Cibula J, Helveston W, et al. Electroencephalographic findings in Hashimoto's encephalopathy. Neurology 1995;45(5):977–81.
[76] Bohnen NI, Parnell KJ, Harper CM. Reversible MRI findings in a patient with Hashimoto's encephalopathy. Neurology 1997;49(1):246–7.
[77] Schwartz MA, Selhorst JB, Ochs AL, et al. Oculomasticatory myorhythmia: a unique movement disorder occurring in Whipple's disease. Ann Neurol 1986;20(6):677–83.
[78] McCabe DJ, Burke T, Connolly S, et al. Amnesic syndrome with bilateral mesial temporal lobe involvement in Hashimoto's encephalopathy. Neurology 2000;54(3):737–9.
[79] Shein M, Apter A, Dickerman Z, et al. Encephalopathy in compensated Hashimoto thyroiditis: a clinical expression of autoimmune cerebral vasculitis. Brain Dev 1986; 8(1):60–4.
[80] Peschen-Rosin R, Schabet M, Dichgans J. Manifestation of Hashimoto's encephalopathy years before onset of thyroid disease. Eur Neurol 1999;41(2):79–84.
[81] Nieuwenhuis L, Santens P, Vanwalleghem P, et al. Subacute Hashimoto's encephalopathy, treated with plasmapheresis. Acta Neurol Belg 2004;104(2):80–3.

[82] Harkness KA, Coles A, Pohl U, et al. Rapidly reversible dementia in cerebral amyloid inflammatory vasculopathy. Eur J Neurol 2004;11(1):59–62.
[83] Moore PM, Richardson B. Neurology of the vasculitides and connective tissue diseases. J Neurol Neurosurg Psychiatry 1998;65(1):10–22.
[84] Younger DS, Hays AP, Brust JC, et al. Granulomatous angiitis of the brain. An inflammatory reaction of diverse etiology. Arch Neurol 1988;45(5):514–8.
[85] Younger DS, Kass RM. Vasculitis and the nervous system. Historical perspective and overview. Neurol Clin 1997;15(4):737–58.
[86] Ferro JM. Vasculitis of the central nervous system. J Neurol 1998;245(12):766–76.
[87] Yazici H, Yurdakul S, Hamuryudan V. Behcet disease. Curr Opin Rheumatol 2001;13(1): 18–22.
[88] Briani C, Baracchini C, Zanette G, et al. Rapidly progressive dementia in hypereosinophilic syndrome. Eur J Neurol 2001;8(3):279–80.
[89] Bruzelius M, Liedholm L, Hellblom M. Celiac disease can be associated with severe neurological symptoms. Analysis of gliadin antibodies should be considered in suspected cases[Swedish]. Lakartidningen 2001;98(34):3538–42.
[90] Caselli RJ, Boeve BF, Scheithauer BW, et al. Nonvasculitic autoimmune inflammatory meningoencephalitis (NAIM): a reversible form of encephalopathy. Neurology 1999;53(7): 1579–81.
[91] Schielke E, Nolte C, Muller W, et al. Sarcoidosis presenting as rapidly progressive dementia: clinical and neuropathological evaluation. J Neurol 2001;248(6):522–4.
[92] Rabinstein AA, Romano JG, Forteza AM, et al. Rapidly progressive dementia due to bilateral internal carotid artery occlusion with infarction of the total length of the corpus callosum. J Neuroimaging 2004;14(2):176–9.
[93] Auchus AP, Chen CP, Sodagar SN, et al. Single stroke dementia: insights from 12 cases in Singapore. J Neurol Sci 2002;203–4:85–9.
[94] Hunder GG, Arend WP, Bloch DA, et al. The American College of Rheumatology 1990 criteria for the classification of vasculitis. Introduction. Arthritis Rheum 1990;33(8): 1065–7.
[95] American College of Rheumatology. Bibliography of criteria, guidelines, and health status assessments used in rheumatology. American College of Rheumatology. Available at: http://rheumatology.org/publications/abbreviations/. Accessed October 10, 2005.
[96] Josephson SA, Papanastassiou AM, Berger MS, et al. The diagnostic utility of brain biopsy procedures in patients with rapidly deteriorating neurological conditions or dementia. J Neurosurg 2007;106(1):72–5.
[97] Wynne PJ, Younger DS, Khandji A, et al. Radiographic features of central nervous system vasculitis. Neurol Clin 1997;15(4):779–804.
[98] Heinrich A, Vogelgesang S, Kirsch M, et al. Intravascular lymphomatosis presenting as rapidly progressive dementia. Eur Neurol 2005;54(1):55–8.
[99] Menendez Calderon MJ, Segui Riesco ME, Arguelles M, et al. Intravascular lymphomatosis. A report of three cases [Spanish]. An Med Interna 2005;22(1):31–4.
[100] Brew BJ. AIDS dementia complex. Neurol Clin 1999;17(4):861–81.
[101] Wallace MR, Nelson JA, McCutchan JA, et al. Symptomatic HIV seroconverting illness is associated with more rapid neurological impairment. Sex Transm Infect 2001;77(3): 199–201.
[102] Nath A, Maragos WF, Avison MJ, et al. Acceleration of HIV dementia with methamphetamine and cocaine. J Neurovirol 2001;7(1):66–71.
[103] Navia BA, Price RW. The acquired immunodeficiency syndrome: dementia as the presenting sole manifestation of human immunodeficiency virus infection. Arch Neurol 1987;44: 65–9.
[104] Ala TA, Doss RC, Sullivan CJ. Reversible dementia: a case of cryptococcal meningitis masquerading as Alzheimer's disease. J Alzheimers Dis 2004;6(5):503–8.

[105] Heckman GA, Hawkins C, Morris A, et al. Rapidly progressive dementia due to Mycobacterium neoaurum meningoencephalitis. Emerg Infect Dis 2004;10(5):924–7.
[106] Glaser CA, Honarmand S, Anderson LJ, et al. Beyond viruses: clinical profiles and etiologies associated with encephalitis. Clin Infect Dis 2006;43(12):1565–77.
[107] Timmermans M, Carr J. Neurosyphilis in the modern era. J Neurol Neurosurg Psychiatry 2004;75(12):1727–30.
[108] Fox PA, Hawkins DA, Dawson S. Dementia following an acute presentation of meningovascular neurosyphilis in an HIV-1 positive patient. AIDS 2000;14(13):2062–3.
[109] Kaplan RF, Jones-Woodward L. Lyme encephalopathy: a neuropsychological perspective. Semin Neurol 1997;17(1):31–7.
[110] Waniek C, Prohovnik I, Kaufman MA, et al. Rapidly progressive frontal-type dementia associated with Lyme disease. J Neuropsychiatry Clin Neurosci 1995;7(3):345–7.
[111] Andersson C, Nyberg C, Nyman D. Rapid development of dementia of an elderly person, diagnosis and successful treatment [Finnish]. Duodecim 2004;120(15):1893–6.
[112] Wormser G, Dattwyler R, Nowakowski J, et al. Diagnosis and treatment of Lyme disease in the United States. Resid Staff Physician April, 2001;15–25.
[113] Kouyoumdjian JA. Subacute sclerosing panencephalitis in an adult: report of a case [Portuguese]. Arq Neuropsiquiatr 1985;43(3):312–5.
[114] Espay AJ, Lang AE. Infectious etiologies of movement disorders. In: Roos KL, editor. Principles of Neurologic Infectious Diseases. New York: McGraw-HilL; 2005. p. 383–408.
[115] Anderson M. Neurology of Whipple's disease. J Neurol Neurosurg Psychiatry 2000;68(1): 2–5.
[116] Durand DV, Lecomte C, Cathebras P, et al. Whipple disease. Clinical review of 52 cases. The SNFMI Research Group on Whipple disease. Societe Nationale Francaise de Medecine Interne. Medicine (Baltimore) 1997;76(3):170–84.
[117] Louis ED, Lynch T, Kaufmann P, et al. Diagnostic guidelines in central nervous system Whipple's disease. Ann Neurol 1996;40(4):561–8.
[118] Matthews BR, Jones LK, Saad DA, et al. Cerebellar ataxia and central nervous system whipple disease. Arch Neurol 2005;62(4):618–20.
[119] Singer R. Diagnosis and treatment of Whipple's disease. Drugs 1998;55(5):699–704.
[120] Ramzan NN, Loftus E Jr, Burgart LJ, et al. Diagnosis and monitoring of Whipple disease by polymerase chain reaction. Ann Intern Med 1997;126(7):520–7.
[121] Bataille B, Delwail V, Menet E, et al. Primary intracerebral malignant lymphoma: report of 248 cases. J Neurosurg 2000;92(2):261–6.
[122] Bakshi R, Mazziotta JC, Mischel PS, et al. Lymphomatosis cerebri presenting as a rapidly progressive dementia: clinical, neuroimaging and pathologic findings. Dement Geriatr Cogn Disord 1999;10(2):152–7.
[123] Carlson BA. Rapidly progressive dementia caused by nonenhancing primary lymphoma of the central nervous system. AJNR Am J Neuroradiol 1996;17(9):1695–7.
[124] Rollins KE, Kleinschmidt-DeMasters BK, Corboy JR, et al. Lymphomatosis cerebri as a cause of white matter dementia. Hum Pathol 2005;36(3):282–90.
[125] Haman A, DeArmond S, Johnson JK, et al. When CJD is not CJD. Paper Presented at the 131st Annual Meeting of the American Neurological Association. Chicago (IL), October 8–11, 2006.
[126] Batchelor T, Loeffler JS. Primary CNS lymphoma. J Clin Oncol 2006;24(8):1281–8.
[127] Fetell MR. Lymphomas. In: Rowland L, editor. Merrit's textbook of neurology. 9th edition. Baltimore (MD): Williams & Wilkins; 1995. p. 351–9.
[128] Kuker W, Nagele T, Korfel A, et al. Primary central nervous system lymphomas (PCNSL): MRI features at presentation in 100 patients. J Neurooncol 2005;72(2): 169–77.
[129] Abrey LE, DeAngelis LM, Yahalom J. Long-term survival in primary CNS lymphoma. J Clin Oncol 1998;16(3):859–63.

[130] Zuckerman D, Seliem R, Hochberg E. Intravascular lymphoma: the oncologist's "great imitator". Oncologist 2006;11(5):496–502.

[131] Balmaceda CM. Lymphomas. In: Rowland LP, editor. Merritt's Neurology. 10th edition. New York: Lippincott Williams & Wilkins; 2001. p. 344–50.

[132] Vieren M, Sciot R, Robberecht W. Intravascular lymphomatosis of the brain: a diagnostic problem. Clin Neurol Neurosurg 1999;101(1):33–6.

[133] Chapin JE, Davis LE, Kornfeld M, et al. Neurologic manifestations of intravascular lymphomatosis. Acta Neurol Scand 1995;91(6):494–9.

[134] Rivas E, Sanchez-Herrero J, Alonso M, et al. Miliary brain metastases presenting as rapidly progressive dementia. Neuropathology 2005;25(2):153–8.

[135] Kinsella LJ, Riley DE. Nutritional deficiencies and syndromes associated with alcoholism. In: Goetz C, editor. Textbook of Clinical Neurology. Chapter 40, 2nd edition. St. Louis, MO: Saunders; 2003.

[136] Cummings JL, Benson DF. Dementia in vascular and infectious disorders. Dementia: a clinical approach. Boston: Butterworths; 1983. p. 125–67.

[137] Ishii N, Nishihara Y. Pellagra among chronic alcoholics: clinical and pathological study of 20 necropsy cases. J Neurol Neurosurg Psychiatry 1981;44(3):209–15.

[138] Geschwind MD, Jay C. Assessment of rapidly progressive dementias. Concise review related to chapter 362: Alzheimer's disease and other primary dementias in Harrison's Textbook of Internal Medicine. New York: McGraw Hill. Available at: http://harrisons.accessmedicine.com/. Accessed June 6, 2007.

[139] Kertesz SG. Pellagra in 2 homeless men. Mayo Clin Proc 2001;76(3):315–8.

[140] Chu K, Kang DW, Kim HJ, et al. Diffusion-weighted imaging abnormalities in wernicke encephalopathy: reversible cytotoxic edema? Arch Neurol 2002;59(1):123–7.

[141] Unlu E, Cakir B, Asil T. MRI findings of Wernicke encephalopathy revisited due to hunger strike. Eur J Radiol 2006;57(1):43–53.

[142] Halavaara J, Brander A, Lyytinen J, et al. Wernicke's encephalopathy: is diffusion-weighted MRI useful? Neuroradiology 2003;45(8):519–23.

[143] Marcao AM, Wiest R, Schindler K, et al. Adult onset metachromatic leukodystrophy without electroclinical peripheral nervous system involvement: a new mutation in the ARSA gene. Arch Neurol 2005;62(2):309–13.

[144] Letournel F, Etcharry-Bouyx F, Verny C, et al. Two clinicopathological cases of a dominantly inherited, adult onset orthochromatic leucodystrophy. J Neurol Neurosurg Psychiatry 2003;74(5):671–3.

[145] Hinkebein JH, Callahan CD. The neuropsychology of Kuf's Disease: a case of atypical early onset dementia. Arch Clin Neuropsychol 1997;12(1):81–9.

[146] Gorbach SL. Bismuth therapy in gastrointestinal diseases. Gastroenterology 1990;99(3): 863–75.

[147] Jungreis AC, Schaumburg HH. Encephalopathy from abuse of bismuth subsalicylate (Pepto-Bismol). Neurology 1993;43(6):1265.

[148] Gordon MF, Abrams RI, Rubin DB, et al. Bismuth toxicity. Neurology 1994;44(12):2418.

[149] Benet LZ. Safety and pharmacokinetics: colloidal bismuth subcitrate. Scand J Gastroenterol Suppl 1991;185:29–35.

[150] Hampel H, Berger C, Muller N. A case of Ganser's state presenting as a dementia syndrome. Psychopathology 1996;29(4):236–41.

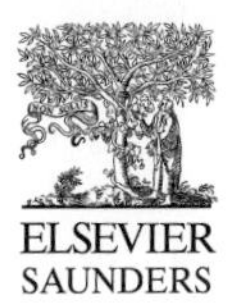

ELSEVIER
SAUNDERS

Neurol Clin 25 (2007) 809–832

NEUROLOGIC
CLINICS

Normal Pressure Hydrocephalus

Neill R. Graff-Radford, MBBCh, FRCP

Mayo Clinic Jacksonville, 4500 San Pablo Road, Jacksonville, FL 32224, USA

Epidemiology

At this time, there is no definitive information on the incidence or prevalence of normal pressure hydrocephalus (NPH). There are a few studies in the literature that address this issue. In one involving the evaluation of all elderly persons in Republic of San Marino (smallest independent country; in Italy), the researchers found that 2 of 396 persons had idiopathic NPH (INPH), a 0.5% prevalence of persons over age 65 [1]. In a door-to-door survey of parkinsonism, Trenkwalder and colleagues [2] found 4 of 982 people who had NPH, again a prevalence of 0.5%. In the 2000 United States census, there were 35 million persons ages 65 and older. Based on the two studies mentioned previously, there is an estimated prevalence of 175,000 persons who have NPH in the United States. Another way to estimate the United States prevalence is from the study by Clarfield [3], who report, in a meta-analysis of 37 dementia studies, a 1% NPH prevalence in more than 5000 dementia patients. Based on this study and the estimated 4 to 6 million persons in the United States who have dementia [4], there would be approximately 40,000 to 60,000 persons who have NPH.

Vanneste and colleagues [5] estimated the incidence in Holland to be 1.3 to 2.2 per million per year, whereas Krauss and Halve [6], in a survey of neurosurgeons, calculated NPH incidence in Germany to be 1.8 per 100,000 per year. They note that this probably is an underestimate because it is based on referrals.

Why the diagnosis is difficult

Doctors find the diagnosis and treatment of patients who have NPH particularly difficult. The reasons for this are that no combinations of the

This study was funded in part by grant P50 AG16574 and by the Robert and Clarice Smith and Abigail Van Buren Alzheimer's Disease Research Program.

This chapter is based in part on the chapter, "Normal Pressure Hydrocephalus" by Dr. Graff-Radford published in the April 2007 Dementia issue of Continuum: Lifelong Learning in Neurology (13[2]:144–164) and is used with permission from the American Academy of Neurology.

E-mail address: graffradford.neill@mayo.edu

doi:10.1016/j.ncl.2007.03.004 *neurologic.theclinics.com*

cardinal findings (gait difficulty, cognitive decline, incontinence of urine, and enlarged ventricles) are pathognomonic for the diagnosis; each of the cardinal symptoms is common in the elderly and has many causes (discussed later); all of the diagnostic tests described give false-positive and false-negative results; the surgical treatment carries significant short- and long-term risks, and the cause or pathogenesis of many NPH cases is not known.

Discussing the cardinal features:

1. Gait difficulty: one study found that 20% of persons ages 75 and older had gait abnormality and this was related to future development of dementia [7].
2. Cognitive decline: one study estimated that 4.5 million persons over age 65 had Alzheimer's disease in the United States in 2000 [4].
3. Incontinence: in 2006, Anger and colleagues [8] reported the overall prevalence of incontinence in older women as 38% and Stothers and colleagues [9] reported a prevalence of 17% in men over age 60.
4. Enlarged ventricles: Barron and colleagues [10] showed that ventricle size increases with age, and Jack and colleagues [11] have shown ventricle size increases faster in patients who have AD compared with controls.

Thus, all the cardinal features are common in the elderly and have many causes.

Differential diagnosis

When evaluating patients, keep in mind a practical differential diagnosis (Box 1), which helps focus the history and examination.

Box 1. Differential diagnosis of normal pressure hydrocephalus

- Combinations of ventriculomegaly, dementia, and factors affecting gait (eg, cervical spondylosis, large joint arthritis, peripheral neuropathy, impaired vision, vestibular dysfunction, and antipsychotics)
- Vascular dementia, including subcortical ischemic encephalopathy or Binswanger's disease
- Parkinson's disease dementia and enlarged ventricles
- Parkinsonian syndromes (Lewy body disease, corticobasal ganglionic degeneration, progressive supranuclear palsy, and multiple system atrophy) and enlarged ventricles
- Frontotemporal dementia with caudate atrophy

Clinical evaluation

General factors

Clinicians should evaluate patients' general medical health because this may be important when considering surgery. Factors theoretically that could aggravate hydrocephalus include systemic hypertension (see discussion later of hydrocephalus association with hypertension) and a recent head injury (which is pertinent particularly in individuals who have gait difficulty). Evaluate for sleep apnea, congestive heart failure, lung disease, and obesity, all of which could increase jugular venous pressure and decrease cerebrospinal fluid (CSF) flow into the cerebral venous sinuses. If patients are on long-term anticoagulants, such as coumadin for atrial fibrillation, take this into account for the theoretic increased risk for brain hemorrhage during and after surgery. Look for evidence of arthritis of the hips and knees, cervical myelopathy, lumbar stenosis and radiculopathy, visual impairment, vestibular dysfunction, and peripheral neuropathy, all of which could impair gait.

History related to hydrocephalus

There are several specific questions that should be asked when taking a history from these patients and their families.

Ask how long patients have been demented. If this is more than 2 years, it is less likely that patients will respond to surgery [12,13]. Note that the question is not how long patients have had gait abnormality but how long patients have been demented. In the author and colleagues' series, this question predicted 5 of 7 unimproved and 21 of 23 improved patients [12].

Ask which started first, gait abnormality or dementia. If the gait abnormality began before or at the same time as dementia, then there is a better chance for successful surgery, whereas if dementia started before gait abnormality, shunting is less likely to help. In the author and colleagues' series this question predicted 3 of 7 unimproved and 23 of 23 improved patients [12]. This observation has been reported previously by Fisher [14].

Ask if patients abused alcohol, because alcohol abuse is a poor prognostic indicator [15].

Ask if there are secondary causes for hydrocephalus, such as subarachnoid hemorrhage, meningitis, prior brain surgery, and head injury. If any of these is present, the chances of improvement with surgery are better [13,15,16].

Ask if patients have a large head size, as evidenced by needing a large hat. This may indicate that patients suffer from congenital hydrocephalus that has become symptomatic in later life [17,18]. The author and colleagues have found that 10% to 20% of persons diagnosed with so-called "INPH" have large heads, indicating that they may have congenital hydrocephalus that becomes symptomatic in later life [17,18].

Examination

On examination, the following issues should be addressed.

Measure the head circumference. If greater than 59 cm in males or 57.5 cm in females, suspect that patients could have an element of congenital hydrocephalus that has become symptomatic in later life [17,18].

Look for signs of diseases that may mimic NPH (see Box 1). These include AD with extrapyramidal features, Parkinson's disease dementia, parkinsonian syndromes (progressive supranuclear palsy, corticobasal degeneration, and multiple system atrophy), diffuse Lewy body disease, frontotemporal dementia, cerebrovascular disease, and phenothiazine use. Also, look for cervical spondylosis with spinal cord compression, lumbar stenosis or radiculopathy, arthritis of the hips and knees, and multiple factors that impair gait abnormality (as might occur in diabetics who have peripheral neuropathy and visual impairment, alcoholics who have peripheral neuropathy and cerebellar atrophy, or the elderly who have vestibular and visual dysfunction and arthritis).

Neuropsychology

Look for evidence of aphasia. If there is evidence of aphasia (eg, anomia), this is a poor prognostic indicator for surgical success [12,15]. Ogino and colleagues recently reported the typical neuropsychology pattern of patients who have NPH compared with those who have AD [19]. Of 42 patients who had AD and 21 who had NPH who were matched for age, gender, and Mini–Mental State Examination [20], the patients who had NPH scored better on orientation and on the delayed recall of the Wechsler Memory Scale–Revised (WMS-R) [21] but significantly lower on the attention and concentration subtests of the WMS-R and on the digit span, arithmetic, block design, and digit symbol substitution subtest of the Wechsler Adult Intelligence Scale–Revised [22]. In summary, the cognitive deficits are characterized by psychomotor slowing, memory impairment, and impaired executive function with preserved cortical tests, such as naming.

Radiologic evaluation

CT

Since the advent of CT, the documentation of ventriculomegaly has become easier. Patients have ventriculomegaly (above the 95th percentile) when the modified Evan's index (maximum width of the frontal horns/measure of the inner table at the same place) is greater than 0.31 [23]. The ventricles normally enlarge with age [10], a point to be taken into account when diagnosing hydrocephalus. There is slow ventricular enlargement to age 60 years and then the rate of enlargement increases. In Barron and colleagues' study [10], the mean ventricular size was 5.2% (percent of intracranial area) in the decade 50 to 59 years, 6.4% in 60 to 69 years, 11.5% in 70 to 79 years, and 14.1% in 80 to 89 years.

In one study, the greater the sulcal enlargement, the less the chance of improvement with surgery [24]. Patients still might improve with surgery, however, even if there is sulcal enlargement and hydrocephalus. Borgesen and Gjerris [24] measured the largest sulcus in the high frontal or parietal region and found that if the cortical sulci were less than 1.9 mm, 17 of 17 patients shunted improved; if the sulci were 1.9 to 5 mm, 17 of 20 shunted improved; and if the sulci were 5 mm or more, 15 of 27 shunted improved.

MRI

Detecting congenital hydrocephalus. MRI is an excellent method for evaluating patients who have possible symptomatic hydrocephalus and is the neuroimaging study of choice in patients who have NPH. It has the advantage of being able to visualize relevant structures in the posterior fossa, including cerebral aqueduct stenosis, cerebellar tonsil herniation, and infarctions in the brainstem. Further, MRI can be used to obtain volumetric measures of medial temporal lobe structures, a technique that has been shown to be useful in separating patients who have AD from normal elderly controls [25].

Approximately 10% to 20% of patients who have symptomatic hydrocephalus after age 60 years may have congenital hydrocephalus that becomes symptomatic in later years [17,18]. A clinical clue to this is that patients have a large head size. On MRI, the ventricular enlargement shows no or little associated periventricular increased signal on T2-weighted imaging, indicating a chronic process. In addition, a cause for the congenital hydrocephalus rarely is found, such as an Arnold-Chiari malformation or aqueductal stenosis.

White matter lesions and normal pressure hydrocephalus. Although some early reports using CT indicated the presence of transependymal flow may be related to a good surgical prognosis [24] (Borgesen and Gjerris' study reported that 16 of 16 who had periventricular hypodensity on CT improved with surgery), later studies did not confirm this or found the opposite. Bradley [26] reported that on MRI the presence or extent of deep white matter changes did not correlate with outcome, whereas Krauss and colleagues [27] reported that the degree of improvement after shunt surgery depends on the extent and severity of white matter lesions (ie, the more extensive the white matter lesions, the less the improvement). In a subsequent report [28], they compared the MRI findings in NPH to an age-matched controlled group and found that in both groups the periventricular white matter lesions correlated with the deep white matter lesions. In the control group, the white matter lesions correlated significantly with age and the anterior horn index (frontal horn width divided by the horizontal intracranial width). In contrast, in the NPH group, there was no correlation of white matter lesions with age and there was a significant negative correlation between the white matter lesions and the frontal horn index (ie, the wider the frontal horns, the fewer white matter lesions present). They argue that the white matter lesions do not cause the hydrocephalus but that the common link between the frequent coexistence of INPH and vascular encephalopathy (as evidenced by white matter lesions) is arterial hypertension (the association of systemic hypertension and NPH is discussed later).

In a postmortem MRI study of autopsied brains and a histologic analysis of the same brains, Munoz and colleagues [29] found the white matter changes seen on MRI correlate with decreased density of axons and myelinated fibers, diffuse vacuolation of white matter (so-called "spongiosis"), and decreased density of glia. Infarctions were not common in these areas. Although this study does not necessarily apply to the white matter changes seen in hydrocephalic patients, it does indicate that white matter MRI findings do not necessarily indicate irreversible periventricular infarctions, which would make shunt surgery unlikely to be effective.

MRI differentiation of normal pressure hydrocephalus and Alzheimer's disease. Traditionally, the presence of ventriculomegaly without sulcal enlargement has been a radiologic finding believed to indicate NPH when accompanied by the typical clinical triad. Studies by Holodny and colleagues [30] and Kitagaki and colleagues [31], however, have pointed out the occasional occurrence of focally dilated sulci over the convexity or medial surface of a hemisphere in patients who have NPH, unlike the diffuse sulcal enlargement seen in AD (Fig. 1). Kitagaki and colleagues' report [31] also indicated significantly greater sylvian CSF volume in patients who had INPH compared with AD. He believed this was a sign supportive of NPH, indicating a "suprasylvian block."

An area where MRI has the potential to be helpful for surgical prognosis is volumetric measurements of certain structures in the temporal lobe. There is enlargement of the temporal horns of the lateral ventricles in patients who have NPH and those who have AD. Jack and colleagues [25] developed a technique for measuring the volumes of structures in the anterior temporal lobe and hippocampal formation. Holodny and colleagues [32] measured the CSF volumes of the perihippocampal fissures and the ventricular volumes. They showed that the perihippocampal fissures were enlarged significantly in patients who had AD compared with patients who had NPH, whereas the ventricles were larger in NPH. This was detectable by visible inspection and computer volumetrics.

MR-based volumetric measurements of the hippocampal formation have been shown to be useful in discriminating between AD and normal elderly controls [25]. Although Golomb and colleagues [33] found smaller hippocampal volumes in patients who had NPH compared with controls, Savolainen and colleagues [34] found only a minor left-side decrease. Savolainen and colleagues, however, detected significantly larger hippocampi in patients who had NPH compared with patients who had AD.

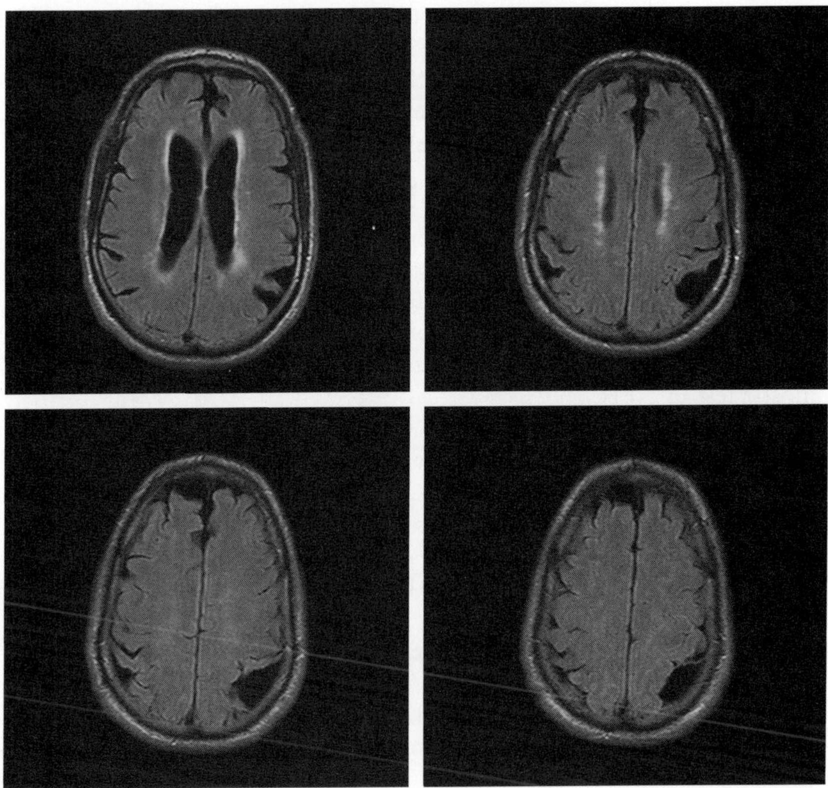

Fig. 1. MRI demonstrating enlarged sulci with entrapped CSF. This is not atrophy but part of the so-called "suprasylvian block" sometimes seen in hydrocephalus.

Flow void on MRI as a predictive test of surgical outcome. In 1991, Bradley and coworkers [35] retrospectively reviewed the MRI scans of 20 patients who had undergone ventriculoperitoneal shunt surgery for NPH. They rated initial surgical outcome as excellent, good, or poor and correlated this with the extent of flow void in the cerebral aqueduct. They found a significant correlation ($P < .003$) between extent of increased aqueduct flow void and initial surgical outcome. More specifically, 8 out of 10 who had an increased CSF flow void score had an excellent or good response to surgery, whereas only 1 out of 9 who had a normal flow void score improved with surgery.

In a subsequent study of 18 patients who had NPH, Bradley and colleagues [36] studied the CSF stroke volume (see article by Bradley and colleagues [36] for methods) and the CSF flow void score. The 12 patients who had a CSF stroke volume of 42 mL all improved, but of those who had a CSF stroke volume less than 42 mL, three improved and three did not. Using the flow void score, 4 of 15 improved patients had false-negative tests and 1 of 3 unimproved patients had a false-positive test.

Krauss and colleagues [37] report that that the flow void in the cerebral aqueduct of 37 patients who had INPH was not significantly different from that in 37 age-matched controls. Further, the extent of the flow void extension into the third, fourth, and lateral ventricles did not correlate with amount of improvement in these patients but correlated with rather the width of the ventricles.

Hakim and Black [38], in a small study of 12 patients of whom 10 improved, found that the MRI-CSF flow studies were correct in six, but five had false negatives and one a false positive.

Dixon and colleagues [39] also found in 49 patients that CSF flow through the cerebral aqueduct did not reliably predict those who improved with shunt surgery. These last three studies cast doubt on CSF flow as a diagnostic test in NPH.

Summary of factors to be addressed when looking at the CT or MRI

Hydrocephalus must be present. The modified Evans ratio should be greater than 0.31 [23]. Is cortical atrophy prominent? If there is extensive cortical atrophy, this reduces but does not eliminate the chance of improvement with surgery [13,24]. Avoid calling entrapped sulci or suprasylvian block brain atrophy [30,31].

The pattern of atrophy may be useful diagnostically (eg, Does it involve the medial temporal lobes as seen in AD?). Although data on this point are lacking, it may be that prominent medial temporal cortical atrophy decreases the chances for surgical cognitive improvement because these patients may have AD [25,30].

Is there evidence of congenital hydrocephalus? For example, is there aqueductal stenosis or an Arnold-Chiari malformation and are the ventricles large with little white matter abnormality indicating a chronic process [17,18]?

Newer MRI techniques, such as cine MRI, involving the analysis of a CSF flow void in the aqueduct of Sylvius, were first believed to be helpful [35,36] but unfortunately have not been found to be so in subsequent studies [37–39].

Regional cerebral blood flow

It has been reported that regional cerebral blood flow (rCBF) is decreased in the frontal areas in hydrocephalus [40] and in the parietotemporal areas in AD [41]. On the presumption that many of the nonimproved group have AD (Bech and colleagues have shown more recently [42] that 25% at time of shunt surgery brain biopsy show AD pathology), the author and colleagues tried to differentiate those who will respond to shunt surgery from those who will not, based on the pattern of preoperative rCBF [43]. To do this, frontal over posterior regional blood flow was calculated, expecting a lower frontal-posterior ratio in true symptomatic hydrocephalus and a higher ratio in pseudosymptomatic hydrocephalus patients who have AD. This has been a good method in predicting surgical outcome: the ratio predicted 5 of 7 unimproved and 22 of 23 improved patients in the author and colleagues' series [12]. Granado and colleagues [44] also found that those suspected of having NPH with and Alzheimer pattern did not improve but those who had frontal hypoperfusion did. Unfortunately, a review of the literature on CBF in NPH shows no clear-cut use at this time [45].

Cisternography

The literature suggests there are many cases of a positive test (radioisotope seen within the ventricles 48 to 72 hours after being injected in the lumber area) with no improvement with surgery and patients who have equivocal or negative tests who do improve. Further, the test itself may be difficult to interpret [46]. Black [46], in a review of his experience with this test, found the following: of 11 patients who had a positive test, nine improved and two did not; of six patients who had mixed results, three improved and three did not; of six who had negative results, four improved and two did not. He suggests a positive test is helpful but an equivocal or negative test is not. A more recent study by Vanneste and colleagues [5] reported, "cisternography did not improve the accuracy of combined clinical and computerized tomography in patients with presumed normal-pressure hydrocephalus."

Cerebrospinal drainage procedures

Lumbar puncture

If a patient's gait improves after removing a large quantity of CSF by lumbar puncture (LP) (30 to 50 mL; this can be repeated daily), this person is a good candidate for shunt surgery [47]. Malm and colleagues [48] found no predictive values of a spinal tap test but Walchenbach and colleagues [49] found a poor sensitivity (9 of 35 cases with a positive test had improvement with shunt surgery) but a good positive predictive value (9 of 9 with a positive test improved). One of the issues is that in both of these studies the gait was evaluated 4 to 6 hours after the LP. In patients who do not leak CSF after the LP, the CSF is replaced at 0.3 mL per minute would be replenished in 2 hours. When the author and coworkers evaluate patients after an LP, they made a videotape of the gait immediately after the LP. Later they compared this to the videotape done prior to the LP. At this time, it is reasonable to presume that a positive LP test has a good positive predictive value but is not sensitive.

External cerebrospinal fluid drainage

A modification of this technique also has been reported and is continuous CSF drainage via a catheter placed in the lumbar CSF space [50]. In the guidelines for the diagnosis and management of INPH [51], the guidelines are based on three studies [48–50]. These studies showed a range of sensitivity from 50% to 100%, specificity 60% to 100%, positive predictive value 80% to 100%, negative predictive value 36% to 100%, and accuracy 58% to 100%. In one study [49], two of 38 developed meningitis and five pulled out their drains. In another study [50], two of 22 had infections, four removed their drains, and three had root irritation.

Although this test is more sensitive than a large-volume spinal tap, the investigators caution that it should be undertaken by an experienced team that can limit the complication rate.

Cerebrospinal fluid infusion tests

There are several ways of measuring the resistance to absorption (Ro) or the reciprocal to this, called the conductance. In Katzman and Hussey's test [52], fluid was infused through an LP needle into the CSF at a known rate until a steady state pressure is reached. The Ro is calculated as the new pressure minus the initial pressure divided by the infused flow rate and is given as mm Hg per mL per minute. Another way of doing this is the bolus method, where 4 mL are infused at 1 mL per second and the new pressure measured. Lastly, Ro can be calculated as described by Borgesen and Gjerris [24]. They called the reciprocal of the Ro the conductance. In this method, CSF absorption is measured at different CSF pressures. The concept is that the greater the pressure needed to obtain an amount of absorption, the better the chances of the patient improving with shunt surgery. Absorption is calculated by infusing fluid through an LP needle for a given time (5 minutes) while catching the overflow from a ventricular catheter. There is some evidence to show that the amount of CSF produced does not vary much at different CSF pressures and is approximately 0.4 mL per minute. Because one knows how much is infused through the LP needle and how much overflows through the ventricular catheter, one can calculate the amount absorbed in this time period. The following equation gives absorption: Absorption = Infused (measured) + Produced (assumed) – Overflow (measured).

The overflow pressure for the ventricular catheter then is raised and absorption then is calculated at this new pressure. Between six and eight absorptions at different pressures are obtained in this way and then absorption is plotted against pressure and the slope of the line calculated (ie, absorption/pressure). The slope of this line is called the conductance. Borgersen and Gjerris reported that a conductance of less than 0.08 predicted a favorable outcome. A conductance of 0.08 = Rcsf of 12.5 mm Hg/mL/min, where Rcsf is resistance to CSF outflow.

Boon and colleagues [53] report the first multiple center randomized study evaluating the predictive value for shunt surgery of measuring Rcsf. They enrolled 101 patients (both idiopathic and secondary, although they note most were idiopathic) and measured the Rcsf by infusing saline through 19-gage LP needle at 1.4 to 1.6 mL per minute until a stable pressure plateau was reached or the pressure exceeded 50 mm Hg. The Rcsf was calculated as the difference between the plateau and the baseline pressure divided by the infusion rate. They randomized the patients to receive either low or medium pressure valves. Outcome measures were an NPH scale (sum of gait and dementia measures) and the modified Rankin scale. Follow-up was at 1, 3, 6, 9, and 12 months. Intention to treat analysis was performed on all 101 patients and 57% showed improvement in the NPH scale and 59% in the modified Rankin scale at 1 year. When all known serious events unrelated to NPH that clearly interfered with neurologic function were excluded, 95 patients were left. In these patients, 76% had a meaningful improvement on the NPH scale and 69% improved one grade on the modified Rankin scale. Using a cutoff of the Rcsf of less than 18 mm Hg per mL per minute, 20 of 59 had no improvement on the NPH scale. Above this cutoff, 3 of 36 had no improvement on the NPH scale.

The investigators conclude that the Rcsf obtained by lumbar CSF infusion is a reliable method for selecting patients for shunt surgery if the Rcsf cutoff is 18 mm Hg per mL per minute or greater. Patients who have an rCBF less than 18 mm Hg per mL per minute should undergo shunt placement only when characteristic clinical features of NPH are present. Unfortunately, the majority of patients (>60%) under consideration for shunt surgery have a Rcsf of less than 18 mm Hg per mL per minute and this diagnostic test is not helpful in this group. In the guidelines [54], they note the data are limited and "the results, methods and thresholds are center specific and subject to wide variation."

Cerebrospinal fluid pressure monitoring

There are reports of a significant relationship between measures of intracranial CSF pressure monitoring and surgical outcome for symptomatic hydrocephalus (eg, in the Borgesen and Gjerris study and in the author and colleagues' study [12,24], the greater the percentage of time B waves were present, the greater the chance of a good outcome). In Williams' and colleagues study, the sensitivity using a threshold of 25% time of B waves the sensitivity in predicting surgical out come was 78% but the specificity was 40%. From all the studies, using only the percentage of time B waves are present would be inadequate in predicting surgical outcome. The consensus guidelines [51] note that there is insufficient evidence to use pressure monitoring for prognostic purposes.

One point to be evaluated in the future is the prognostic value of how long the pressure is high when patients are monitored. In the author and colleagues' series, the longer the pressure was more than 15 mm Hg, the better the chance of successful surgery [12]. This may be important because it implies that increased pressure may be pathogenic in symptomatic hydrocephalus.

These data raise the issue about what is meant by NPH. Does it mean normal pressure at one spinal tap or does it imply the pressure remains normal all the time? It is not known what 24-hour CSF pressure recordings in normal people show. It follows that it is not known if the pressure is normal or abnormal in those who respond to surgery but have CSF pressures greater than 15 mm Hg for a percentage of time. For this reason, some prefer the term, symptomatic hydrocephalus, to NPH but recognize that with the use of the latter term for more than 4 decades, it is unlikely to be replaced.

A summary of prognostic factors related to shunt surgery is given in Box 2.

Probable and possible normal pressure hydocephalus criteria

Relkin and colleagues [55] published criteria for probable and possible INPH. Although these have not been tested prospectively, they are based on an extensive review of the literature (Box 3).

Box 2. Prognostic factors for shunt surgery

Factors favoring clinical improvement in normal pressure hydrocephalus after shunting

Secondary NPH
Gait disturbance preceding cognitive impairment
Mild impairment in cognition
Short duration of cognitive impairment
Clinical improvement (usually in gait) after LP or continuous lumbar CSF drainage
Rcsf outflow of 18 mm Hg/mL/min or greater during continuous lumbar CSF infusion test
Presence of B waves for 50% of the time or greater during continuous lumbar CSF monitoring

Factors weighing against clinical improvement after shunting

Moderate or severe cognitive impairment
Dementia present for 2 or more years
Cognitive impairment preceding gait disturbance
Presence of aphasia
History of ethanol abuse
MRI with significant white matter involvement or diffuse cerebral atrophy

Factors of unproved significance

Long duration of gait abnormality
Absence of aqueductal flow void despite patent aqueduct (on MRI)
No clinical improvement after LP
Cisternography
CBF measurements

Box 3. Criteria for probable and possible normal pressure hydrocephalus

Probable idiopathic normal pressure hydrocephalus

The diagnosis of probable INPH is based on clinical history, brain imaging, physical findings, and physiologic criteria.

1. History

History should be corroborated by an informant.

- A. Insidious onset (versus acute)
- B. Start after 40 years
- C. Minimum duration of 3 to 6 months
- D. No secondary causes (head trauma, intracerebral hemorrhage, meningitis, or other known cause of secondary hydrocephalus)
- E. Progression over time
- F. No other neurologic, psychiatric, or medical condition sufficient to explain the presenting symptoms

2. Brain imaging

Brain imaging study (CT or MRI) after onset must show evidence of

1. Ventricular enlargement not entirely attributable to cerebral atrophy or congenital enlargement (Evans index >0.3 or comparable measure)
2. No macroscopic obstruction of CSF flow
3. At least one of the following supportive features
   - A. Enlargement of the temporal horns of the lateral ventricles not attributable to hippocampal atrophy
   - B. Callosal angle of 40° or more
   - C. Evidence of altered brain water content, including periventricular signal changes on CT and MRI not attributable to microvascular ischemic changes or demyelination
   - D. An aqueductal or fourth ventricular flow void on MRI

Other brain imaging findings

1. Brain imaging study performed before onset of symptoms showing smaller ventricular size or without evidence of hydrocephalus
2. Radionucleotide cisternogram showing delayed clearance of radiotracer over the cerebral convexities after 48–72 h.
3. Cine-MRI study or other technique showing increased ventricular flow rate

4. A single photon emission CT–acetazolamide challenge showing decreased periventricular perfusion that is not altered by acetazolamide

3. Clinical

By classic definitions, findings of gait or balance disturbance must be present plus at least one other area of impairment in cognition and urinary symptoms or both

With respect to gait and balance, at least two of the following should be present and not entirely attributable to other conditions:

A. Decreased step height
B. Decreases step length
C. Decreased cadence
D. Increased trunk sway
E. Widened standing base
F. Toes turned outward on walking
G. Retropulsion (spontaneous or provoked)
H. En bloc turning (turning requires 3 or more steps for 180°)

With respect to cognition, there must be documented impairment (adjusted for age and education) or decrease in performance on a cognitive screening instrument (such as the Mini–Mental State Examination) or evidence of at least two of the following on examination that is not fully attributable to other conditions:

A. Psychomotor slowing
B. Decreased fine motor speed
C. Difficulty dividing or maintaining attention
D. Impaired recall, especially for recent events
E. Executive dysfunction, such as impairment in multistep procedures, working memory, formulation of abstract/similarities, insight
F. Behavioral or personality change

To document symptoms in the domains of urinary continence, either one of the following should be present:

A. Episodic or persistent urinary incontinence and not attributable to urologic disorders
B. Persistence of urinary incontinence
C. Persistence of fecal incontinence

Or any two of the following be present:

A. Urinary urgency as defined by perception of a pressing need to void
B. Urinary frequency as defined by more than six episodes in an average 12-hour period despite normal fluid intake

C. Nocturia as defined by need to urinate more that 2 times in an average night

4. Physiologic

CSF pressure opening in the range of 5 to 18 mm Hg (or 70–245 mm H_2O) as determined by a LP or a comparable procedure. Appropriately measure pressures that are significantly higher or lower are not consistent with a probable NPH diagnosis.

Possible idiopathic normal pressure hydrocephalus

1. History

Reported symptoms may

A. Have a subacute or indeterminate mode of onset
B. Begin at any age after childhood
C. May have less than 3 months of indeterminate duration
D. May follow events, such as mild head trauma, remote history of intracerebral hemorrhage, or childhood and adolescent meningitis, or other conditions that in the judgment of the clinician are not likely to be casually related
E. Coexist with other neurologic, psychiatric, or general medical disorders but in the judgment of a clinician not be entirely attributed to these conditions
F. Be nonprogressive or not clearly progressive

2. Brain imaging

Ventricular enlargement consistent with hydrocephalus but associated with either of the following:

A. Evidence of cerebral atrophy of sufficient severity to potentially explain ventricular size
B. Structural lesions that may influence ventricular size

3. Clinical

Symptoms of either

A. Incontinence or cognitive impairment in the absence of an observable gait or balance disturbance
B. Gait disturbance or dementia alone

4. Physiologic

Opening pressure not available or pressure outside the range of required for probable INPH.

Unlikely idiopathic normal pressure hydrocephaloathty

1. No evidence of ventriculomegaly
2. Signs of increased intracranial pressure, such as papilledema
3. No component of the clinical triad of INPH
4. Symptoms explained by other causes (eg, spinal stenosis)

Based on the published guidelines for NPH in Relkin N, Marmarou A, Klinge P, et al. Diagnosing idiopathic normal-pressure hydrocephalus. Neurosurgery 2005; 57(3 Suppl):S4–16; [discussion: ii–v].

How to assess patient improvement

Older studies measure patient improvement on a five-point rating scale [24,46]. This may be problematic, because levels on the scale overlap and it is a subjective judgment into which level patients fall. More recently, measures of outcome have included more objective measures of gait change [12,53]—scales measuring change in activities of daily living, such as the Katz index [12] or the Rankin scale [53], both of which are sensitive to deficits in NPH.

One of the crucial unknowns in NPH is if patients improve, how long do they stay improved? One study addressing this issue was published by Malm and colleagues [56]. They found when they prospectively followed 84 surgically treated patients who had INPH, 64% were improved at 3 months but only 26% remained improved at 3 years. In Aygok and colleagues' [54], study they followed 50 patients who had INPH and noted a decline in gait improvement from 90% at 3 months to 75% at 3 years, but cognitive improvement remained steady at 80% at 3 months and 3 years, and incontinence improved from 70% at 3 months to 82.5% at 3 years.

Shunts

There is no good guidance in the literature to advise patients on the complication rate and the type of shunt that should be used. Some of the older studies report a complication rate from 30% to 40% [13,16]. The best way for doctors to be able to advise patients about the complication rate of shunt surgery is for them to become familiar with the complication rate at the center they practice. All complications are important but some effect patients more. A list of the complications encountered more commonly is given is Box 4 and is based on the surgical management article in the INPH guidelines [57]. Before adjustable valves becoming available, one prospective study compared low and medium pressure valves. In this study, 35 of 49 patients receiving low pressure and 16 of 47 patients receiving medium pressure valves developed subdural collections. More patients in the LPV group improved compared with the MPV group ($P<.06$). In recent years, the use of adjustable shunts has made the management of subdural hygromas and hematomas easier and allowed adjustment down of the opening pressure if patients do not improve. Accurate information on shunt complications and which shunt to use is sorely needed.

Histopathology of the brains of patients who have idiopathic normal pressure hydrocephalus

In a unique study, Bech and colleagues [42] reported their experience with 38 consecutive patients who had INPH. They monitored and performed

Box 4. Complications of shunt surgery

Complications related to surgery and anesthesia, such as myocardial infarction and deep vein thrombosis
Acute intracerebral hemorrhage
Infection of the shunt
Subdural hematoma
Subdural hygroma (sometimes these my have a small hemorrhagic component)
Seizures
Shunt malfunction
Headache
Hearing loss
Tinnitis
Oculomotor palsies
Damage to intra-abdominal organs

absorption tests on all, but most importantly they performed brain biopsies on all. Twenty-nine of 38 patients fulfilled hydrodynamic criteria for shunt surgery (Rcsf of 10 mm Hg per mL per minute with or without B activity for more than 50% of the monitoring period). Of 29 individuals shunted, 27 had follow-up and of these nine (33.3%) improved, 10 (37%) remained stable and eight (29.6%) deteriorated. These results are not necessarily representative of all series in which patients who had INPH undergo shunt surgery (eg, in the author and colleagues' series, more than 70% improved [12], and in Boon and colleagues' series [53], 53% of the medium-pressure valve group and 74% of the low-pressure valve group improved). Nonetheless, the biopsy findings are of great interest; only 12 of 25 had arachnoid fibrosis (not all biopsies had arachnoid tissue), 17 had normal parenchyma, 10 had AD, and 8 had vascular disease.

There was no significant association of the presence or absence of arachnoid fibrosis with the hydrodynamic measures.

The Bech study has some important implications. Ten of 38 patients who were believed clinically possibly to have NPH had biopsy-verified AD. The criteria used to diagnose AD were conservative, that is, 10 neuritic plaques per high-power field in the frontal lobe. It is possible that at autopsy, several additional patients may have had AD. In a follow-up article [58], Bech and colleagues found no correlation between clinical outcome after shunting patients who had NPH and the presence or absence of AD pathology. Further, he also found that vascular disease and arachnoid fibrosis did not correlate with outcome. Golomb and coworkers [59] found AD pathology in 23 of 56 (41%) patients who had biopsied NPH. The patients who had NPH with concomitant AD had more impairment of gait and cognition than the patients who had "pure" NPH. Only 18% of the patients who had Global Deterioration Scores of 3 and below had AD-positive biopsies, whereas 75% of those who had Global Deterioration Scores 6 or above were AD positive. There was comparable improvement in gait velocity in patients who had NPH regardless of the presence of AD pathology. No consistent cognitive improvement occurred in either group after shunting. Savolainen and colleagues [60] found concomitant AD pathology by biopsy in 31% of 51 consecutive patients who had NPH.

These three studies [42,59,60] show that AD pathology is frequent in patients diagnosed with INPH. Further, some of these patients have gait improvement after shunting. The implication is that NPH and AD may occur simultaneously in the same patient, and families should be made aware of this. In Braak and Braak's classic study [61] of autopsies of more than 2000 persons from the medical examiner, the prevalence of AD pathology in the age group 71 to 75 was 30% and 76 to 80 was 40%, so the AD biopsy rate of patients who have NPH is similar to that patients not selected for being demented (ie, from the medical examiner). Future studies should investigate if CSF markers, such as the amyloid-beta protein 1-42 and tau protein [62], may be helpful in these cases.

The relationship of idiopathic normal pressure hydrocephalus and systemic hypertension

Several lines of evidence in the literature now point to a relationship between hydrocephalus and systemic hypertension.

Clinical and autopsy studies of normal pressure hydrocephalus patients

Several postmortem examinations of patients who had NPH and case control studies have reported the association of systemic hypertension and NPH [42,63–67]. In the author and Godersky's series [68], a significantly higher prevalence of systemic hypertension was found in patients who had INPH compared with matched, demented controls and to the published prevalence of hypertension in the United States population, matched for age. A more recent, much larger case control study [27] of 65 patients who had INPH versus 70 matched control patients found a prevalence of 83% of systemic hypertension in the patients who had NPH compared with 36% in the control group. This was highly significant ($P < .001$).

Boon and colleagues [69] showed that cerebrovascular risk factors (hypertension, diabetes mellitus, cardiac disease, peripheral vascular disease, male gender, and advancing age) did not influence outcome after shunt placement. The presence of cerebrovascular disease (history of stroke, cerebral infarction noted on CT, or moderate-to-severe white matter hypodense lesions on CT), however, was an important predictor of poor outcome. Nonetheless, even though 74% of those who did not have concomitant cerebrovascular disease improved with shunting, 49% who had it also improved. Four of the seven patients who had the most severe white matter hypodense lesions responded favorably to shunting.

At this time, regarding hypertension, subcortical arteriosclerotic encephalopathy, and NPH, there are more questions than answers. Are hypertension, white matter changes, and cerebrovascular disease merely frequent concomitants of NPH? Do NPH and subcortical arteriosclerotic encephalopathy represent a spectrum (as suggested by Gallassi and colleagues) [70]? Is one causative of the other?

Hydrocephalus after subarachnoid hemorrhage

Another line of evidence showing that systemic hypertension and hydrocephalus may be related comes from the Cooperative Aneurysm Study [71]. In more than 3000 patients who had subarachnoid hemorrhage, it was found that a preoperative history of hypertension, the admission blood pressure measurement, and sustained hypertension during hospitalization after surgery, all were highly significantly related to patients developing hydrocephalus.

Hypertension in patients who have aqueductal stenosis

Greitz and colleagues [72] found a high prevalence of systemic hypertension in patients who had hydrocephalus from aqueductal stenosis.

Hydrocephalus in the spontaneously hypertensive rat

The association of hypertension and hydrocephalus is corroborated by reports in the animal literature. Ritter and Dinh [72] showed that the spontaneously hypertensive rat develops hydrocephalus.

Experimental models of hydrocephalus, ventricular pulse pressure, and systemic hypertension

Portnoy and colleagues [73] showed, in dogs, that infusing dopamine and norepinephrine led to increased systemic blood pressure, which, in turn, resulted in an increased CSF pressure and pulse pressure. Experimentally creating an increased CSF pulse pressure with an inflatable balloon in the lateral ventricle of sheep leads to hydrocephalus within hours [74]. Bering and Salibi [75] performed seminal work on hydrocephalus in dogs. They tied off the jugular veins in the dogs and measured the intraventricular pulse pressure. They concluded that the mechanism involved in the ventricular enlargement seemed to be a combination of at least two factors: "One was the possible failure of CSF absorption in the face of increased superior sagittal sinus venous pressure, and the other the increased intraventricular pulse pressure from the choroid plexus."

Thus, a body of information is accumulating that systemic hypertension and hydrocephalus are associated. It remains to be shown whether or not hypertension causes hydrocephalus or hydrocephalus causes hypertension, or both.

Large head size and hydrocephalus

Approximately 10% to 20% of patients diagnosed with INPH have a large head size [17,18]. This raises the possibility that one of the causes of so-called "INPH" may be patients born with hydrocephalus who become symptomatic late in life.

Summary

When confronted with patients who have possible NPH, use the following systematic approach. Keeping in mind the differential diagnosis, look for pertinent factors in the history and examination and neuropsychologic evaluation that have a bearing on diagnosis and surgical prognosis. On the MRI, look at the amount and pattern of atrophy and white matter changes. Perform between one and three spinal taps and evaluate the effect of this on the gait. Consider sending the CSF for AD markers (tau and amyloid beta 1-42). At this time you may wish to advise about surgery. If your center performs external CSF drainage or intracranial pressure monitoring, this may be helpful. Patients and families must be aware of the possible benefits and the risks for the surgery. If they choose surgery, follow patients carefully to see if there is improvement and to detect possible surgical complications. If you are uncertain whether or not patients should undergo surgery or if families and patients choose that a patient should not undergo surgery, make sure you have established a baseline from which you can follow the patient. Ideally, this includes a video of the gait, a brain MRI, and neuropsychologic testing. Follow patients at 3-month intervals with serial videotaping of gait. Stability or deterioration of the gait often helps families and doctors decide on further action.

References

[1] Casmiro M, Benassi G, Cacciatore FM, et al. Frequency of idiopathic normal pressure hydrocephalus. Arch Neurol 1989;46(6):608.

[2] Trenkwalder C, Schwarz J, Gebhard J, et al. Starnberg trial on epidemiology of Parkinsonism and hypertension in the elderly. Prevalence of Parkinson's disease and related disorders assessed by a door-to-door survey of inhabitants older than 65 years. Arch Neurol 1995; 52(10):1017–22.

[3] Clarfield AM. The decreasing prevalence of reversible dementias: an updated meta-analysis. Arch Intern Med 2003;163(18):2219–29.

[4] Hebert LE, Scherr PA, Bienias JL, et al. Alzheimer Disease in the US population: prevalence estimates using the 2000 census. Arch Neurol 2003;60(8):1119–22.
[5] Vanneste J, Augustijn P, Dirven C, et al. Shunting normal-pressure hydrocephalus: do the benefits outweigh the risks? A multicenter study and literature review. Neurology 1992; 42(1):54–9.
[6] Krauss JK, Halve B. Normal pressure hydrocephalus: survey on contemporary diagnostic algorithms and therapeutic decision-making in clinical practice. Acta Neurochir (Wien) 2004;146(4):379–88 [discussion: 388].
[7] Verghese J, Lipton RB, Hall CB, et al. Abnormality of gait as a predictor of non-Alzheimer's dementia. N Engl J Med 2002;347(22):1761–8.
[8] Anger JT, Saigal CS, Litwin MS. The prevalence of urinary incontinence among community dwelling adult women: results from the National Health and Nutrition Examination Survey. J Urol 2006;175(2):601–4.
[9] Stothers L, Thom D, Calhoun E. Urologic diseases in America project: urinary incontinence in males–demographics and economic burden. J Urol 2005;173(4):1302–8.
[10] Barron SA, Jacobs L, Kinkel WR. Changes in size of normal lateral ventricles during aging determined by computerized tomography. Neurology 1976;26(11):1011–3.
[11] Jack CR Jr, Shiung MM, Gunter JL, et al. Comparison of different MRI brain atrophy rate measures with clinical disease progression in AD. Neurology 2004;62(4):591–600.
[12] Graff-Radford NR, Godersky JC, Jones M. Variables predicting surgical outcome in symptomatic hydrocephalus in the elderly. Neurology 1989;39:1601–4.
[13] Petersen RC, Mokri B, Laws ER Jr. Surgical treatment of idiopathic hydrocephalus in elderly patients. Neurology 1985;35(3):307–11.
[14] Fisher CM. The clinical picture in occult hydrocephalus. Clin Neurosurg 1977;24:270–84.
[15] De Mol J. Prognostic factors for therapeutic outcome in normal-pressure hydrocephalus. Review of the literature and personal study [French]. Acta Neurol Belg 1985;85(1):13–29.
[16] Black PM, Ojemann RG, Tzouras A. CSF shunts for dementia, incontinence, and gait disturbance. Clin Neurosurg 1985;32:632–51.
[17] Graff-Radford NR, Godersky JC. Symptomatic congenital hydrocephalus in the elderly simulating normal pressure hydrocephalus. Neurology 1989;39(12):1596–600.
[18] Krefft TA, Graff-Radford NR, Lucas JA, et al. Normal pressure hydrocephalus and large head size. Alzheimer Dis Assoc Disord 2004;18(1):35–7.
[19] Ogino A, Kazui H, Miyoshi N, et al. Cognitive impairment in patients with idiopathic normal pressure hydrocephalus. Dement Geriatr Cogn Disord 2006;21(2):113–9.
[20] Folstein MF, Folstein SE, McHugh PR. "Mini-mental state". A practical method for grading the cognitive state of patients for the clinician. J Psychiatr Res 1975;12(3):189–98.
[21] Wechsler D. Wechsler Memory Scale-Revised. New York: The Psychological Corporation; 1987.
[22] Wechsler D. Wechsler Adult Intelligence Scale, 3rd Edition administration and scoring manual. Orlando: The Psychological Corporation; 1997.
[23] Gyldenstad C. Measurements of the normal ventricular system and hemispheric sulci of 100 adults with computerizes tomography. Neuroradiology 1977;14:183–92.
[24] Borgesen SE, Gjerris F. The predictive value of conductance to outflow of CSF in normal pressure hydrocephalus. Brain 1982;105(Pt 1):65–86.
[25] Jack CR Jr, Petersen RC, O'Brien PC, et al. MR-based hippocampal volumetry in the diagnosis of Alzheimer's disease. Neurology 1992;42(1):183–8.
[26] Bradley WG. Normal pressure hydrocephalus and deep white matter ischemia: which is the chicken, and which is the egg? AJNR Am J Neuroradiol 2001;22(9):1638–40.
[27] Krauss JK, Regel JP, Vach W, et al. Vascular risk factors and arteriosclerotic disease in idiopathic normal-pressure hydrocephalus of the elderly. Stroke 1996;27(1):24–9.
[28] Krauss JK, Regel JP, Vach W, et al. White matter lesions in patients with idiopathic normal pressure hydrocephalus and in an age-matched control group: a comparative study. Neurosurgery 1997;40(3):491–5 [discussion: 495–6].

[29] Munoz DG, Hastak SM, Harper B, et al. Pathologic correlates of increased signals of the centrum ovale on magnetic resonance imaging. Arch Neurol 1993;50(5):492–7.
[30] Holodny AI, George AE, de Leon MJ, et al. Focal dilation and paradoxical collapse of cortical fissures and sulci in patients with normal-pressure hydrocephalus. J Neurosurg 1998;89(5):742–7.
[31] Kitagaki H, Mori E, Ishii K, et al. CSF spaces in idiopathic normal pressure hydrocephalus: morphology and volumetry. AJNR Am J Neuroradiol 1998;19(7):1277–84.
[32] Holodny AI, Waxman R, George AE, et al. MR differential diagnosis of normal-pressure hydrocephalus and Alzheimer disease: significance of perihippocampal fissures. AJNR Am J Neuroradiol 1998;19(5):813–9.
[33] Golomb J, de Leon MJ, George AE, et al. Hippocampal atrophy correlates with severe cognitive impairment in elderly patients with suspected normal pressure hydrocephalus. J Neurol Neurosurg Psychiatry 1994;57(5):590–3.
[34] Savolainen S, Laakso MP, Paljarvi L, et al. MR imaging of the hippocampus in normal pressure hydrocephalus: correlations with cortical Alzheimer's disease confirmed by pathologic analysis. AJNR Am J Neuroradiol 2000;21(2):409–14.
[35] Bradley WG Jr, Whittemore AR, Kortman KE, et al. Marked cerebrospinal fluid void: indicator of successful shunt in patients with suspected normal-pressure hydrocephalus. Radiology 1991;178(2):459–66.
[36] Bradley WG Jr, Scalzo D, Queralt J, et al. Normal-pressure hydrocephalus: evaluation with cerebrospinal fluid flow measurements at MR imaging. Radiology 1996;198(2):523–9.
[37] Krauss JK, Regel JP, Vach W, et al. Flow void of cerebrospinal fluid in idiopathic normal pressure hydrocephalus of the elderly: can it predict outcome after shunting? Neurosurgery 1997;40(1):67–73 [discussion: 73–4].
[38] Hakim R, Black PM. Correlation between lumbo-ventricular perfusion and MRI-CSF flow studies in idiopathic normal pressure hydrocephalus. Surg Neurol 1998;49(1):14–9 [discussion: 19–20].
[39] Dixon GR, Friedman JA, Luetmer PH, et al. Use of cerebrospinal fluid flow rates measured by phase-contrast MR to predict outcome of ventriculoperitoneal shunting for idiopathic normal-pressure hydrocephalus. Mayo Clin Proc 2002;77(6):509–14.
[40] Jagust WJ, Friedland RP, Budinger TF. Positron emission tomography with [18F] fluorodeoxyglucose differentiates normal pressure hydrocephalus from Alzheimer-type dementia. J Neurol Neurosurg Psychiatry 1985;48(11):1091–6.
[41] Mosconi L. Brain glucose metabolism in the early and specific diagnosis of Alzheimer's disease. FDG-PET studies in MCI and AD. Eur J Nucl Med Mol Imaging 2005;32(4): 486–510.
[42] Bech RA, Juhler M, Waldemar G, et al. Frontal brain and leptomeningeal biopsy specimens correlated with cerebrospinal fluid outflow resistance and B-wave activity in patients suspected of normal-pressure hydrocephalus. Neurosurgery 1997;40(3):497–502.
[43] Graff-Radford NR, Rezai K, Godersky JC, et al. Regional cerebral blood flow in normal pressure hydrocephalus. J Neurol Neurosurg Psychiatry 1987;50(12):1589–96.
[44] Granado JM, Diaz F, Alday R. Evaluation of brain SPECT in the diagnosis and prognosis of the normal pressure hydrocephalus syndrome. Acta Neurochir (Wien) 1991;112(3–4): 88–91.
[45] Owler BK, Pickard JD. Normal pressure hydrocephalus and cerebral blood flow: a review. Acta Neurol Scand 2001;104(6):325–42.
[46] Black PM. Normal-pressure hydrocephalus: current understanding of diagnostic tests and shunting. Postgrad Med 1982;71(2):57–61, 65–7.
[47] Wikkelso C, Andersson H, Blomstrand C, et al. Normal pressure hydrocephalus. Predictive value of the cerebrospinal fluid tap-test. Acta Neurol Scand 1986;73(6):566–73.
[48] Malm J, Kristensen B, Karlsson T, et al. The predictive value of cerebrospinal fluid dynamic tests in patients with th idiopathic adult hydrocephalus syndrome. Arch Neurol 1995;52(8): 783–9.

[49] Walchenbach R, Geiger E, Thomeer RT, et al. The value of temporary external lumbar CSF drainage in predicting the outcome of shunting on normal pressure hydrocephalus. J Neurol Neurosurg Psychiatry 2002;72(4):503–6.
[50] Haan J, Thomeer RT. Predictive value of temporary external lumbar drainage in normal pressure hydrocephalus. Neurosurgery 1988;22(2):388–91.
[51] Marmarou A, Bergsneider M, Klinge P, et al. The value of supplemental prognostic tests for the preoperative assessment of idiopathic normal-pressure hydrocephalus. Neurosurgery 2005;57(3 Suppl):S17–28 [discussion: ii–v].
[52] Katzman R, Hussey F. A simple constant-infusion manometric test for measurement of CSF absorption. I. Rationale and method. Neurology 1970;20(6):534–44.
[53] Boon AJ, Tans JT, Delwel EJ, et al. Dutch normal-pressure hydrocephalus study: prediction of outcome after shunting by resistance to outflow of cerebrospinal fluid. J Neurosurg 1997; 87(5):687–93.
[54] Aygok G, Marmarou A, Young HF. Three-year outcome of shunted idiopathic NPH patients. Acta Neurochir Suppl 2005;95:241–5.
[55] Relkin N, Marmarou A, Klinge P, et al. Diagnosing idiopathic normal-pressure hydrocephalus. Neurosurgery 2005;57(3 Suppl):S4–16 [discussion: ii–v].
[56] Malm J, Kristensen B, Stegmayr B, et al. Three-year survival and functional outcome of patients with idiopathic adult hydrocephalus syndrome. Neurology 2000;55(4):576–8.
[57] Bergsneider M, Black PM, Klinge P, et al. Surgical management of idiopathic normal-pressure hydrocephalus. Neurosurgery 2005;57(3 Suppl):S29–39 [discussion: ii–v].
[58] Bech RA, Waldemar G, Gjerris F, et al. Shunting effects in patients with idiopathic normal pressure hydrocephalus; correlation with cerebral and leptomeningeal biopsy findings. Acta Neurochir (Wien) 1999;141(6):633–9.
[59] Golomb J, Wisoff J, Miller DC, et al. Alzheimer's disease comorbidity in normal pressure hydrocephalus: prevalence and shunt response. J Neurol Neurosurg Psychiatry 2000; 68(6):778–81.
[60] Savolainen S, Paljarvi L, Vapalahti M. Prevalence of Alzheimer's disease in patients investigated for presumed normal pressure hydrocephalus: a clinical and neuropathological study. Acta Neurochir (Wien) 1999;141(8):849–53.
[61] Braak H, Braak E. Frequency of stages of Alzheimer-related lesions in different age categories. Neurobiol Aging 1997;18(4):351–7.
[62] Blennow K, Hampel H. CSF markers for incipient Alzheimer's disease [review]. Lancet Neurol 2003;2:605–13.
[63] Koto A, Rosenberg G, Zingesser LH, et al. Syndrome of normal pressure hydrocephalus: possible relation to hypertensive and arteriosclerotic vasculopathy. J Neurol Neurosurg Psychiatry 1977;40(1):73–9.
[64] Earnest MP, Fahn S, Karp JH, et al. Normal pressure hydrocephalus and hypertensive cerebrovascular disease. Arch Neurol 1974;31(4):262–6.
[65] Haidri NH, Modi SM. Normal pressure hydrocephalus and hypertensive cerebrovascular disease. Dis Nerv Syst 1977;38(11):918–21.
[66] Shukla D, Singh BM, Strobos RJ. Hypertensive cerebrovascular disease and normal pressure hydrocephalus. Neurology 1980;30(9):998–1000.
[67] Casmiro M, D'Alessandro R, Cacciatore FM, et al. Risk factors for the syndrome of ventricular enlargement with gait apraxia (idiopathic normal pressure hydrocephalus): a case-control study. J Neurol Neurosurg Psychiatry 1989;52(7):847–52.
[68] Graff-Radford NR, Godersky JC. Idiopathic normal pressure hydrocephalus and systemic hypertension. Neurology 1987;37(5):868–71.
[69] Boon AJ, Tans JT, Delwel EJ, et al. Dutch Normal-Pressure Hydrocephalus Study: the role of cerebrovascular disease. J Neurosurg 1999;90(2):221–6.
[70] Gallassi R, Morreale A, Montagna P, et al. Binswanger's disease and normal-pressure hydrocephalus. Clinical and neuropsychological comparison. Arch Neurol 1991;48(11): 1156–9.

[71] Graff-Radford NR, Torner J, Adams HP Jr, et al. Factors associated with hydrocephalus after subarachnoid hemorrhage. A report of the Cooperative Aneurysm Study. Arch Neurol 1989;46(7):744–52.
[72] Ritter S, Dinah TT. Progressive postnatal dilation of brain ventricles in spontaneously hypertensive rats. Brain Res 1986;340:327–32.
[73] Portnoy HD, Chopp M, Branch C. Hydraulic model of myogenic autoregulation and the cerebrovascular bed: the effects of altering systemic arterial pressure. Neurosurgery 1983; 13(5):482–98.
[74] Pettorossi V, Di Rocci C, Mancinelli R, et al. Communicating hydrocephalus induced by mechanically increased amplitude of the intraventricular cerebrospinal fluid pulse pressure; rationale and method. Exp Neurol 1978;59:30–9.
[75] Bering RJ, Salibi B. Production of hydrocephalus by increased cephalic-venous pressure. Arch Neurol Psychiatry 1959;81:693–8.

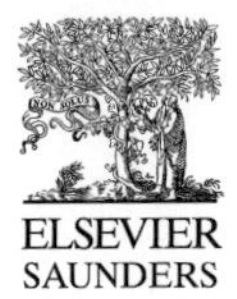

ELSEVIER
SAUNDERS

Neurol Clin 25 (2007) 833–842

NEUROLOGIC
CLINICS

Prion Disease

Eric Eggenberger, DO, FAAN

Department of Neurology and Ophthalmology, Michigan State University, A217 Clinical Center, 138 Service, East Lansing, MI 48824, USA

Transmissible spongiform encephalopathies are a unique category of diseases related to abnormalities in the prion protein. These diseases affect animal and human hosts, produce neurologic symptoms, and uniformly are fatal according to current understanding. They have become the subject of increasing media and popular interest since the emergence of "mad cow disease" (bovine spongiform encephalopathy [BSE]) in 1986 and the related subsequent human consequences in the form of new variant Creutzfeldt-Jakob disease (vCJD) in 1996. Although rare, prion diseases have a well worked-out pathophysiology that may hold lessons applicable to other neurodegenerative conditions.

Biology

The protein-only theory is the main theory regarding the pathophysiology of prion diseases [1]. This theory holds that the exclusive (or primary) agent in Creutzfeldt-Jakob disease (CJD) is the abnormal prion protein form and that this agent acts in an "auto"-enzymatic fashion to convert normal host prion into the abnormal isoform. Although prior protein cellular (PrP^C) and the abnormal protease resistant scrapie form of PrP (PrP^{Sc}) have identical amino acid sequences (chemically identical), PrP^{Sc} is distinguished from PrP^C by several characteristics: unique 3-D conformational structure, enhanced stability, greater hydrophobic character, protease resistance, insolubility after detergent extraction, deposition in lysosomes, posttranslational synthesis, and polymerization into rod-like structures with the characteristics of amyloid. Prions are resistant to normal sterilization methods, organic solvents, formalin fixation, irradiation, and heat; however, prions are inactivated by exposure to hypochlorite solutions or by prolonged high-temperature sterilization. Procedures that normally denature protein may diminish but not eliminate infectivity completely.

E-mail address: eeggenberger@yahoo.com

doi:10.1016/j.ncl.2007.03.006 *neurologic.theclinics.com*

Species barrier and strains

Different strains of CJD can be distinguished by differences in incubation times, clinical manifestations, transmissibility, and pathology (pattern of vacuolation and PrP accumulation) when tested in experimental animals. The different strains of PrP demonstrate varying degrees of "infectivity"; this strain difference accounts for a degree of the species barrier, whereby PrP^{sc} from one species is more difficult to inoculate successfully into a different species. Greater homology between the abnormal prion and the native prion is associated with greater chances of successful transmission and disease development; nonetheless, there probably is no absolute species barrier when taking dose, route, and host genome factors into account. Strain specificity may be related to prion conformation in addition to route of inoculation, glycoform ratios, aggregation state, and degree of protease resistance. Different classification schema of prion protein strains have been proposed based on the configuration of the protein (as detected by the remnants of PrP postproteinase digestion) and the clinical characteristic caused by that PrP.

Animal prion diseases

Scrapie, a disease of goats and sheep first recognized in the 1700s, is perhaps the most common animal prion disease. Scrapie occurs in most regions throughout the world and is endemic in several countries, including France and the United Kingdom. This disease causes incoordination, twitching, irritability, and pruritis, often so intense that animals literally may scrape their fur and skin off by itching, hence the name, "scrapie." The disease ultimately produces paralysis and death. Although the disease first was shown to be transmissible in 1936 by Cuille and Chelle [2], the majority of cases of scrapie seem to result from genetic defects, but oral transmission is well known. Other animal prion diseases include chronic wasting disease of elk and deer (Western states and Canada), transmissible mink encephalopathy, and many more.

BSE, or mad cow disease, focused world attention on prion diseases. BSE is characterized by insidious onset of incoordination and apprehension, and was described first in 1986 in Great Britain. The source of the disease was traced to a bovine food supplement derived from meat and bone meal prepared from dead sheep and cattle by a modified rendering process. Rendering previously had included prolonged, high-temperature solvent exposure and superheated steam; however, the process was changed to exclude these steps in the late 1970s and consequently did not attenuate the prion agent, presumably because the tissue no longer was exposed to prolonged, high temperatures. The altered rendering process was banned by the British government in 1988, and subsequent regulations prohibited ruminants from entering animal feed ("neocannibalism"). More than 150,000 cattle and approximately 50% of British herds were affected by BSE, which peaked in 1992. The human consequences of BSE subsequently became evident when BSE was linked to the emergence of vCJD.

Human prion diseases

Human prion diseases take sporadic, iatrogenic, and genetic forms. Most cases of CJD are sporadic (sCJD), whereas approximately 15% are inherited in an autosomal-dominant fashion, and less than 2% of cases currently are transmitted iatrogenically. The genetic forms include Gerstmann-Straüssler-Schenker disease and fatal familial insomnia (these are not discussed further in this article).

Kuru

Kuru (from the Fore word for "shiver") occurs among the Fore highlanders of Papua New Guinea. Kuru affected persons primarily between the ages of 5 and 60 years, with an equal gender ratio among preadolescents but a striking excess in female adults. The disease uniformly is fatal after an average duration of 12 months.

Kuru once was the most common cause of death among Fore women; however, the number of deaths per year related to Kuru has declined steadily since the 1950s, and there have been fewer than 15 deaths from Kuru per year since 1985. This decline in Kuru incidence is attributable to the cessation of ritual cannibalism—the consumption of dead kinsmen that was practiced as a rite of mourning, primarily by women and small children. No one born since cannibalism ceased in a given village has died of kuru [3]. Field surveillance among the Fore tribes has documented 11 cases of Kuru occurring between 1996 and 2004. All the victims were born before the late 1950s, and 8 of 10 were heterozygous at the codon 129. The investigators calculated the minimal incubation as 34 to 41 years, and the "likely" incubation as 39 to 56 (±7 years). This data fits with the hypothesis that intraspecies transmission with codon 129 heterogeneous status occurs late and that cross-species transmission with codon 129 heterogeneous status occurs even later [4]. The disease seems to be transmissible orally and by peripheral inoculation but not through casual contact. Kuru produces rapidly progressive cerebellar dysfunction with cortical and brainstem symptoms after an insidious onset The ataxia is associated with a shivering tremor (accounting for the Fore name of the disease) that affects the head, trunk, and legs more than the arms. Extrapyramidal and cerebellar signs worsen gradually until patients are unable to ambulate or even move without disabling ataxic tremors; this is accompanied by decline in mentation and behavior, ultimately producing severe dementia and dysphagia and dysarthria. Patients eventually die of inanition, pneumonia, or respiratory failure 3 to 24 months after onset of symptoms.

Creutzfeldt-Jakob disease

In the 1920s, H.G. Creutzfeldt published the case of a 22-year-old woman who had dementia, tremor, spasticity, and startle myoclonus, and Alfons Maria Jakob published "About Peculiar Diseases of the Central Nervous System with Remarkable Anatomical Findings" [5,6]. Pathology from these cases suggests that Creutzfeldt's patient (1920) was atypical, whereas two of Jakob's cases satisfied modern-era CJD criteria [7]; however, the CJD moniker remains engrained in the literature.

Gajdusek and colleagues [8] transmitted the disease to chimps via intracerebral inoculation of a human brain homogenate, with later investigators demonstrating transmissibility from humans to nonhuman primates and other animals.

Epidemiology

The events leading to sCJD remain an enigma. sCJD occurs throughout the world with a prevalence, annual incidence, and yearly mortality rate of 0.5 to1 per million. There is no gender predilection, and most cases occur between the ages of 55 and 75 (mean 61.5 years) [9].

Genetic polymorphisms

The PRNP gene is highly conserved but has two common polymorphisms (codons 129 and 219). The codon 129 position of PRNP gene is the site of an important polymorphism with either methionine (Met) or valine (Val) and seems to be a primary determinant of prion susceptibility [10]. Windl and colleagues [11] calculated the sCJD relative risk among the three genotypes (Met-Met, Val-Val, or Met-Val) as 11:4:1 for the Met/Met:Val/Val:Met/Val genotypes (Table 1).

Genetic Creutzfeldt-Jakob disease

Approximately 15% of cases of CJD are familial and associated with several different mutations of various codons on chromosome 20, including point mutations and insertion repeats between codons 51 and 91 (the open reading frame) of the PRNP gene. Each mutation is associated with

Table 1
Codon 129 status in Creutzfeldt-Jakob disease and controls

Codon 129 status	Caucasian	Creutzfeldt-Jakob disease	Relative risk
Val homo	11%	92%–95%	4
Met homo	38%		11
Val/met hetero	51%	—	1

an approximately 1-million–fold increase in the probability of a configurational change to the pathologic form, PrP^{Sc}.

Iatrogenic Creutzfeldt-Jakob disease

Iatrogenic CJD first was reported in 1974 in a patient who had received a corneal transplant; in addition to corneal tissue, the disease can be transmitted through postmortem pituitary tissue (used for extraction of human growth hormone [HGH] or gonadotropins), cadaveric dural or other grafts, and inadequately sterilized neurosurgical instruments.

HGH-related and other iatrogenic CJD acquired through a peripheral route usually present with progressive ataxia and later dementia; this contrasts to CJD acquired centrally (eg, contaminated neurosurgical instruments or electroencephalographic [EEG] electrodes) that usually presents with cognitive decline. In a study of HGH-derived CJD, ataxia was a presenting feature in 94% [12]. Myoclonic jerks were present in 82% of patients. EEG generally was not useful in making the diagnosis; pseudoperiodic bursts were present in only nine patients, and classic triphasic waves were noted in only two patients.

Clinical: sporadic Creutzfeldt-Jakob disease

sCJD usually is insidious in onset with a nonspecific prodrome in approximately one third of patients (asthenia, anxiety, changes in sleep pattern, anorexia, weight loss, fatigue, dizziness, vague difficulties with memory, changes in mood or behavior, weakness, or problems with locomotion). During this time, patients typically develop increasing difficulties with higher-order mental functioning, including problems with calculation, abstract thought, memory, reasoning, and judgment; subsequent progressive aphasia, apraxia, pyramidal signs, myoclonus, and choreiform-athetoid movements often intervene. The Heidenhain variant of CJD is characterized by a visual presentation, most commonly a homonymous visual field defect leading to cerebral blindness early in the course of the disease. MRI typically shows hyperintensity on diffusion-weighted imaging (DWI) within the parietal-occipital cortex. The initial EEG often is normal; however, EEG abnormalities emerge in almost all patients who have this form of CJD. The classic clinical triad of dementia, typical EEG changes, and myoclonus are components of the current diagnostic criteria (discussed later). Patients become severely demented within 6 months, with death usually within 12 months of the onset of symptoms, typically resulting from intercurrent infection [13].

Diagnosis

The diagnosis of sCJD often is difficult, especially early, and the differential diagnosis includes such varied disorders as Alzheimer's disease, paraneoplastic conditions, stroke, or encephalopathy. EEG, MRI, and cerebrospinal fluid (CSF) analysis are the most helpful investigatory tests.

Classic EEG changes with pseudoperiodic discharges are present in approximately 70% of patients who have sCJD but may require 3 months to develop. MRI findings usually appear as bilateral increased signal intensity in the basal ganglia, corpus striatum, or thalamus, visualized best on DWI, and are less evident on fluid-attenuated inversion recovery (FLAIR) or T2-weighted scans (Fig. 1) [14]. Approximately two thirds of patients who have CJD exhibit basal ganglia MRI hyperintensity [15], although advances in imaging protocols likely will increase this figure. The MRI findings of basal ganglia hyperintensity in an appropriate clinical setting is relatively specific for CJD. vCJD exhibits a distinct and specific pattern of MRI abnormality, with approximately 80% of patients demonstrating prominent high signal in the posterior thalamus (pulvinar sign); this is part of current vCJD diagnostic criteria [16]. CSF routine analysis may demonstrate minimal pleocytosis (<10 cells/mL) but otherwise is normal. The 14-3-3 protein is a sensitive and useful surrogate marker of relatively rapid and extensive neuronal damage. CSF 14-3-3 protein elevation is a sensitive maker of prion disease but also occurs in several other conditions, such as cerebral infarction, neoplasm, inflammation, and paraneoplastic disorders, or post seizures, mandating incorporation of the clinical circumstances in interpretation. Several studies have demonstrated the usefulness of the 14-3-3 marker in the diagnosis of sCJD. Occasionally, repeat CSF analysis more than 2 weeks separated from the initial lumbar puncture is helpful, demonstrating increasing 14-3-3 levels in CJD compared with other acute events associated with an elevated 14-3-3 level (Table 2) [15,17].

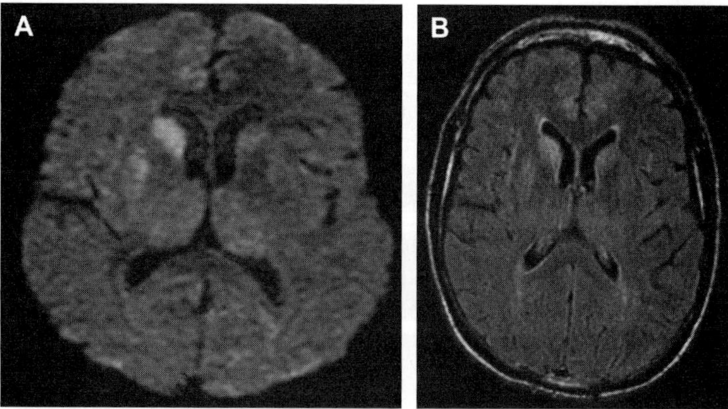

Fig. 1. Diffusion-weighted MRI (*left*) and FLAIR MRI (*right*) sequences demonstrate increased signal in the caudate and lenticular nuclei (right greater than left) in a case of CJD. (*Courtesy of* Neill R. Graff-Radford, MD, Jacksonville, FL.)

Table 2
CSF 14-3-3 abnormality by prion disease state

Disease	n positive/N total	Percentage
CJD (path confirmed)	311/329	95%
Iatrogenic	6/10	60%
Genetic	35/57	61%
vCJD	5/11	45%

From Zerr I, Pocchiari M, Collins S. Analysis of EEG and CSF 14-3-3 proteins as aids to the diagnosis of Creutzfeldt-Jakob disease. Neurology 2000;55(6):811–5; with permission.

Clinical criteria of sporadic Creutzfeldt-Jakob disease

1. Progressive dementia and
2. At least two of the following four:
   A. Myoclonus
   B. Visual or cerebellar signs or symptoms
   C. Pyramidal or extrapyramidal signs or symptoms
   D. Akinetic mutism

Probable CJD is defined by these criteria and periodic slow wave complexes in EEG or 14-3-3 CSF protein in patients who have disease duration for less than 2 years. Possible CJD is defined by these criteria and the absence of EEG or CSF changes.

Variant Creutzfeldt-Jakob disease

In 1995, a new and distinct variation of human CJD emerged in the United Kingdom known as vCJD. Several features contributed to its distinct clinical picture, including appearance in younger patients than in traditional CJD and initial prominent psychiatric symptoms. The disease has been linked convincingly to BSE, although the exact mechanism of transmission remains enigmatic; one theory speculates that human exposure to high concentrations of BSE-contaminated products in the late 1980s led to the BSE prion agent crossing the species barrier into humans, producing the vCJD epidemic.

The average age at onset in vCJD is 29 years, contrasting to the sCJD average age of 65 years. vCJD typically presents with psychiatric symptoms, with later emergence of more typical CJD features, such as ataxia, dementia, and involuntary movements (dystonia, myoclonus, or chorea) approximately 6 months post onset. Death occurs after a median duration of 13 months (compared with approximately 4 months in sCJD). In contrast to sCJD, vCJD may be blood transmissible. There are three documented cases of transfusion-related transmission in vCJD in the "Transfusion Medicine Epidemiological Review" (United Kingdom) [18]. The blood recipients developed vCJD symptoms 6.5 and 7.8 years after transfusion from vCJD donor in two cases, whereas the third recipient had no symptoms of vCJD, but vCJD-related prion evidence was discovered in lymph nodes on autopsy examination (the patient died of unrelated causes). The symptoms in the donors occurred 18 to 40 months pretransfusion [19].

As of September 2006, a total of 156 cases of vCJD have been recorded, all in patients who have codon 129 Met-Met homozygous status. Although some early trend data suggests the disease may have peaked, models vary widely on this point, and it is possible that a second peak will emerge related to transfusions or in codon 129 heterozygous subjects.

Current World Health Organization criteria for vCJD diagnosis include

I. A. Progressive psychiatric disorder
   B. Duration greater than 6 months
   C. Routine investigations that do not suggest alternative diagnosis
   D. No history of iatrogenic exposure
   E. No evidence of familial prion disease
II. A. Early psychiatric symptoms
   B. Persistent painful sensory symptoms
   C. Ataxia
   D. Myoclonus, chorea, or dystonia
   E. Dementia
III. A. EEG without typical periodic slow wave changes
   B. Bilateral pulvinar high signal on MRI
IV. A. positive tonsillar biopsy

Definite diagnosis of vCJD requires IA and neuropathologic confirmation; probable diagnosis requires I and 4 of 5 of II and IIIA and IIIB, or I and IVA, and possible diagnosis consists of I and 4 of 5 of II and IIIA [20].

Therapy

In order for a prion therapy to be useful, an agent would have to be effective against prion accumulation or pathophysiology, be delivered to the required sites in a timely manner, and be tolerable. This is challenging because there is evidence that significant CNS damage and PrP accumulation occur long before clinical signs and symptoms develop, and current diagnostic testing does not reliably allow early or presymptomatic diagnosis. The limited knowledge about the variety of prion diseases and strains and the exact pathophysiology of the prion agent are additional hurdles in the investigation of treatments. Prophylactic therapy in high-risk populations (eg, prion genetic aberrations or recipients of contaminated materials) may be the earliest application for any prion therapy, but this represents a limited number of cases.

Prion in context

Prion diseases are a serious condition, albeit rare. They have been covered extensively by the media, and mad cow disease has become a common lay term. Despite the dire consequences of individual prion diseases, they have not emerged as a serious population threat. This paradigm perhaps is addressed best through the philosophy of risk assessment pioneered by Peter Sandman, which hypothesizes that risk assessment is based on the actual hazard of the condition and the level of perceived "outrage" concerning the issue [21]; prions do not represent a widespread hazard (although they are hazardous in the rare patients so afflicted), but the degree of outrage drives the public's perceived risk.

Summary

Prions are an important and fatal group of neurologic animal and human diseases. The protein-only pathophysiology theory seems to be unique in medical diseases but may find parallels in other conditions. The BSE and vCJD epidemics have taught us important lessons about the food chain. Although knowledge of prions has grown tremendously in the past 2 decades, this has not translated into prophylactic or therapeutic measures, and much about basic prion biology remains enigmatic.

References

[1] Prusiner SB. Novel proteinaceous infectious particles cause scrapie. Science 1982;216(4542): 136–44.
[2] Cuillé J, Chelle P-L. La maladie dite "tremblante" du mouton est-elle inoculable? Compte Rend Acad Sci 1936;203:1552.
[3] Liberski PP, Gajdusek DC. Kuru: forty years later, a historical note. Brain Pathol 1997;7(1): 555–60.
[4] Collinge J, Whitfield J, McKintosh E, et al. Kuru in the 21st century—an acquired human prion disease with very long incubation periods. Lancet 2006;367(9528):2068–74.
[5] Creutzfeldt H. Über eine eigenartige Erkrankung des Zentralnervensystems. In: Nissl F, Alzheimer A, editors. Histologische und Histopathologische Arbeiten über die Grosshirnrinde. Berlin: Springer; 1921 [in German].
[6] Jakob A. Über eigenartige Erkrankungen des Zentralnervensystems mit bemerkenswerten anatomischen Befunde (spastische Pseudosklerose Encephalomyelopathie mit disseminierten Degenerationsherden). Z Gesamte Neurol Psychiatr 1921;64:147–228 [in German].
[7] Richardson EP, Masters CL. The nosology of Creutzfeldt-Jakob Disease and conditions related to the accumulation of PrP^{CJD} in the nervous system. Brain Pathol 1995;5:33–41.
[8] Gajdusek DC, Gibbs CJ, Alpers M. Experimental transmission of a kuru-like syndrome to chimpanzees. National Institute of Neurological Diseases and Blindness, National Institutes of Health, Bethesda, Maryland. Nature 1966;209(5025):794–6.
[9] Ironside JW. Review: Creutzfeldt-Jakob disease. Brain Pathol 1996;6(4):379–88.
[10] Prusiner SB, Hsiao KK. Human prion diseases. Ann Neurol 1994;35:385–95.
[11] Windl O, Dempster M, Estibeiro JP, et al. Genetic basis of Creutzfeldt-Jakob disease in the United Kingdom: a systematic analysis of predisposing mutations and allelic variation in the PRNP gene. Hum Genet 1996;98:259–64.

[12] Billette de Villemeur T, Deslys JP, Pradel A, et al. Creutzfeldt-Jakob disease from contaminated growth hormone extracts in France. Neurology 1996;47(3):690–5.
[13] Brown P, Cathala F, Castaigne P, et al. Creutzfeldt-Jakob disease: clinical analysis of a consecutive series of 230 neuropathologically verified cases. Ann Neurol 1986;20(5):597–602.
[14] Collie DA, Sellar RJ, Zeidler M, et al. MRI of Creutzfeldt-Jakob disease: imaging features and recommended MRI protocol. Clin Radiol 2001;56(9):726–39.
[15] Zerr I, Poser S. Clinical diagnosis and differential diagnosis of CJD and vCJD. With special emphasis on laboratory tests. APMIS 2002;110(1):88–98.
[16] Zeidler M, Sellar RJ, Collie DA, et al. The pulvinar sign on magnetic resonance imaging in variant Creutzfeldt-Jakob disease. Lancet 2000;355(9213):1412–8.
[17] Zerr I, Pocchiari M, Collins S, et al. Analysis of EEG and CSF 14-3-3 proteins as aids to the diagnosis of Creutzfeldt-Jakob disease. Neurology 2000;55(6):811–5.
[18] Transfusion Medicine Epidemiological Review. United Kingdom. Available at: http://www.cjd.ed.ac.uk/TMER/TMER.htm.
[19] Hewitt PE, Llewelyn CA, Mackenzie J, et al. Three reported cases of variant Creutzfeldt–Jakob disease transmission following transfusion of labile blood components. Vox Sang 2006;91(4):348.
[20] Will RG, Zeidler M, Stewart GE, et al. Diagnosis of new variant Creutzfeldt-Jakob disease. Ann Neurol 2000;47(5):575–82.
[21] Available at: http://www.psandman.com/articles/facing.htm. Accessed June 12, 2007.

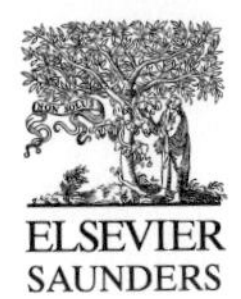

ELSEVIER
SAUNDERS

Neurol Clin 25 (2007) 843–857

NEUROLOGIC
CLINICS

Neuroimaging in Dementia

Jennifer L. Whitwell, PhD*, Clifford R. Jack, Jr, MD

Department of Radiology, Mayo Clinic, 200 1st Street SW, Rochester, MN 55905, USA

Structural neuroimaging

The traditional role of structural imaging is to identify structural and potentially treatable causes of cognitive impairment, for example brain tumors, hydrocephalus, and subdural haematomas. X-ray CT and MRI scanning detect most of these pathologies. Structural imaging also increasingly has been recognized as an important tool in the diagnosis of degenerative dementias. A CT or MRI scan has become a routine part of the clinical workup to aid in differential diagnosis. Recommendations from the American Academy of Neurology are that at least one structural scan be performed in all patients who have dementia. CT scans are widely available, cheap, relatively rapid, and appropriate for patients who present acutely with impaired cognition or an acute decline from a previous level. The improved tissue contrast and the ability to detect focal temporal lobe abnormalities, however, mean MRI has several advantages in evaluating brain structures and is more appropriate for nonemergent evaluation. MRI also avoids ionizing radiation. Hence, MRI is one of the most widely used imaging techniques in the assessment of the degenerative dementias.

Different patterns of atrophy can be identified on visual inspection of MRI in different neurodegenerative conditions. Alzheimer's disease (AD) is the most common neurodegenerative disorder, affecting approximately 4.5 million people in the United States, and, therefore, has received the most attention. Patients who have AD often show patterns of cerebral atrophy involving the medial temporal lobe, in particular the hippocampus and entorhinal cortex, and the posterior cingulate, precuneus, and the temporoparietal association neocortex, with concurrent expansion of the ventricles. There is a relative sparing of the sensorimotor cortex, visual cortex, and cerebellum. The first structural changes seem to occur in the

* Corresponding author.
E-mail address: whitwell.jennifer@mayo.edu (J.L. Whitwell).

0733-8619/07/$ - see front matter
doi:10.1016/j.ncl.2007.03.003 *neurologic.theclinics.com*

medial temporal lobe, with early volume loss of the hippocampus and entorhinal cortex (Fig. 1). This matches the progression of neurofibrillary pathology in AD, which starts in the entorhinal cortex and medial temporal lobe, before spreading to other limbic areas and out into the neocortex. Visual qualitative rating scales have been developed for the medial temporal lobe, which are quick and easy to apply in clinical practice. These assessments can differentiate patients who have AD from controls with a sensitivity ranging from 40% to 95% and a specificity of 90% [1]. More specific measurements of medial temporal structures also have been performed, particularly of the hippocampus and entorhinal cortex, which again have shown good separation of patients who have AD from controls. Hippocampal atrophy is shown to be a sensitive marker to pathologic AD stage and consequent cognitive status [2]. Medial temporal lobe atrophy is not specific to AD, however, and is seen commonly in other dementias, which limits its usefulness for differential diagnosis of AD. In addition, although the presence of medial temporal atrophy makes the diagnosis of AD more likely, the absence of atrophy does not exclude the diagnosis.

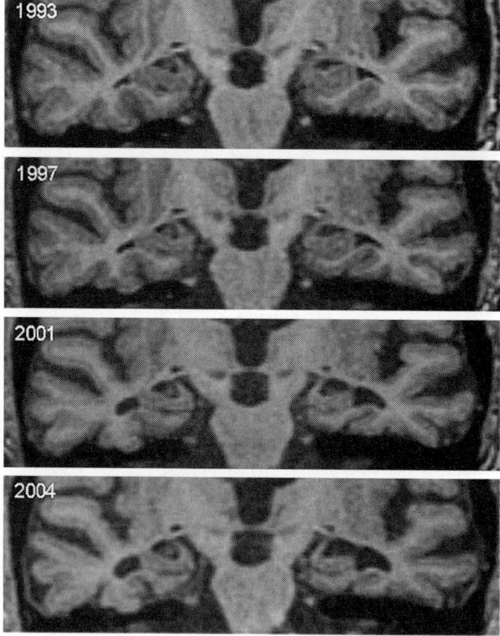

Fig. 1. Serial MRI sections showing progressive atrophy of the hippocampus throughout the disease course in a patient who began normal and then progressed to a diagnosis of AD. The patient clinically was normal in 1993, diagnosed with MCI in 1997, and then diagnosed with AD in 2001. Note the progressive atrophy of the hippocampus and widening of the temporal horn of the lateral ventricle.

Automated assessment techniques also have been used recently to investigate patterns of cerebral atrophy on MRI in AD and other dementias. One of the most common techniques is voxel-based morphometry (VBM), which compares groups of patients and identifies differences in the patterns of cerebral atrophy across the whole brain. This has advantages over region-of-interest based techniques in that it does not require any a priori decisions concerning which structures to assess and can provide more detailed information about cortical changes. VBM studies show that although the regions of greatest loss occur most often in the medial temporal lobe, there also is extensive atrophy throughout the temporal lobe, parietal lobe, posterior cingulate and precuneus, insula, temporoparietal association neocortex, and prefrontal gyri in subjects who have a clinical diagnosis of AD compared with controls (Fig. 2) [3]. Structures in the central gray matter also are

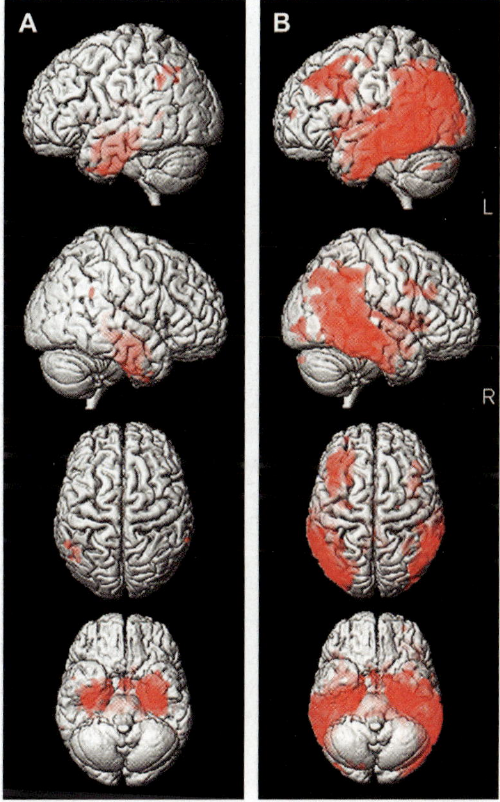

Fig. 2. 3-D surface renders generated using VBM showing regions of gray matter loss in groups of patients who had amnestic MCI (*A*) or AD (*B*) compared with a group of controls. Notice the relatively restricted patterns of loss in the anteromedial temporal lobes in MCI compared with a more widespread pattern of loss affecting the temporoparietal association neocortex in AD.

involved, including the caudate, putamen, thalamus, and hypothalamus. VBM studies show a difference in the patterns of atrophy in patients who have an early ($\leq$65 years) versus late ($>$65-year) disease onset. Patients who have late onset tend to show a pattern of loss relatively restricted to the medial temporal lobes, whereas patients who have early onset show a more widespread pattern of atrophy involving the temporoparietal association neocortex, precuneus, and frontal lobes [4]. This technique, therefore, provides useful information about the disease process. It is a tool designed primarily for group level studies, however. Although it has been applied to assess patterns of atrophy in single patients, it has not yet been optimized fully for single-patient comparisons. Once these optimizations have occurred, VBM could be a powerful tool in the differential diagnosis of individual patients.

Hippocampal atrophy also is shown to occur several years before patients are diagnosed with AD [5]. Patterns similar to those observed in AD also are present in patients who have mild cognitive impairment (MCI). This syndrome is considered a transitional period between normal ageing and a diagnosis of AD, with patients showing early deficits in memory but not fulfilling criteria for dementia. These patients show atrophy of the medial temporal lobe structures, usually at a level intermediate between those of controls and AD (see Fig. 1). Patients who have MCI and are at greater genetic risk have smaller hippocampal volumes [6], and atrophy of hippocampus and amygdala can predict progression to dementia in cognitively intact elderly individuals and in patients who have MCI [7], although the overlap is too large to have a prognostic value in individual patients.

Structural MRI also can help in the differential diagnosis of AD from other neurodegenerative dementias, especially frontotemporal lobar degeneration (FTLD). There is some overlap in the clinical features of the two dementias, which increases the importance of imaging in the clinical assessment. Patients who have FTLD show more severe atrophy in the frontal lobe and anterior temporal poles than patients who have AD, with little involvement of the temporoparietal association neocortex. This anterior-posterior gradient of atrophy in the brains of patients who have FTLD can help distinguish them from subjects with AD, who show a more posterior bias [8]. Asymmetry also is a common feature that is relatively specific to FTLD and can be useful diagnostically. FTLD can be divided into several different syndromic variants that show different, although overlapping, patterns of atrophy [9,10]. The behavioral variant of frontotemporal dementia (bvFTD) presents with early behavioral abnormalities and is associated with atrophy of the frontal and temporal lobes, although the frontal lobes often show the greatest loss. In contrast, the other two variants present with early language deficits. Patients who have semantic dementia present with a loss of memory for words and show a well-defined pattern of atrophy affecting the anterior temporal lobes most predominantly (Fig. 3) [11]. The patterns often are asymmetric, affecting the left temporal lobe in particular, although the right temporal lobes also

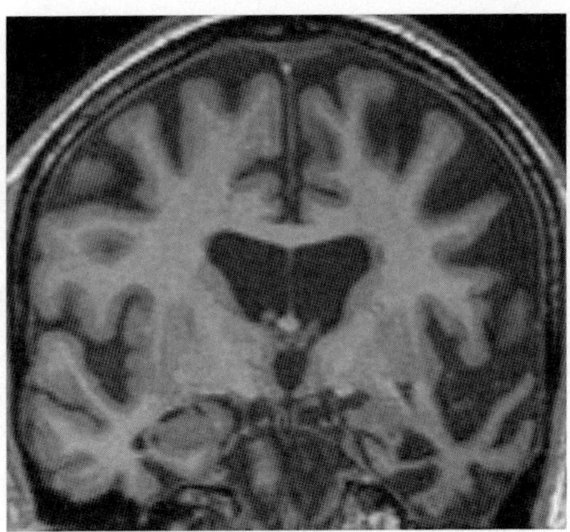

Fig. 3. Coronal MRI section through the brain of a subject who had semantic dementia. Note the severe atrophy of the left temporal lobe and the left frontal gyri.

can show the brunt of the loss. The patterns observed in progressive nonfluent aphasia, the other language variant, are more variable but generally involve almost exclusively the left hemisphere, in particular the regions of the brain surrounding the perisylvian fissure, including the inferior frontal lobe and insula [10].

The patterns of atrophy present in patients who have dementia with Lewy bodies (DLB) are not as well established and visual inspection of individual magnetic resonance scans for a specific atrophy pattern typically is not used to aid clinical diagnosis of DLB. Some group studies have shown patterns of atrophy similar to those observed in AD, although others have observed a more focal pattern of loss in the basal forebrain in DLB. Patients who have DLB do seem to show less atrophy of the medial temporal lobe, which may prove diagnostically useful [12]. Imaging, however, is necessary for the diagnosis of vascular dementia (VaD) [12]. MRI, in particular, is more sensitive to vascular changes than CT, especially in subcortical regions. The features characteristic of VaD include cortical infarctions, lacunar infarctions, and diffuse white matter hyperintensities, also known as leukariosis, that appear bright on a T2-weighted or fluid-attenuated inversion recovery (FLAIR) sequence and reflect regions of demyelination and enlargement of perivascular spaces (Fig. 4). Although the presence of lacunar infarctions and white matter hyperintensities defines VaD, they also often are present, although to a lesser degree, in healthy elderly controls and in patients who have AD and FTLD. The presence of high signal abnormalities themselves, therefore, is not particularly diagnostically useful, and can correctly classify only 42% of patients who have VaD on visual inspection [13]. Cerebral atrophy does occur in patients who have VaD, although not to the same degree as brain losses in AD. No specific patterns of atrophy have been observed, with mild losses

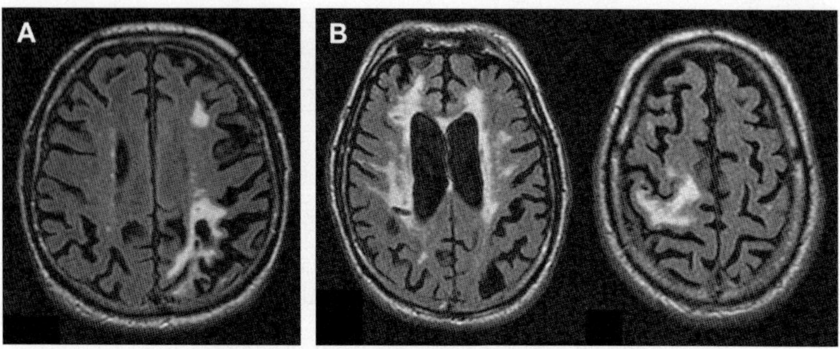

Fig. 4. Axial sections through FLAIR images from (*A*) a patient who had VaD showing multiple cortical infarctions, and (*B*) a patient who had VaD showing extensive white matter disease (*left*) and a large cortical infarction (*right*).

reported in the frontal, lateral temporal, medial temporal, and parietal lobes [14]. Characteristic imaging features also can be identified in patients who have Creutzfeldt-Jakob disease. Increased signal intensity often is observed bilaterally in the basal ganglia and cortical ribbon on a FLAIR sequence (Fig. 5).

There is increasing interest in studying change in the brain over multiple serial MRI scans in patients who have dementia. Rates of atrophy can be calculated from pairs of scans that have been matched positionally or registered. There is some evidence that rates of cerebral atrophy may aid in the differentiation of different neurodegenerative dementias [15]. Rates of cerebral atrophy in AD are reported in the range of 1.5% to 3% per year, with rates of hippocampal atrophy approximately 4% to 6% per year. Rates of hippocampal atrophy can differentiate AD from controls with a high sensitivity and specificity and have a greater discriminatory power than baseline volumes [16]. There also is evidence that high rates of atrophy in patients who have MCI help predict conversion to AD [17]. Although these

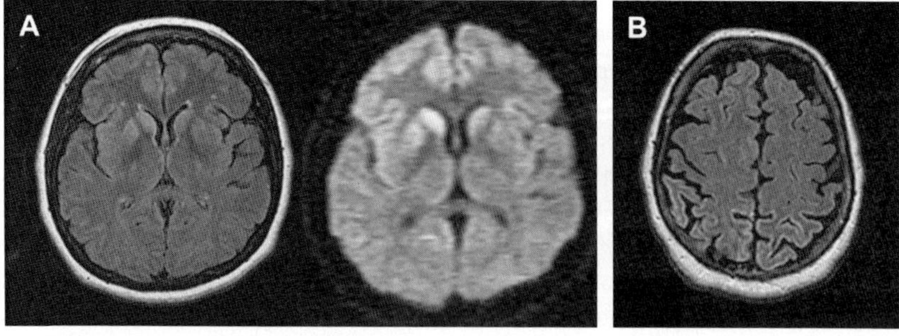

Fig. 5. Images from subjects who had Creutzfeldt-Jakob disease showing (*A*) increased signal in the basal ganglia on FLAIR and DWI sequences and (*B*) increased signal in the cortical ribbon on FLAIR.

techniques currently are not used in clinical practice, the procedures are relatively simple and could be applied if the technique was made easy to use and automated. Rates of whole brain and regional atrophy increasingly are incorporated into clinical drug trials as one of the primary outcome measures. More complex registration methods also have been developed that can provide detailed information concerning exactly where in the brain change has occurred over time. These techniques show widespread patterns of tissue loss in the temporal and parietal lobes, with a relative sparing of the sensorimotor cortices, over time in patients who have AD [18,19]. These techniques are not widely available, however they are automated, would be relatively easy to apply in a clinical setting, and would provide invaluable diagnostic information about the progression of brain atrophy in individual patients.

Functional nuclear medicine

In contrast to structural imaging, functional nuclear medicine techniques measure glucose uptake or cerebral blood flow. It is hypothesized that functional losses may precede structural changes in the brain and, therefore, may provide more sensitive markers of early disease progression. There are two main techniques that this article considers. F18-fluorodeoxyglucose–positron emission tomography (FDG-PET) measures the local cerebral metabolic rate of glucose uptake. In contrast, single photon emission CT (SPECT) measures blood flow alterations, or perfusion. Both techniques require the injection of radioactive tracers. Imaging using PET has a higher sensitivity and greater spatial resolution than SPECT. The Centers for Medicare and Medicaid Services have approved FDG-PET imaging as a routine examination tool for the early and differential diagnosis of AD specifically to differentiate AD from FTLD. This was based on evidence showing that adding PET to a clinical examination increases diagnostic sensitivity in AD.

It is well established that by the time a patient presents with clinical dementia symptoms, a reduction in glucose uptake already has occurred. FDG-PET shows a pattern of abnormally low uptake in the posterior cingulate, precuneus, temporoparietal regions, and frontal cortex in AD when compared with controls (Fig. 6). Hypometabolism also can be observed in the medial temporal lobe [20]. These patterns can differentiate patients who have pathologically confirmed AD from controls with sensitivities and specificities of approximately 86%, although they are as high as 100% in some studies [21]. Similar patterns of hypoperfusion have been identified on SPECT in patients who have AD, although it has been shown that PET provides better differentiation between AD and control patients.

FDG-PET also can detect very early changes in uptake. Reports of patients at increased risk for AD, either because of family history or genetic susceptibility, show reductions in glucose uptake before the onset of clinical

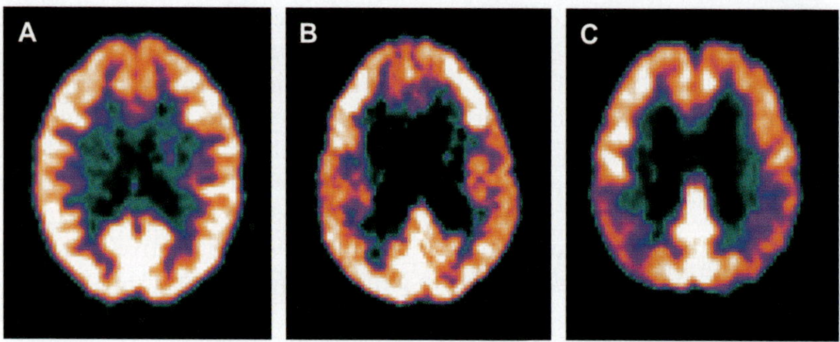

Fig. 6. FDG-PET images from a healthy control (*A*), a patient who had MCI (*B*), and a patient who had AD (*C*).

symptoms [22]. Studies in MCI show medial temporal and temporoparietal hypometabolism on FDG-PET (see Fig. 6). Visual assessments of the medial temporal lobe can distinguish patients who have MCI from controls at a sensitivity of 77% and a specificity of 71% [20]. Temporoparietal hypometabolism in MCI also is shown to predict conversion to AD with an accuracy of 75% to 100% [21]. Hypoperfusion has been demonstrated in patients who have MCI on SPECT, particularly in the posterior cingulate, although only minor changes can be observed on visual inspection.

A significant value of PET is expected to be in the differential diagnosis of AD and other neurodegenerative conditions. The patterns of metabolic and perfusion abnormalities in AD are different from those observed in patients who have FTD, which show early and more severe frontal and anterior/mesial temporal hypometabolism and increased perfusion [23,24]. These patterns often are asymmetric in patients who have FTLD [14]. The signal of decreased perfusion in the posterior cingulate that is useful in the diagnosis of AD is not present in FTLD on SPECT [25]. There also is some evidence that the different syndromic variants of FTLD show different patterns of hypometabolism and hypoperfusion. There are some trends for left inferior frontal changes in progressive nonfluent aphasia [26], left anterior temporal changes in semantic dementia, and frontal lobe changes in bvFTD [27], although there is considerable overlap between the different variants and the value of these trends in differential diagnosis is unknown. The patterns of hypometabolism and hypoperfusion observed in patients who have DLB closely mirror those observed in AD, although patients who have DLB seem to have greater reductions in the occipital lobe, particularly in the primary visual cortex, compared with AD [28,29]. Patterns of brain metabolic activity are less well defined for patients who have VaD. Hypometabolism has been observed in cortical regions but also in subcortical regions and the cerebellum, which usually are spared in AD [30], although others have found no characteristic patterns in patients who have VaD.

Functional MRI

Functional MRI (fMRI) uses the paramagnetic properties of oxygenated versus deoxygenated blood to visualize areas of cortex engaged in specific activation tasks. Neural activation causes a proportionately greater increase in regional blood flow than in oxygen consumption. This produces an increase in the local cerebral blood oxygenation level and a decrease in deoxyhemoglobin. The magnetic resonance signal of blood is slightly different depending on the level of oxygenation. The magnitude of the signal difference, however, is too small to be identified on single images; therefore, multiple scans are performed and summed. This technique has higher spatial resolution and is less expensive and invasive than PET; however, at the moment it remains largely a research tool.

Studies show reduced activation in regions, including the medial temporal lobes, during memory tasks in patients who have MCI or AD compared with groups of control subjects [31], reflecting neuronal loss or dysfunction in these regions [32,33]. Differences in activity pattern also are observed between patients who are at risk for AD and those who are not [34,35]. There are suggestions that patients who have FTLD show reduced activation in the frontal lobes and patients who have DLB show reduced activation in the occipital lobes during a variety of cognitive tasks compared with AD. Although most fMRI studies aim to identify areas of increased activation related to specific tasks, several recent studies have identified a network of regions that are more active during periods of mental rest from specific cognitive tasks (ie, the "default network"). Default activation patterns in young adults correspond to regions that show amyloid deposition, atrophy, or hypometabolism on PET [36]. Patients who have AD or MCI show decreased activation in the default network, in regions including the hippocampus, posterior cingulate, and precuneus [37].

^{1}H magnetic resonance spectroscopy

^{1}H magnetic resonance spectroscopy (MRS) is a noninvasive technique that allows assessment of specific brain metabolites. It is unique among diagnostic imaging techniques in that it allows the signals from several different metabolites to be measured within a single measurement period, with each metabolite in turn sensitive to a different aspect of in vivo pathologic processes at the molecular or cellular level. The metabolites measured most commonly include N-acetylaspartate (NAA), which provides a marker of neuronal density; myoinositol (mI), which provides a marker of glial cell activity; and choline (Cho), which is believed to reflect the level of membrane turnover.

It is well established that patients who have AD show a decrease in the level of NAA in several brain regions, including the posterior cingulate, temporal, and parietal and frontal lobes, compared with control subjects. In contrast, the levels of mI increase in patients who have AD. The clinical specificity of the NAA decline is poor, but a decrease in the ratio of the NAA to mI is robust in discriminating patients who have AD from healthy controls. The metabolite changes in patients who have MCI generally are intermediate between normal elderly controls and patients who have AD [38] and can predict the rate at which those patients will progress to AD [39]. Longitudinal studies also show progressive decreases in NAA over time, which seem to correlate to clinical decline in AD [40]. Differences in the profile and regional distribution of metabolites are observed in other dementias, which may aid in the differential diagnosis [41]. Patients who have FTLD show decreased levels of NAA and Cho and increased levels of mI in the frontal lobes, and decreased levels of NAA in the temporal lobes, compared with subjects who have AD [42,43]. In contrast to AD and FTLD, the levels of NAA are not decreased in the gray matter of patients who have DLB; the only difference from controls is in the Cho levels that are elevated [41], probably reflecting the fact that severe cholinergic deficits are a feature of DLB. Patients who have VaD show decreased levels of NAA, as in AD and FTLD, although the mI and Cho levels usually are not elevated [41]. MRS, therefore, could contribute to the differential diagnosis and early detection of AD and monitoring disease progression. Results from serial MRS studies, however, are mixed and need further validation before MRS can be considered a biomarker for disease progression.

Diffusion-weighted imaging

The technique of diffusion-weighted imaging (DWI) allows the measurement of the microscopic random motion of water molecules in the brain. The more modern version of DWI is diffusion tensor imaging. DWI and diffusion tensor imaging produce measures of a variety of features of water diffusion but the two studied most widely are apparent diffusion coefficient (ADC) and fractional anisotropy. Both are scalar parameters. ADC is a measure of diffusion magnitude, whereas fractional anisotropy is an indication of the directionality of water diffusion. Increases occur in ADC and decreases in fractional anisotropy in degenerative brains as a result of an assumed loss or disruption of barriers restricting water motion, such as the membranes of cell bodies, axons, and myelin. Patients who have AD and MCI show elevated ADC in brain regions that typically are involved in AD. In addition, hippocampal diffusivity is greater in patients who have MCI and who convert to dementia compared with those who remain stable and may provide better prediction of rate of conversion than hippocampal volumes measured on MRI [44]. Diffusion-weighted imaging has potential, therefore, to be clinically useful but as with other imaging techniques, it remains purely a research tool at the present time.

Amyloid imaging

A recent major advance in the field of neuroimaging is the development of a technique to image amyloid in the human brain [45]. The presence of amyloid plaques and neurofibrillary tangles are the hallmark pathologic features of AD and are required to give a definite pathologic diagnosis of AD. The ability to identify plaques in living patients has the potential to revolutionize patient diagnosis and management.

Several amyloid-binding compounds have been developed and studied in humans [46–48]. The compound studied the most extensively is Pittsburgh Compound-B (PIB). PIB binds to aggregated fibrillar amyloid-beta deposits with high affinity and can be detected by PET imaging [47]. A robust signal has been identified in patients who have AD that is different from that seen in healthy controls (Fig. 7). In patients who have AD, PIB binding is most prominent in cortical association areas, including the frontal lobes, temporal lobes, parietal lobes, parts of occipital lobe, and striatum [47,49]. Amyloid deposition is found commonly on pathology in all these regions in patients who have AD. Particularly severe binding has been observed in the frontal lobes [47] and precuneus [49], with low levels observed in the sensorimotor strip, primary visual cortex, and medial temporal lobe [49]. An absence of binding has been observed in the cerebellum, pons, and subcortical white matter, areas that do not show amyloid deposition on pathology. These changes are present in practically but not all patients who have clinically evident AD. It is possible that the few patients who do not show PIB retention may have a different underlying cause for their dementia. Similar patterns of retention have been observed in sporadic and familial patients who have AD, although there is some evidence that neostriatal PIB binding is higher

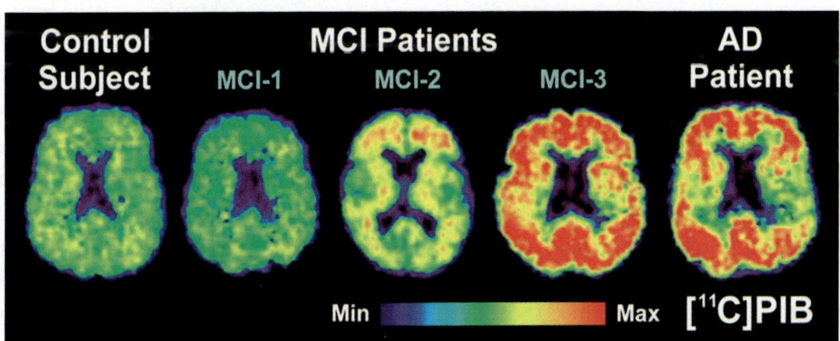

Fig. 7. PET images obtained with the amyloid-imaging agent, [^{11}C]PIB, in a normal control, three different patients who had MCI, and a patient who had mild AD. Some patients who have MCI have control-like levels of amyloid, some have AD-like levels of amyloid, and some have intermediate levels. (*Courtesy of* William Klunk, MD, PhD, Pittsburgh, PA. *Adapted from* Lopresti BJ, Klunk WE, Mathis CA, et al. Simplified quantification of Pittsburgh compound B amyloid imaging PET studies: a comparative analysis. J Nucl Med 2005; 46(12):1967; with permission from the Society of Nuclear Medicine.)

in familial patients. The levels of PIB retention, however, seem stable over time, even in patients who have declined cognitively [50].

In comparison, the majority of healthy controls show little or no retention in cortical areas [47]. Some studies, however, have reported healthy controls who do show positive PIB binding, sometimes at a similar level to that found in AD. This is consistent with the fact that neuropathologic AD is present in some nondemented elderly subjects and may suggest that the pathologic changes of AD can be detected before any clinical evidence of dementia. In support of this hypothesis is neocortical PIB binding that has been observed in presymptomatic subjects who have familial AD. PIB retention seems to vary greatly in MCI, with patients often showing a pattern of binding similar to AD or similar to controls. Patients rarely show intermediate levels of PIB binding (see Fig. 7) [51].

The assessment of PIB imaging also may prove highly useful in the differential diagnosis of dementia, especially in differentiating AD from FTLD. Recent work suggests that no PIB binding is found in patients who have FTLD [52]. A pattern of binding similar to that found in AD is observed in DLB, although it is present in only 89% of patients [52]. This most likely reflects the fact that the majority of DLB patients have concomitant AD pathology.

Therefore, although research in amyloid imaging in humans is in its infancy, it shows huge promise as a sensitive and specific marker of AD amyloid pathology. It has the potential to revolutionize clinical practice and the conduct of clinical trials completely, as a measure of amyloid reduction and as a potential inclusion criterion. It is still important, however, to be cautious, because large studies with long clinical follow-up, or extensive postmortem confirmation, have not yet been performed. This validation will be crucial before PIB can be integrated into clinical practice.

Summary

Over the past decade there has been an exponential increase in the number of studies applying neuroimaging techniques to the study of degenerative dementia. A diverse range of techniques is available, some of which already are used routinely in clinical practice, whereas others still are research tools but hold significant promise for the future. Structural images already are an important component of the clinical assessment, as they allow the identification and exclusion of potentially treatable causes of cognitive impairment. They also highlight structural changes in the brain, which can be useful diagnostically. Many other techniques also have been developed to measure aspects of brain function, such as rates of glucose uptake or cerebral blood flow and the levels of certain brain metabolites. Imaging amyloid in the brain of living patients also is possible now and is likely to revolutionize patient diagnosis and management. A huge amount of imaging work has focused on patients who have AD, although increasingly research also is beginning to focus on the non-AD dementias, such as FTLD, DLB, and VaD. There are several key aspects of clinical practice for which imaging can play an important role: first, in the differential diagnosis of the different dementias; second, in allowing early detection and prediction of patients who will develop dementia; and third, in monitoring progression of the disease over time. In addition to clinical usefulness, an important aim is to develop surrogate markers of disease progression that can be used in the assessment of potentially disease-modifying therapies.

References

[1] Wahlund LO, Julin P, Johansson SE, et al. Visual rating and volumetry of the medial temporal lobe on magnetic resonance imaging in dementia: a comparative study. J Neurol Neurosurg Psychiatry 2000;69(5):630–5.
[2] Jack CR Jr, Dickson DW, Parisi JE, et al. Antemortem MRI findings correlate with hippocampal neuropathology in typical aging and dementia. Neurology 2002;58(5): 750–7.
[3] Whitwell JL, Jack CR Jr. Comparisons between Alzheimer's disease, frontotemporal lobar degeneration, and normal ageing with brain mapping. Top Magn Reson Imaging 2006;16: 409–25.
[4] Frisoni GB, Testa C, Sabattoli F, et al. Structural correlates of early and late onset Alzheimer's disease: voxel based morphometric study. J Neurol Neurosurg Psychiatry 2005; 76(1):112–4.
[5] Fox NC, Warrington EK, Freeborough PA, et al. Presymptomatic hippocampal atrophy in Alzheimer's disease. A longitudinal MRI study. Brain 1996;119(Pt 6):2001–7.
[6] Farlow MR, He Y, Tekin S, et al. Impact of APOE in mild cognitive impairment. Neurology 2004;63(10):1898–901.
[7] Jack CR Jr, Petersen RC, Xu YC, et al. Prediction of AD with MRI-based hippocampal volume in mild cognitive impairment. Neurology 1999;52(7):1397–403.
[8] Likeman M, Anderson VM, Stevens JM, et al. Visual assessment of atrophy on magnetic resonance imaging in the diagnosis of pathologically confirmed young-onset dementias. Arch Neurol 2005;62(9):1410–5.
[9] Rosen HJ, Gorno-Tempini ML, Goldman WP, et al. Patterns of brain atrophy in frontotemporal dementia and semantic dementia. Neurology 2002;58(2):198–208.
[10] Josephs KA, Duffy JR, Strand EA, et al. Clinicopathological and imaging correlates of progressive aphasia and apraxia of speech. Brain 2006;129:1385–98.
[11] Chan D, Fox NC, Scahill RI, et al. Patterns of temporal lobe atrophy in semantic dementia and Alzheimer's disease. Ann Neurol 2001;49(4):433–42.
[12] Whitwell JL, Weigand SD, Shiung MM, et al. Focal atrophy in dementia with Lewy bodies on MRI: a distinct pattern from Alzheimer's disease. Brain 2007;130:708–19.
[13] Varma AR, Laitt R, Lloyd JJ, et al. Diagnostic value of high signal abnormalities on T2 weighted MRI in the differentiation of Alzheimer's, frontotemporal and vascular dementias. Acta Neurol Scand 2002;105(5):355–64.
[14] Varma AR, Adams W, Lloyd JJ, et al. Diagnostic patterns of regional atrophy on MRI and regional cerebral blood flow change on SPECT in young onset patients with Alzheimer's disease, frontotemporal dementia and vascular dementia. Acta Neurol Scand 2002;105(4): 261–9.
[15] Whitwell JL, Jack CR, et al. Rates of cerebral atrophy differ in different degenerative pathologies. Brain 2007;130:1148–58.

[16] Barnes J, Scahill RI, Boyes RG, et al. Differentiating AD from aging using semiautomated measurement of hippocampal atrophy rates. Neuroimage 2004;23(2):574–81.

[17] Jack CR Jr, Shiung MM, Weigand SD, et al. Brain atrophy rates predict subsequent clinical conversion in normal elderly and amnestic MCI. Neurology 2005;65(8):1227–31.

[18] Fox NC, Crum WR, Scahill RI, et al. Imaging of onset and progression of Alzheimer's disease with voxel-compression mapping of serial magnetic resonance images. Lancet 2001; 358(9277):201–5.

[19] Thompson PM, Hayashi KM, de Zubicaray G, et al. Dynamics of gray matter loss in Alzheimer's disease. J Neurosci 2003;23(3):994–1005.

[20] Mosconi L, De Santi S, Li Y, et al. Visual rating of medial temporal lobe metabolism in mild cognitive impairment and Alzheimer's disease using FDG-PET. Eur J Nucl Med Mol Imaging 2006;33(2):210–21.

[21] Mosconi L. Brain glucose metabolism in the early and specific diagnosis of Alzheimer's disease. FDG-PET studies in MCI and AD. Eur J Nucl Med Mol Imaging 2005;32(4): 486–510.

[22] Jagust W, Gitcho A, Sun F, et al. Brain imaging evidence of preclinical Alzheimer's disease in normal aging. Ann Neurol 2006;59(4):673–81.

[23] Ibach B, Poljansky S, Marienhagen J, et al. Contrasting metabolic impairment in frontotemporal degeneration and early onset Alzheimer's disease. Neuroimage 2004;23(2):739–43.

[24] Jeong Y, Cho SS, Park JM, et al. 18F-FDG PET findings in frontotemporal dementia: an SPM analysis of 29 patients. J Nucl Med 2005;46(2):233–9.

[25] Bonte FJ, Harris TS, Roney CA, et al. Differential diagnosis between Alzheimer's and frontotemporal disease by the posterior cingulate sign. J Nucl Med 2004;45(5):771–4.

[26] Zahn R, Buechert M, Overmans J, et al. Mapping of temporal and parietal cortex in progressive nonfluent aphasia and Alzheimer's disease using chemical shift imaging, voxel-based morphometry and positron emission tomography. Psychiatry Res 2005;140(2):115–31.

[27] McMurtray AM, Chen AK, Shapira JS, et al. Variations in regional SPECT hypoperfusion and clinical features in frontotemporal dementia. Neurology 2006;66(4):517–22.

[28] Minoshima S, Foster NL, Sima AA, et al. Alzheimer's disease versus dementia with Lewy bodies: cerebral metabolic distinction with autopsy confirmation. Ann Neurol 2001;50(3): 358–65.

[29] Gilman S, Koeppe RA, Little R, et al. Differentiation of Alzheimer's disease from dementia with Lewy bodies utilizing positron emission tomography with [18F]fluorodeoxyglucose and neuropsychological testing. Exp Neurol 2005;191(Suppl 1):S95–103.

[30] Kerrouche N, Herholz K, Mielke R, et al. (18)FDG PET in vascular dementia: differentiation from Alzheimer's disease using voxel-based multivariate analysis. J Cereb Blood Flow Metab 2006;26(9):1213–21.

[31] Sperling RA, Bates JF, Chua EF, et al. fMRI studies of associative encoding in young and elderly controls and mild Alzheimer's disease. J Neurol Neurosurg Psychiatry 2003;74(1):44–50.

[32] Machulda MM, Ward HA, Borowski B, et al. Comparison of memory fMRI response among normal, MCI, and Alzheimer's patients. Neurology 2003;61(4):500–6.

[33] Johnson SC, Schmitz TW, Moritz CH, et al. Activation of brain regions vulnerable to Alzheimer's disease: the effect of mild cognitive impairment. Neurobiol Aging 2005;27(11): 1604–12.

[34] Bookheimer SY, Strojwas MH, Cohen MS, et al. Patterns of brain activation in people at risk for Alzheimer's disease. N Engl J Med 2000;343(7):450–6.

[35] Johnson SC, Schmitz TW, Trivedi MA, et al. The influence of Alzheimer disease family history and apolipoprotein E epsilon4 on mesial temporal lobe activation. J Neurosci 2006; 26(22):6069–76.

[36] Buckner RL, Snyder AZ, Shannon BJ, et al. Molecular, structural, and functional characterization of Alzheimer's disease: evidence for a relationship between default activity, amyloid, and memory. J Neurosci 2005;25(34):7709–17.

[37] Rombouts SA, Barkhof F, Goekoop R, et al. Altered resting state networks in mild cognitive impairment and mild Alzheimer's disease: an fMRI study. Hum Brain Mapp 2005;26(4): 231–9.

[38] Kantarci K, Jack CR Jr, Xu YC, et al. Regional metabolic patterns in mild cognitive impairment and Alzheimer's disease: a 1H MRS study. Neurology 2000;55(2):210–7.

[39] Modrego PJ, Fayed N, Pina MA. Conversion from mild cognitive impairment to probable Alzheimer's disease predicted by brain magnetic resonance spectroscopy. Am J Psychiatry 2005;162(4):667–75.

[40] Kantarci K, Weigand SD, Petersen RC, et al. Longitudinal (1)H MRS changes in mild cognitive impairment and Alzheimer's disease. [Epub] Neurobiol Aging 2006;129(11):2856–66.

[41] Kantarci K, Petersen RC, Boeve BF, et al. 1H MR spectroscopy in common dementias. Neurology 2004;63(8):1393–8.

[42] Mihara M, Hattori N, Abe K, et al. Magnetic resonance spectroscopic study of Alzheimer's disease and frontotemporal dementia/Pick complex. Neuroreport 2006;17(4):413–6.

[43] Coulthard E, Firbank M, English P, et al. Proton magnetic resonance spectroscopy in frontotemporal dementia. J Neurol 2006;253(7):861–8.

[44] Kantarci K, Petersen RC, Boeve BF, et al. DWI predicts future progression to Alzheimer disease in amnestic mild cognitive impairment. Neurology 2005;64(5):902–4.

[45] Nordberg A. PET imaging of amyloid in Alzheimer's disease. Lancet Neurol 2004;3(9): 519–27.

[46] Shoghi-Jadid K, Small GW, Agdeppa ED, et al. Localization of neurofibrillary tangles and beta-amyloid plaques in the brains of living patients with Alzheimer disease. Am J Geriatr Psychiatry 2002;10(1):24–35.

[47] Klunk WE, Engler H, Nordberg A, et al. Imaging brain amyloid in Alzheimer's disease with Pittsburgh Compound-B. Ann Neurol 2004;55(3):306–19.

[48] Newberg AB, Wintering NA, Plossl K, et al. Safety, biodistribution, and dosimetry of 123I-IMPY: a novel amyloid plaque-imaging agent for the diagnosis of Alzheimer's disease. J Nucl Med 2006;47(5):748–54.

[49] Mintun MA, Larossa GN, Sheline YI, et al. [11C] PIB in a nondemented population: potential antecedent marker of Alzheimer disease. Neurology 2006;67(3):446–52.

[50] Engler H, Forsberg A, Almkvist O, et al. Two-year follow-up of amyloid deposition in patients with Alzheimer's disease. Brain Jul 19 2006.

[51] Lopresti BJ, Klunk WE, Mathis CA, et al. Simplified quantification of Pittsburgh compound B amyloid imaging PET studies: a comparative analysis. J Nucl Med 2005;46(12):1959–72.

[52] Rowe CR, Ng S, Gong SJ, et al. C-11 PIB PET amyloid imaging in aging and dementia. Alzheimer's & Dementia 2006;2(3):S66.

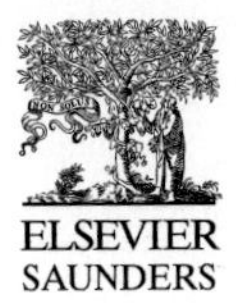

ELSEVIER
SAUNDERS

NEUROLOGIC CLINICS

Neurol Clin 25 (2007) 859–865

Index

Note: Page numbers of article titles are in **boldface** type.

A

ADAS. See *Alzhemier's Disease Assessment Scale (ADAS).*

ADAS-Cog. See *Alzheimer's Disease Assessment Scale–Cognitive Subscale (ADAS-Cog).*

Aging
- as factor in ß-amyloid peptide levels, 674
- normal, cognitive changes in, 578–579

Agitation, in Alzheimer's disease, 600

Alzheimer's disease
- agitation in, 600
- apathy in, 599
- as common disorder, public impact of, 611–612
- assessment of, 597
- clinical-neuropathologic correlations in, 675
- clinicopathologic correlates in, 748–749
- costs related to, 612
- depression in, 598
- described, 579, 669
- Down syndrome and, 671
- environment and, 612–613
- epidemiology of, 579
- evaluation of
  - biomarkers in, 584
  - clinical diagnosis in, 580
  - genetic testing in, 583–584
  - laboratory tests in, 581–582
  - lumbar puncture in, 583
  - neuroimaging in, 582
  - neurologic examination in, 581
  - neuropsychologic testing in, 583
- genetics of, 672–674
  - amyloid precrusor protein in, 618–619
  - apolipoprotein E in, 621–628
  - autosomal dominant mutations in, 619–621
  - candidate gene studies in, 655–659
  - centennial review of, **611–667**
  - early-onset, 618–621
  - familial aggregation studies, 613–615
  - late-onset, 621–628
    - risk loci for, detection methods, 653–655
  - link to chromosome 21, 671
- mild cognitive impairment and, **577–609**
- neuropathology of, 670–671
- noncognitive symptoms of, 596–600
- NPH and, MRI differentiation of, 814
- pathophysiology of, 584–585
- presenilins in, 619
- prevalence of, 577, 611–612, 669
- psychosis in, 598–599
- symptomatic, treatment of, 591–594
- symptoms of, 597
- testing in, 583–584
- transmission pattern studies, 615–616
- treatment of, 591–600
  - agents under investigation in, 594–596
  - amyloid therapy in, 595–596
  - anti-inflammatory drugs in, 594–595
  - behavioral management in, 597
  - disease-modifying agents in, 594
  - donepezil in, 592–593
  - ERT in, 595
  - galantamine in, 593
  - pharmacologic, 597–598
  - rivastigmine in, 593
  - tacrine in, 591
- twin studies, 616–617
- whole-genome linkage in, studies of, 628–655
  - characteristics of, 628–629
  - chromosome 6 in, 650

doi:10.1016/S0733-8619(07)00068-0

Alzheimer's (*continued*)
chromosome 9 in, 652–653
chromosome 10 in, 650–651
chromosome 12 in, 652
results of, 629–655
incidence of, 611–612

Alzheimer's Disease Assessment Scale (ADAS), 736

Alzheimer's Disease Assessment Scale–Cognitive Subscale (ADAS-Cog), 592

American Academy of Neurology, 577

ß-Amyloid, identification of, neuropathology of Alzheimer's disease and, 670–671

Amyloid hypothesis, update on, **669–682**

Amyloid imaging, in dementia, 853–854

ß-Amyloid peptide
increased levels of, causes of, 674–675
levels of, aging effects on, 674
toxicity of, 675–678

Amyloid precrusor protein, in Alzheimer's disease, 618–619

ß-Amyloid precursor protein, metabolism of, 671–672

Amyloid therapy, for Alzheimer's disease, 595–596

Anti-inflammatory drugs, for Alzheimer's disease, 594–595

Apathy, Alzheimer's disease and, 599

Aphasia(s), progressive nonfluent, 685

Apolipoprotein E, in Alzheimer's disease, 621–628

Apraxia of speech, frontotemporal lobar degeneration and, 687

Aqueductal stenosis, hypertension in patients with, 827

Atherosclerosis Risk in Communities study, 727, 732–734

Atrophy, multiple system, 770–773. See also *Multiple system atrophy (MSA).*

Austrian Stroke Prevention Study, 735

Autoimmune encephalopathies, RPD and, 790–794

Autosomal dominant mutations, in Alzheimer's disease, 619–621

B

Binswanger's syndrome, 718

Biomarker(s)
in Alzheimer's disease evaluation, 584
in mild cognitive impairment evaluation, 590

Brain–behavior correlations, in SIVD, 725–732

C

CADASIL. See *Cerebral autosomal dominant arteriopathy with subcortical infarctions and leukoencephalopathy (CADASIL).*

Cancer(s), lung, small cell, RPD and, 790–791

Cardiovascular Health Cognitive Study (CHCS), 727–728, 735

CBD. See *Corticobasal degeneration (CBD).*

Cerebral autosomal dominant arteriopathy with subcortical infarctions and leukoencephalopathy (CADASIL), 731–732

Cerebral blood flow, regional, NPH and, 816–817

Cerebrospinal fluid (CSF), frontotemporal lobar degeneration and, 687–688

Cerebrospinal fluid (CSF) drainage procedures, for NPH, 817–823. See also *Normal pressure hydrocephalus (NPH), CSF drainage procedures for.*

Cerebrospinal fluid (CSF) infusion tests, in NPH, 818–819

Cerebrospinal fluid (CSF) pressure monitoring, in NPH, 819–820

CHCS. See *Cardiovascular Health Cognitive Study (CHCS).*

Chromatic-modifying protein 2B gene, in FTD, 709–710

Chromosome 6, in whole-genome linkage studies of genetics in Alzheimer's disease, 650

Chromosome 9, in whole-genome linkage studies of genetics in Alzheimer's disease, 652–653

Chromosome 10, in whole-genome linkage studies of genetics in Alzheimer's disease, 650–651

Chromosome 12, in whole-genome linkage studies of genetics in Alzheimer's disease, 652

Chromosome 21, link to Alzheimer's disease and Down syndrome, 671

CIBIC Plus. See *Clinician's Interview-Based Impression of Change (CIBIC Plus).*

Cisternography, in NPH evaluation, 817

Clinician's Interview-Based Impression of Change (CIBIC Plus), 592

Cognition, aging effects on, 578–579

Cognitive impairment
- dementia, 579
- mild, 585–591
  - Alzheimer's disease and, **577–609**
  - clinical criteria for, 585–587
  - conceptual framework of, 585
  - evaluation of, 587–590
    - biomarkers in, 590
    - genetic testing in, 590
    - neuroimaging in, 588–589
    - neuropsychologic testing in, 589
  - neuropathology of, 590–591

Computed tomography (CT), in NPH evaluation

Cooperative Aneurysm Study, 827

Corticobasal degeneration (CBD), 761–767
- clinical features of, 761–763
- management of, 766–767
- neuropathologic features of, 764–765
- neuropsychologic features of, 763
- neuroradiologic features of, 763–764

Corticobasal syndrome, 761–767
- frontotemporal lobar degeneration and, 686

Creutzfeldt-Jakob disease, 836
- genetic, 836–837
- iatrogenic, 837
- RPD and, 783–787
- sporadic, 837
  - diagnosis of, 837–839
- treatment of, 840
- variant, sporadic, 839–840

CSF. See *Cerebrospinal fluid (CSF).*

D

Daytime drowsiness, excessive, DLB and, 745–746

Degenerative dementias
- as RPDs, 787–794
- typically chronic, RPD and, 788–790

Dementia(s), 579
- degenerative
  - as RPD, 787–794
  - typically chronic, RPD and, 788–790
- frontotemporal, genetics of, **697–715.** See also *Frontotemporal dementia (FTD), genetics of.*
- neuroimaging in, **843–857**
  - amyloid imaging, 853–854
  - diffusion-weighted imaging, 852
  - functional MRI, 851
  - functional nuclear medicine, 849–850
  - ^{1}H MRS, 851–852
  - structural, 843–849
- Parkinson-related, **761–781.** See also specific types and *Parkinson-related dementias.*
- rapidly progressive, **783–807.** See also *Rapidly progressive dementia (RPD).*
- semantic, 685–686
- strategic infarction, 718
- subcortical ischemic vascular, **717–740.** See also *Subcortical ischemic vascular dementia (SIVD).*
- thalamic, 718

Dementia with Lewy bodies (DLB), **741–760**
- cholinergic hypothesis in, 749
- clinical diagnosis of, revised criteria for, 742
- clinicopathologic correlates in, 748–749
- decline due to, 747
- described, 741
- dysautonomia and, 747
- excessive daytime drowsiness with, 745–746
- fluctuations in, 745
- neuropsychologic function in, 741–743
- pathology in, 747–748
- REM sleep behavior disorder with, 746–747
- treatment of
  - nonpharmacologic, 751
  - pharmacologic, 749–751
- visual hallucinations in, 744

Depression, in Alzheimer's disease, 598

Diffusion-weighted imaging, in dementia, 852

DLB. See *Dementia with Lewy bodies (DLB).*

Donepezil, for Alzheimer's disease, 592–593

Down syndrome, Alzheimer's disease and, 671

Drowsiness, excessive daytime, DLB and, 745–746

Dysautonomia, DLB and, 747

E

EEG. See *Electroencephalogram (EEG).*

Electroencephalogram (EEG), in frontotemporal lobar degeneration evaluation, 688

Encephalopathy(ies), autoimmune, RPD and, 790–794

Environment, as factor in Alzheimer's disease, 612–613

Epidemiology of Vascular Aging study, 735

ERT. See *Estrogen replacement therapy (ERT).*

Estrogen replacement therapy (ERT), for Alzheimer's disease, 595

Excessive daytime drowsiness, DLB and, 745–746

F

Familial aggregation studies, in Alzheimer's disease, 613–615

FDA. See *Food and Drug Administration (FDA).*

Fluctuation(s), DLB and, 745

Food and Drug Administration (FDA), 591–593

Framingham Heart Study, 734

Frontotemporal dementia (FTD)
- as complex trait, 700–707
- as heterogeneous clinical syndrome, 698
- described, 697
- genetics of, **697–715**
  - chromatic-modifying protein 2B gene, 709–710
  - *MAPT* mutations used to generate transgenic mouse models of tauopathy, 707–709
  - microtubule-associated protein tau gene, 704–707
  - progranulin, 701–704
  - valosin-containing protein gene, 710
- neuropathology of, 698–700

Frontotemporal dementia with parkinsonism linked to chromosome 17 (FTDP-17), **773–778**
- clinical features of, 773–774
- management of, 778
- neuropathologic features of, 775–778
- neuropsychologic features of, 774
- neuroradiologic features of, 774–775

Frontotemporal lobar degeneration, **683–696**
- ancillary testing of, 687–688
- apraxia of speech and, 687
- behavioral variant of, 684–685
- corticobasal syndrome and, 686
- CSF in, 687–688
- EEG in, 688
- genetics of, 692
- historical perspective of, 683–684
- motor neuron disease and, 686–687
- neuroimaging in, 688–690
- pathology of, 690–692
- progressive nonfluent aphasia and, 685
- progressive supranuclear palsy and, 686
- semantic dementia, 685–686
- syndromic diagnosis of, 684–687
- treatment of, 692–693

FTDP-17. See *Frontotemporal dementia with parkinsonism linked to chromosome 17 (FTDP-17).*

Functional MRI, in dementia, 851

Functional nuclear medicine, in dementia, 849–850

G

Galantamine, for Alzheimer's disease, 593

Gene(s)
- chromatic-modifying protein 2B, in FTD, 709–710
- microtubule-associated protein tau, FTD and, 704–707
- valosin-containing protein, in FTD, 710

Genetic(s)
- in mild cognitive impairment, 590
- of Alzheimer's disease, 672–674
  - centennial review of, **611–667.** See also *Alzheimer's disease, genetics of.*
- of frontotemporal dementia, **697–715.** See also *Frontotemporal dementia (FTD), genetics of.*
- of frontotemporal lobar degeneration, 692

H

^{1}H MRS, in dementia, 851–852

Hallucination(s), visual, DLB and, 744

Head, large size, hydrocephalus and, 828

Hemorrhage, subarachnoid, NPH after, 827

Honolulu Asia Aging Study, 735

Hydrocephalus
- after subarachnoid hemorrhage, 827
- in spontaneously hypertensive rat, 827
- large size head and, 828
- normal pressure, **809–832.** See also *Normal pressure hydrocephalus (NPH).*

Hypertension
- aqueductal stenosis and, 827
- systemic, idiopathic NPH and, relationship between, 826–828

I

Idiopathic NPH. See *Normal pressure hydrocephalus (NPH), idiopathic.*

K

Kuru, 835

L

Lesion(s), white matter, NPH and, 813–814

Lewy bodies, dementia with, **741–760.** See also *Dementia with Lewy bodies (DLB).*

Lumbar puncture, in Alzheimer's disease evaluation, 583

Lung cancer, small cell, RPD and, 790–791

M

Magnetic resonance imaging (MRI)
- functional, in dementia, 851
- in NPH and Alzheimer's disease differentiation, 814
- in NPH evaluation, 813–816

Magnetic resonance spectroscopy (MRS), ^{1}H, in dementia, 851–852

Malignancy(ies), RPD due to, 797–798

MAPT mutations, in generation of transgenic mouse models of tauopathy, in FTD, 707–709

Microtubule-associated protein tau gene, FTD and, 704–707

Motor neuron disease, frontotemporal lobar degeneration and, 686–687

MRI. See *Magnetic resonance imaging (MRI).*

MRS. See *Magnetic resonance spectroscopy (MRS).*

MSA. See *Multiple system atrophy (MSA).*

Multiple system atrophy (MSA), 770–773
- clinical features of, 770
- management of, 773
- neuropathologic features of, 773
- neuropsychologic features of, 770–773
- neuroradiologic features of, 773

Mutation(s)
- autosomal dominant, in Alzheimer's disease, 619–621
- *MAPT,* in generation of trangenic mouse models of tauopathy in FTD, 707–709

N

Neuroimaging
- in Alzheimer's disease evaluation, 582
- in dementia, **843–857.** See also *Dementia(s), neuroimaging in.*
- in mild cognitive impairment evaluation, 588–589

Neuropsychologic testing
- in Alzheimer's disease evaluation, 583
- in mild cognitive impairment evaluation, 589

Normal pressure hydrocephalus (NPH), **809–832**
- after subarachnoid hemorrhage, 827
- Alzheimer's disease and, MRI differentiation of, 814
- cisternography in, 817
- clinical and autopsy studies of patients with, 826–827
- clinical evaluation of, 842
  - general factors in, 811
  - neuropsychologic, 812
  - patient history related to hydrocephalus in, 811
  - physical examination in, 812
- CSF drainage procedures for, 817–823
  - CSF infusion tests, 818–819
  - CSF pressure monitoring, 819–820
  - external procedure, 817–818
  - lumbar puncture, 817
- diagnosis of, difficulty of, 809–810
- differential diagnosis of, 810
- epidemiology of, 809

Normal pressure (*continued*)
idiopathic
brains of patients with, histopathology of, 824–826
criteria for, 821–823
systemic hypertension and, relationship between, 826–828
patient improvement in, assessment of, 824
radiologic evaluation of, 812–816
CT in, 812–813
MRI in, 813–816
regional cerebral blood flow in, 816–817
shunt surgery for, 824
complications of, 825
prognostic factors for, 820
surgical outcome of, flow void on MRI as predictive test of, 815–816
white matter lesions and, 813–814

NPH. See *Normal pressure hydrocephalus (NPH).*

Nun Study, 590

P

Paraneoplastic neurologic disorders (PNDs), RPD and, 790

Parkinsonism, spontaneous motor features of, 744

Parkinson-related dementias, **761–781.** See also specific types.
CBD, 761–767
corticobasal syndrome, 761–767
FTDP-17, 773–778
MSA, 770–773
overview of, 761
PSP, 767–770

Peptide(s), ß-amyloid
increased levels of, causes of, 674–675
levels of, aging effects on, 674
toxicity of, 675–678

Perindopril Protection Against Recurrent Stroke Study (PROGRESS), 736

PNDs. See *Paraneoplastic neurologic disorders (PNDs).*

Pogranulin, FTD and, 701–704

Presenilin(s), in Alzheimer's disease, 619

Prion disease, **833–842**
animal, 834–835
biology of, 833
Creutzfeldt-Jakob disease, 836
described, 833
diagnosis of, 837–840
epidemiology of, 836
genetic polymorphisms in, 836–837
human, 835–836
in context, 841
kuru, 835
RPD and, 787–788
species barrier and strains in, 834
treatment of, 840

PROGRESS. See *Perindopril Protection Against Recurrent Stroke Study (PROGRESS).*

Progressive nonfluent aphasia, 685

Progressive supranuclear palsy (PSP), 767–770
clinical features of, 767–769
frontotemporal lobar degeneration and, 686
management of, 769–770
neuropathologic features of, 769
neuropsychologic features of, 769
neuroradiologic features of, 769

Protein(s), amyloid precrusor, in Alzheimer's disease, 618–619

Protein gene, valosin-containing, in FTD, 710

PSP. See *Progressive supranuclear palsy (PSP).*

Psychosis(es), in Alzheimer's disease, 598–599

Puncture, lumbar, in Alzheimer's disease evaluation, 583

R

Radiology, in NPH evaluation, 812–816

Rapid eye movement (REM) sleep behavior disorder, DLB and, 746–747

Rapidly progressive dementia (RPD), **783–807**
autoimmune encephalopathies and, 790–794
causes of
infectious, 795–797
malignancies, 797–798
nonorganic, 800
toxic-metabolic, 799–800
vascular, 794–795
Creutzfeldt-Jakob disease and, 783–787
degenerative dementias as, 787–794
differential diagnosis of, 785–786
mnemonic for categories of conditions causing, 784

PNDs and, 790
prion diseases and, 787–788
small cell lung cancer and, 790–791
typically chronic degenerative dementias and, 788–790

Regional cerebral blood flow, NPH and, 816–817

Religious Orders Study, 590

REM. See *Rapid eye movement (REM).*

Rivastigmine, for Alzheimer's disease, 593

Rotterdam Scan Study, in SIVD, 727, 734

RPD. See *Rapidly progressive dementia (RPD).*

S

Sandoz Clinical Assessment–Geriatric scale, 736

Semantic dementia, 685–686

Shunt surgery, for NPH, 824
complications of, 825
prognostic factors for, 820

SIVD. See *Subcortical ischemic vascular dementia (SIVD).*

Small cell lung cancer, RPD and, 790–791

Speech, apraxia of, frontotemporal lobar degeneration and, 687

Stenosis(es), aqueductal, hypertension in patients with, 827

Strategic infarction dementia, 718

Subarachnoid hemorrhage
hydrocephalus after, 827
NPH after, 827

Subcortical ischemic vascular dementia (SIVD), **717–740**
Binswanger's syndrome, 718
brain–behavior correlations in, 725–732
conceptualization of, 717–725
diagnostic criteria for, 722–725
epidemiology of, 732–735
evidence for, 718–719
hypotheses for, 719–722
lacunar state in, 718
patient history in, 717–719
prevention of, 732–736
strategic infarction dementia, 718
treatment of, 732–736

Subcortical ischemic vascular dementia (SIVD) program project, 728

Systemic hypertension, idiopathic NPH and, relationship between, 826–828

T

Tacrine, for Alzheimer's disease, 591

Thalamic dementia, 718

Toxicity, of ß-amyloid peptide, 675–678

Transmission pattern studies, in Alzheimer's disease, 615–616

Twin studies, in Alzheimer's disease, 616–617

V

Valosin-containing protein gene, in FTD, 710

Visual hallucinations, DLB and, 744

Vitamin E, for Alzheimer's disease, 594

VITAMINS mnemonic, for categories of conditions causing RPD, 784

W

Washington University Study, 591

White matter lesions, NPH and, 813–814

Women's Health Initiative Memory Study, 595

Moving?

Make sure your subscription moves with you!

To notify us of your new address, find your **Clinics Account Number** (located on your mailing label above your name), and contact customer service at:

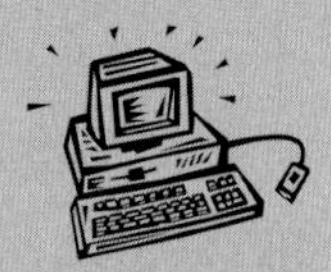

E-mail: elspcs@elsevier.com

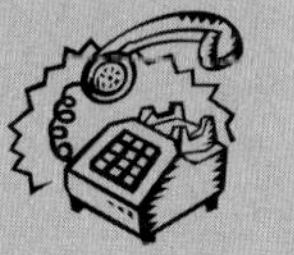

800-654-2452 (subscribers in the U.S. & Canada)
407-345-4000 (subscribers outside of the U.S. & Canada)

Fax number: 407-363-9661

Elsevier Periodicals Customer Service
6277 Sea Harbor Drive
Orlando, FL 32887-4800

*To ensure uninterrupted delivery of your subscription, please notify us at least 4 weeks in advance of move.

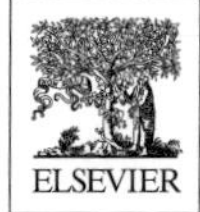